Probability Modeling and Statistical Inference in Cancer Screening

Cancer screening has been carried out for six decades – however, there are many unsolved problems: how to estimate key parameters involved in screenings, such as sensitivity, the time duration in the preclinical state (i.e., sojourn time), and time duration in the disease-free state; how to estimate the distribution of lead time, the diagnosis time advanced by screening; how to evaluate the long-term outcomes of screening, including the probability of overdiagnosis among the screen-detected; when to schedule the first exam based on one's current age and risk tolerance; and when to schedule the upcoming exam based on one's screening history, age, and risk tolerance. These problems need proper probability models and statistical methods in order to be dealt with.

Features:

- This book gives a concise account of the analysis of cancer screening data, using probability models and statistical methods.
- Real data sets are provided so that cancer researchers and statisticians can apply the methods in the learning process.
- It develops statistical methods in the commonly used disease progressive model.
- It provides solutions to practical problems and introduces open problems.
- It provides a framework for the most recent developments based on the author's research.

The book is primarily aimed at researchers and practitioners from biostatistics and cancer research. Readers should have the prerequisite knowledge of calculus, probability, and statistical inference. The book could be used as a one-semester textbook on the topic of cancer screening methodology for a graduate-level course.

Dongfeng Wu is a full professor in the Department of Bioinformatics and Biostatistics, School of Public Health and Information Sciences, University of Louisville. She got her PhD in Statistics and MS in Computer Science from the University of California, Santa Barbara in 1999. She worked at Mississippi State University and MD Anderson Cancer Center before joining the University of Louisville.

Chapman & Hall/CRC Biostatistics Series

Recently Published Titles

Quantitative Methods for Precision Medicine
Pharmacogenomics in Action
Rongling Wu

Drug Development for Rare Diseases
Edited by Bo Yang, Yang Song and Yijie Zhou

Case Studies in Bayesian Methods for Biopharmaceutical CMC
Edited by Paul Faya and Tony Pourmohamad

Statistical Analytics for Health Data Science with SAS and R
Jeffrey Wilson, Ding-Geng Chen and Karl E. Peace

Design and Analysis of Pragmatic Trials
Song Zhang, Chul Ahn and Hong Zhu

ROC Analysis for Classification and Prediction in Practice
Christos Nakas, Leonidas Bantis and Constantine Gatsonis

Controlled Epidemiological Studies
Marie Reilly

Statistical Methods in Health Disparity Research
J. Sunil Rao, Ph.D.

Case Studies in Innovative Clinical Trials
Edited by Binbing Yu and Kristine Broglio

Value of Information for Healthcare Decision Making
Edited by Anna Heath, Natalia Kunst, and Christopher Jackson

Probability Modeling and Statistical Inference in Cancer Screening
Dongfeng Wu

For more information about this series, please visit: https://www.routledge.com/Chapman--Hall-CRC-Biostatistics-Series/book-series/CHBIOSTATIS

Probability Modeling and Statistical Inference in Cancer Screening

Dongfeng Wu

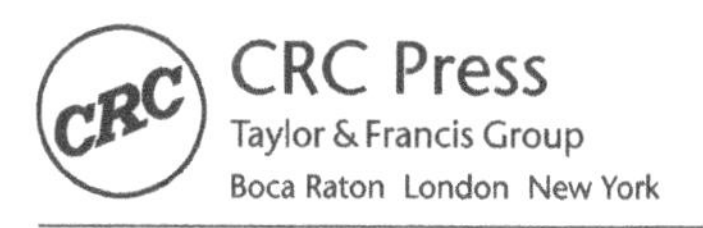

CRC Press is an imprint of the
Taylor & Francis Group, an **informa** business
A CHAPMAN & HALL BOOK

First edition published 2024
by CRC Press
2385 Executive Center Drive, Suite 320, Boca Raton, FL 33431, U.S.A.

and by CRC Press
4 Park Square, Milton Park, Abingdon, Oxon, OX14 4RN

CRC Press is an imprint of Taylor & Francis Group, LLC

ISBN: 978-1-032-51330-0 (hbk)
ISBN: 978-1-032-51831-2 (pbk)
ISBN: 978-1-003-40412-5 (ebk)

DOI: 10.1201/9781003404125

Typeset in CMR10
by KnowledgeWorks Global Ltd.

Publisher's note: This book has been prepared from camera-ready copy provided by the authors.

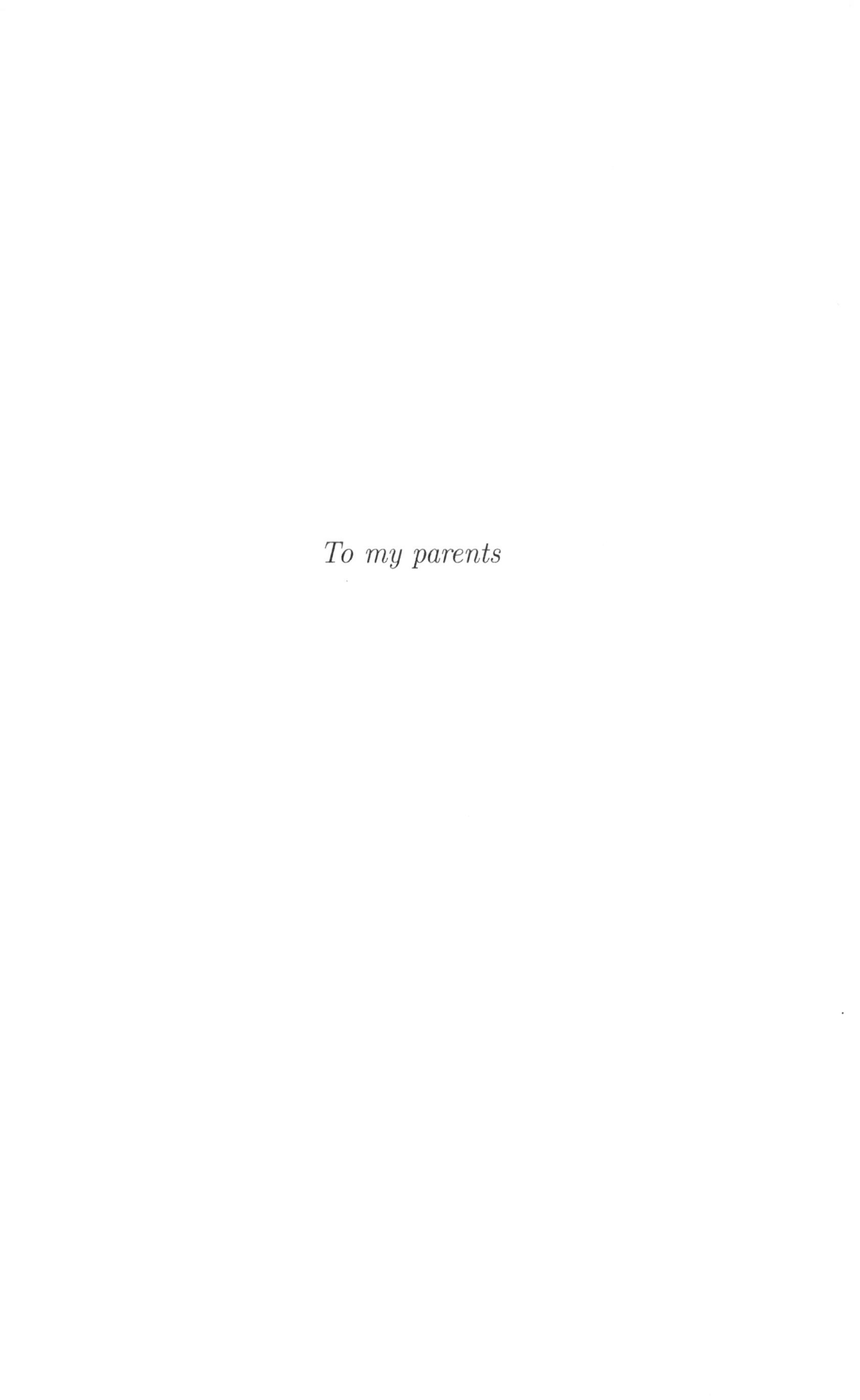

To my parents

Contents

Preface

Cancer screening has been carried out for six decades; however, there are many unsolved problems:

(i) how to estimate key parameters involved in screening exams, such as screening sensitivity, time duration in the preclinical state (i.e., sojourn time), and time duration in the disease-free state;

(ii) how to estimate the distribution of lead time, the diagnosis time advanced by screening;

(iii) how to evaluate the long-term outcomes of screening, including the probability of overdiagnosis, true-early-detection, and disease-free-life;

(iv) when to schedule the first exam based on one's current age and risk tolerance; and

(v) when to schedule the upcoming exam based on one's screening history, age, and risk tolerance.

(vi) These problems need proper probability models and statistical methods to deal with. Also, this is an area that is under development and needs more researchers to get involved.

The objective of this book is to give a concise account of the analysis of cancer screening data, using probability models and statistical methods. Some real data sets are provided, so that cancer researchers and statisticians can apply the methods in the learning process. The main focus is to develop statistical methods in the commonly used disease progressive model, provide solutions to some practical problems, and introduce some open problems. The book does not cover every method in this area due to the limited knowledge of the author, although it provides a framework of the most recent developments based on the author's research. It is assumed that readers have the prerequisite knowledge of calculus, probability, and statistical inference. The book could be used as a one-semester text on the topic of cancer screening methodology for a graduate-level course.

The book is organized into seven chapters: Chapter 1 is a quick review of probability concepts, definitions, the Markov Chain Monte Carlo (MCMC) algorithms that will be used, and some screening data.

Chapter 2 starts with an introduction to cancer screening terminologies, such as the progressive disease model (i.e., disease-free state, preclinical state, and clinical state), screening sensitivity, specificity, sojourn time in the preclinical state, transition probability density, lead time, and overdiagnosis. Then it focuses on deriving the probability of screen-detected and interval incident cases, and using the likelihood method and Bayesian inference to estimate the three key parameters: the sensitivity, the sojourn time distribution, and the transition density from the disease-free state to the preclinical state. The three key parameters are considered building blocks in cancer screening, as all other terms are functions of the three.

Chapter 3 is on the testing of dependence/independence of two screening modalities, where the sensitivity was considered either fixed (or stable) or changing with one's age. This is a short chapter and can be skipped in the learning process.

Chapter 4 focuses on the lead time distribution when the human lifetime is either fixed or random. The distribution is derived under a few different situations depending on whether an asymptomatic individual has a screening history or not and whether the sensitivity is a function of one's age or a function of the sojourn time. In all cases, the lead time distribution is a function of the three key parameters.

Chapter 5 is on the evaluation of the long-term outcomes of cancer screening. All participants in a screening program would eventually fall into one of the four mutually exclusive groups: symptom-free-life, no-early-detection, true-early-detection, and overdiagnosis. The probability of each case was derived to estimate future outcomes with and without a screening history. The probability of overdiagnosis among the screen-detected cases can be estimated as well. This is the probability that the general public was really concerned. All these probabilities are functions of the three key parameters.

Chapter 6 addresses the problem of when to schedule the first exam for an asymptomatic individual, based on the current age and risk tolerance. The first screening time is chosen so that the probability of incidence from the current to the first exam is limited to some pre-selected small value.

Chapter 7 is on the dynamic scheduling of the upcoming exams based on one's screening history, current age, and risk tolerance. The probability of incidence is used as the criterion similar to Chapter 6. The upcoming exam time is chosen such that the probability of incidence is controlled by some pre-selected small value (risk). The sensitivity can be a function of either one's age or the sojourn time in the model. Individuals or physicians may use this information for the planning of the next exam.

Each chapter starts with a clear probability model and statistical methods, then simulations and applications are presented using the methods. The materials are arranged in a way that readers can read Chapters 1 and 2, then followed by any chapters they are interested in. Since Chapters 6 and 7 are closely related, it is beneficial to read Chapter 6 first.

I want to thank my collaborators for their help and support over the years – specifically, Gary L. Rosner, Karen Kafadar, Lyle D. Broemeling, Seongho Kim, Adriana Perez, Guy Brock, Shesh Rai, Jeremy Gaskins, and

Ruiqi Liu. I want to thank Diane Erwin and Beth Levitt for organizing the screening data into the format that I usually use. I want to thank Rob Calver, senior publisher of Chapman & Hall/CRC Press, for his patience and support in publishing this book. Finally, I want to thank my family members for their support over the years.

Dongfeng Wu
University of Louisville

List of Figures

List of Tables

Symbols

Symbol Description

Symbol	Description
P	Probability.
∞	Positive infinity.
$-\infty$	Negative infinity.
$\mathcal{R}^1$	The real line $(-\infty, \infty)$.
$\sum x_i$	Summation notation, add all x_i.
$\prod x_i$	Multiplication notation, multiply all x_i.
$A \cup B$	Union of A and B means elements that belong to either A or B or both.
$A \cap B$	Intersection of A and B means elements that belong to both A and B.
A^c	Complement of A means elements that do not belong to A.
$A\|B$	Event A happens given that event B happened.
PMF	Probability mass function.
PDF	Probability density function.
CDF	Cumulative distribution function.
MCMC	Markov Chain Monte Carlo, a simulation algorithm or procedure.
HPD	Highest posterior density.
$\int$	Integration.
$\propto$	Is proportional to.

1

A Brief Review of Probability and Examples of Screening Data

CONTENTS

We will briefly review probability theory and Bayes inference that will be used in this book. Important concepts, such as random variable, distribution function, joint and conditional probability, correlation, likelihood function, prior and posterior distribution, Markov Chain Monte Carlo algorithms including Metropolis-Hastings algorithm and Gibbs sampler, etc. are provided. For those who are familiar with the topics, you can simply skip the first few sections; for those who are not familiar with these or who need a refresh of memory, you can learn basic concepts, and algorithms, and use this chapter as a reference. We will also introduce the screening data format and provide a few examples of real screening data.

1.1 Sample space, event, and probability

When an experiment is carried out, there are many possible outcomes. A *sample space* S of an experiment includes all possible outcomes of this specific experiment. An *event* E is some possible outcome of an experiment, and it is a subset of the sample space, $E \subseteq S$. *Probability* is a function defined for each

DOI: 10.1201/9781003404125-1

outcome in the sample space, and it satisfies the three axioms as follows:

(i) For any event $E, P(E) \geq 0$;

(ii) The probability for the whole sample space $S, P(S) = 1$;

(iii) For any sequence of *mutually exclusive events* $A_1, A_2, \ldots,$ (1.1)

$$P(\bigcup_{i=1}^{\infty} A_i) = \sum_{i=1}^{\infty} P(A_i).$$

Therefore, the probability of any event always takes a value in (0,1). There are some rules that a probability must follow. For any two events A and B,

$$P(A \cup B) = P(A) + P(B) - P(A \cap B). \tag{1.2}$$

If A^c is the *complement* of A, which represents all events "not A", then

$$P(A^c) = 1 - P(A). \tag{1.3}$$

An important definition is *conditional probability*: for any two events A and B, if $P(B) > 0$, the conditional probability of event A given that event B has happened is

$$P(A|B) = \frac{P(A \cap B)}{P(B)}. \tag{1.4}$$

And we can use this formula to calculate the *joint probability* of both events A and B happen:

$$P(A \cap B) = P(B)P(A|B) = P(A)P(B|A). \tag{1.5}$$

Two events A and B are *independent*, if

$$P(A \cap B) = P(A)P(B). \tag{1.6}$$

Equivalently, we say A and B are *independent*, if

$$P(A|B) = P(A), \text{ or } P(B|A) = P(B).$$

An intuitive meaning of independence is: whether A happens or not, does not have any effect on B happens or not, and vice versa.

A collection of events $\{A_1, A_2, \ldots\}$ is called a *partition* of the sample space S, if the events are *disjoint* (or mutually exclusive) and satisfy

$$\bigcup_i A_i = S.$$

For any event B and a partition $\{A_1, \ldots, A_n\}$ of the sample space S, we can use the *Bayes' rule* to calculate the conditional probability:

$$P(A_i|B) = \frac{P(A_i)P(B|A_i)}{\sum_{j=1}^{n} P(A_j)P(B|A_j)}, \text{ for } i = 1, \ldots, n. \tag{1.7}$$

Exercise 1.1.

Prove that the conditional probability is a probability. That is, the conditional probability $P(A|B)$ satisfies the three axioms defined in (1.1).

1.2 Random variable and distribution function

A *random variable* X is a mapping from a sample space S to some real values. The *distribution function* is used to describe a random variable. There are two types of random variables: *discrete* or *continuous*. A *discrete random variable* can take on (at most) a countable number of possible values. An example of a discrete random variable is when we toss a coin: let $X = 1$ if it is a face, and $X = 0$ if it is a tail; and the X is a discrete random variable. A *continuous random variable* can take on values that are uncountable. An example of a continuous random variable could be one's height or weight, which takes value in an interval (a, b) or in the whole real line $(-\infty, \infty)$, denoted by $\mathcal{R}^1$. We usually use capital letters to represent a random variable, such as X, Y, Z; and use lowercase letters to represent fixed values, such as x, y, z.

We use *probability mass function (PMF)* to describe the distribution of a discrete random variable: $p(a) = P(X = a)$. For example, when tossing a fair coin, $P(X = 1) = P(X = 0) = 1/2$; and $P(X = 1) + P(X = 0) = 1$, this probability is the PMF of X. A PMF satisfies the following two properties:

1. $P(X = x_i) \geq 0$, for $i = 1, 2, \ldots,$
2. $\sum_{i=1}^{\infty} P(X = x_i) = 1.$

We use *probability density function (PDF)* to describe the distribution of a continuous random variable. The PDF is a non-negative function $f(x) \geq 0$, for any $x \in (-\infty, \infty)$, we write $X \sim f(x)$, meaning that a random variable X has a PDF $f(x)$, and the $f(x)$ must satisfy:

1. $P(a < X < b) = \int_a^b f_X(x)dx$, for any $a < b$,
2. $P(-\infty < X < \infty) = \int_{-\infty}^{\infty} f_X(x)dx = 1.$

We use the *cumulative distribution function (CDF)* to describe both discrete and continuous random variables. The CDF of a random variable X is defined for all real numbers by

$$F_X(x) = P(X \leq x), \quad -\infty < x < \infty.$$

The relationship between the PDF and the CDF of a random variable X is

$$F'_X(x) = f_X(x).$$

The *survival function* of a random variable X is defined as

$$Q_X(x) = P(X > x) = 1 - F_X(x), \quad -\infty < x < \infty.$$

And it is easy to prove that

$$f_X(x) = -Q'_X(x).$$

We often deal with two or more random variables at the same time, and we use the *joint probability mass function* or the *joint probability density function* to describe the distribution of the discrete or continuous random variables respectively. For two continuous random variables (X, Y), let $f(x, y)$ represent the joint PDF of (X, Y), that means

1. $P(x_1 < X < x_2, y_1 < Y < y_2) = \int_{y_1}^{y_2} \int_{x_1}^{x_2} f_{X,Y}(x, y)dxdy$, for any $x_1 < x_2$ and $y_1 < y_2$;
2. $\int_{-\infty}^{\infty} \int_{-\infty}^{\infty} f_{X,Y}(x, y)dxdy = 1$.

The *conditional probability density function* of a random variable Y given that $X = x$ is

$$f_{Y|X}(y|x) = \frac{f_{X,Y}(x, y)}{f_X(x)}, \quad \text{provided } f_X(x) > 0. \tag{1.8}$$

If the *joint distribution* of $(X, Y) \sim f_{X,Y}(x, y)$, then the PDF of $(X + Y)$ is

$$f_{X+Y}(s) = \int_{-\infty}^{\infty} f_{X,Y}(x, s - x)dx = \int_{-\infty}^{\infty} f_{X,Y}(s - y, y)dy. \tag{1.9}$$

We say two random variables are *independent* if for any $x \in \mathcal{R}^1$, and $y \in \mathcal{R}^1$,

$$f_{X,Y}(x, y) = f_X(x)f_Y(y). \tag{1.10}$$

If X and Y are two independent continuous random variables, with $X \sim f_X(x), Y \sim f_Y(y)$, then the probability density function of $(X + Y)$ is

$$f_{X+Y}(s) = \int_{-\infty}^{\infty} f_X(x)f_Y(s - x)dx = \int_{-\infty}^{\infty} f_X(s - y)f_Y(y)dy. \tag{1.11}$$

The conditional probability density function of a random variable X given that an event A has happened is

$$f_X(x|A) = \begin{cases} \frac{f_X(x)}{P(A)}, & \text{if } x \in A \\ 0, & \text{if } x \notin A \end{cases} \tag{1.12}$$

Exercise 1.2.
Prove that the function $f_X(x|A)$ defined above is a valid PDF. That is, it satisfies the definition of a PDF.

A *mixture distribution* is simply a mixture of two or more probability distributions. For example, if X_1 is a discrete random variable and X_2 is a continuous random variable, a mixture distribution of X_1 and X_2 could be $Y = aX_1 + (1 - a)X_2$, where $a \in (0, 1)$ is a real number.

1.3 Expectation, moments, and correlation

The *expectation* or *expected value* of a random variable is just the weighted average under its probability distribution. For a random variable X, and any function $g()$, the expected value of $g(X)$ is

$$Eg(X) = \begin{cases} \int_{-\infty}^{\infty} g(x) f_X(x) dx, & \text{if } X \text{ is continuous;} \\ \sum_{i=1}^{\infty} g(x_i) P(X = x_i), & \text{if } X \text{ is discrete.} \end{cases} \quad (1.13)$$

provided that the integral or sum exists. If $E|g(X)| = \infty$, we say that $Eg(X)$ does not exist.

The k-th *moment* of X is defined by $E(X^k)$. For example, the first moment is the *mean* of X, denoted by $\mu = EX$. The k-th *central moment* of X is defined by $E[(X - EX)^k]$. For example, the second central moment usually is called the *variance*, denoted by $\sigma^2 = Var(X) = E[(X - EX)^2]$.

If X and Y are two random variables defined on the same sample space, then the *covariance* of X and Y is defined by

$$Cov(X, Y) = E[(X - EX)(Y - EY)] = E(XY) - E(X)E(Y).$$

where

$$E(XY) = \begin{cases} \int\int xyf(x, y) dx dy, & \text{if } X, Y \text{ are continuous;} \\ \sum_{i=1}^{\infty} \sum_{j=i}^{\infty} x_i y_j P(X = x_i, Y = y_j), & \text{if } X, Y \text{ are discrete.} \end{cases}$$

If $Cov(X, Y) > 0$, we say that X and Y are *positively correlated.* If $Cov(X, Y) < 0$, we say that X and Y are *negatively correlated.* If $Cov(X, Y) = 0$, we say that X and Y are *uncorrelated.*

If X, Y are two random variables with finite variances, that is, $0 < Var(X) < \infty$ and $0 < Var(Y) < \infty$, the *correlation coefficient* of X and Y is defined by

$$\rho(X, Y) = \frac{Cov(X, Y)}{\sqrt{Var(X) Var(Y)}}.$$

Exercise 1.3.
Prove that $|\rho(X, Y)| \leq 1$.

1.4 Frequentist statistics and Bayes inference

We assume that the observed data $\mathbf{X} = \{X_1, X_2, \ldots, X_n\}$ follow some parametric models, that is, $X_i \sim f_X(x|\theta), i = 1, 2, \ldots, n$, are *independently and identically distributed (i.i.d.)* , and θ is some *parameters* that we are interested to estimate. In traditional frequentist statistics, the θ is a fixed unknown value; while in Bayesian statistics, the θ is a random variable. The θ could be one-dimensional or multi-dimensional, i.e., a vector. There are three areas in statistical inference: point estimation, hypothesis testing, and interval estimation.

For point estimation of the θ, traditional statistics use the *maximum likelihood estimate (MLE)* of θ, that is, using a *likelihood function*

$$L(\theta|\mathbf{X}) = \prod_{i=1}^{n} f(x_i|\theta), \tag{1.14}$$

we can find a maximizer $\hat{\theta}$ either mathematically or numerically, such that the likelihood function reaches its maximum at $\hat{\theta}$, and we call $\hat{\theta}$ the MLE of θ.

In the Bayesian approach, θ is assumed to be a random variable, and there is a *prior distribution or prior information* of θ before any data is collected. That is, we assume the *prior* $\theta \sim \pi(\theta)$. After the data collection, we can find the *posterior distribution* of θ by

$$p(\theta|\mathbf{X}) = \frac{\pi(\theta)L(\theta|\mathbf{X})}{\int \pi(\theta)L(\theta|\mathbf{X})d\theta} \propto \pi(\theta) \cdot L(\theta|\mathbf{X}). \tag{1.15}$$

If the prior distribution $\pi(\theta)$ and the posterior distribution $p(\theta|\mathbf{X})$ belong to the same parametric family, then we call $\pi(\theta)$ a *conjugate prior* . The *point estimate* of θ in a Bayes inference could be the *posterior mean* $E(\theta|\mathbf{X})$, the *posterior median* , and the *posterior mode* .

For hypothesis testing, there are two complementary hypotheses: the *null hypothesis* H_0 and the *alternative hypothesis* H_1. The general form of the testing is $H_0 : \theta \in \Theta_0$ versus $H_1 : \theta \in \Theta_0^c$. The hypothesis testing procedure is to find a *test statistic* $T(X)$ and a subset of the sample space of $T(X)$, and when $T(X)$ falls in that subset, the H_0 is rejected; otherwise, the H_0 is accepted. There could be two types of errors in hypothesis testing. The *type I error* is that H_0 is rejected when it is true; The *type II error* is that H_0 is accepted when it is false. The test is usually carried out by limiting the type I error to a small value, which is called *the significance level* α; then try to minimize the type II error. The α should be chosen before carrying out the test, and it usually takes a value of 0.01, 0.05, or 0.1. Another way is to calculate the p-value, and it is the probability of committing a type I error when the H_0 is true.

One commonly used frequentist approach is to use the *likelihood ratio test (LRT)*. The LRT statistic is

$$LR = \frac{\sup_{\Theta_0} L(\theta|\mathbf{x})}{\sup_{\Theta} L(\theta|\mathbf{x})},$$

where Θ is the whole parameter space. The LRT is to reject the H_0 when $LR \leq c$, with some $c \in (0, 1)$. When the sample size is large, under some regularity conditions on the $f(x|\theta)$, the test statistic $-2\log(LR)$ will approximately follows a chi-squared distribution, with the degree of freedom, v, equal to the difference between the number of free parameters specified by Θ_0 and Θ. For a given significance level α, the H_0 is rejected if

$$-2\log(LR) = 2[\sup_{\Theta} \log L(\theta|x) - \sup_{\Theta_0} \log L(\theta|x)] \geq \chi^2_{v,\alpha}.$$

For more details, readers can use the book Casella and Berger 2001 as a reference [5].

The Bayesian approach is easier in one-sided hypothesis testing. If we want to test $H_0 : \theta \leq \theta_0$ versus $H_1 : \theta > \theta_0$, we can calculate the posterior probability $p_0 = P(\theta \leq \theta_0|\mathbf{X})$, and $p_1 = P(\theta > \theta_0|\mathbf{X}) = 1 - p_0$. Then the *Bayes factor*: $BF_{01} = \frac{p_0/p_1}{\pi_0/\pi_1}$, where $\pi_0 = P(\theta \leq \theta_0)$, and $\pi_1 = P(\theta > \theta_0) = 1 - \pi_0$, and it is usually assumed that $\pi_0 = \pi_1 = 1/2$. A large BF_{01} value (> 20) is a strong evidence to support H_0, and a small BF_{01} value ($< 1/20$) is a strong evidence to support H_1.

A two-sided test of $H_0 : \theta = \theta_0$ vs. $H_1 : \theta \neq \theta_0$ is usually more complicated when calculating the Bayes factor. However, there is an alternative to the Bayes factor for the two-sided test, which is Lindley's method, by computing the posterior distribution $p(\theta|\mathbf{x})$, and the $(1 - \alpha)$ *highest posterior density (HPD)* interval (or region) $\mathcal{C}_\alpha(\mathbf{x})$. If $\theta_0 \in \mathcal{C}_\alpha(\mathbf{x})$, then we accept (or fail to reject) H_0. Readers can use the book Christensen et al 2011 as a reference [9].

For interval estimation, the frequentist approach is to construct the $(1-\alpha)$ *confidence interval* of θ, and this is usually achieved by inverting a test statistic in some hypothesis testing.

The Bayes approach uses the posterior probability coverage, such that $P(\theta \in C|\mathbf{X}) = 1 - \alpha$. This is a true probability, and we call it the $(1 - \alpha)$ *credible interval*. We can find the shortest credible interval by using the *highest posterior density (HPD)* method. That is, for a posterior PDF $p(\theta|\mathbf{X})$, we can find the *HPD interval or region* by letting $C_\alpha = \{\theta : p(\theta|\mathbf{X}) \geq k_\alpha\}$, and find the value k_α, such that

$$P(\theta \in C_\alpha|\mathbf{X}) \geq 1 - \alpha. \tag{1.16}$$

There is a built-in function in the free software **R** library *TeachingDemos* called *hpd* to find the *HPD interval* for commonly used parametric distributions. If we only have the posterior samples from the posterior distribution $p(\theta|\mathbf{X})$, which is obtained from simulation, there is also a built-in function called *emp.hpd* for numerical approximation to find the empirical HPD interval.

1.5 Markov Chain Monte Carlo algorithms

For Bayesian analysis, when the likelihood function is complicated, there is no conjugate prior distribution available. In this case, we can use *Markov Chain Monte Carlo (MCMC)* simulations to obtain the *posterior samples* of $p(\theta|\mathbf{X})$, then make inferences based on the posterior samples. We will briefly review the *Gibbs sampler* and the *Metropolis-Hastings algorithm* , and how to use the algorithms to generate the posterior samples. Readers can use other books on Bayesian analysis as references [4, 9, 19, 20].

A sequence of random variables $(X_1, X_2, \ldots, X_{n-1}, X_n, X_{n+1}, \ldots)$ is a *Markov chain* if X_{n+1} and X_{n-1} are independent given X_n for all n. In other words, the distribution of X_{n+1} only depends on the value at the most recent time point X_n.

Suppose we want to generate a p-dimensional random sample $\mathbf{X} = (X_1, \ldots, X_p)$, with $\mathbf{X} \sim f_{\mathbf{X}}(x_1, \ldots, x_p)$; however, the joint density is hard to sample from, but we are able to sample from each of the conditional densities $f_{X_j}(x_j|x_{(-j)})$, where $x_{(-j)} = (x_1, \ldots,\ x_{j-1},\ x_{j+1}, \ldots,\ x_p)$, then we can use the multi-stage *Gibbs sampler* algorithm as the following:

- Pick a starting point $\mathbf{x}^{(0)} = (x_1^{(0)},\ x_2^{(0)}, \ldots,\ x_p^{(0)})$ in the domain of $f_{\mathbf{X}}(x)$.
- Repeat for $n = 1, 2, 3, \ldots$

1. Sample $X_1^{(n)} \sim f_{X_1}(\cdot\,|X_2^{(n-1)}, \ldots,\ X_p^{(n-1)})$
2. Sample $X_2^{(n)} \sim f_{X_2}(\cdot\,|X_1^{(n)},\ X_3^{(n-1)}, \ldots,\ X_p^{(n-1)})$

$\vdots$

j. Sample $X_j^{(n)} \sim f_{X_j}(\cdot\,|X_1^{(n)}, \ldots,\ X_{j-1}^{(n)},\ X_{j+1}^{(n-1)}, \ldots, X_p^{(n-1)})$

$\vdots$

p. Sample $X_p^{(n)} \sim f_{X_p}(\cdot\,|X_1^{(n)}, \ldots,\ X_{p-1}^{(n)})$

The sequence $\mathbf{X}^{(1)}$, $\mathbf{X}^{(2)}, \ldots,\ \mathbf{X}^{(\mathbf{n})}, \ldots$ is a Markov chain. Under some regularity conditions, the distribution of $\mathbf{X}^{(n)} = (X_1^{(n)},\ X_2^{(n)}, \ldots,\ X_p^{(n)})$ goes to $f_{\mathbf{X}}(x_1, \ldots, x_p)$ as $n \to \infty$.

We often face a more difficult situation, where we cannot directly sample from the conditional distributions in the Gibbs sampler. In this case, we have to use the *Metropolis-Hastings (MH) algorithm.* We assume that $f(x)$ is the target PDF that we want to sample from, the MH algorithm is the following:

- Pick a starting point $x^{(0)}$ in the domain of $f_{\mathbf{X}}(x)$, and a *proposal or jumping PDF* $q(\cdot\,|\,\cdot)$.
- Repeat for $n = 1, 2, 3, \ldots$

- Generate a candidate value $x^\star \sim q(\cdot\,|x^{(n-1)})$
- Calculate the MH acceptance probability

$$\alpha(x^{(n-1)}, x^\star) = \min\left\{1,\ \frac{f(x^\star)q(x^{(n-1)}|x^\star)}{f(x^{(n-1)})q(x^\star|x^{(n-1)})}\right\}.$$

- With probability $p^* = \alpha(x^{(n-1)}, x^\star)$, we let $x^{(n)} = x^\star$. Otherwise, with probability $(1-p^*)$, we let $x^{(n)} = x^{(n-1)}$.

To achieve the last step, generate a Bernoulli random variable with probability p^*; if it is 1, then we accept $x^{(n)} = x^*$; if it is 0, then we let $x^{(n)} = x^{(n-1)}$.

We usually pick a symmetric proposal density, so that $q(x|x^*) = q(x^*|x)$. For example, a good choice of proposal distribution is the normal distribution $N(x, \sigma^2)$, or Unif$(x-c, x+c)$, where $x = x^{(n-1)}$ is the current value. This is the original *Metropolis algorithm*. In this case, the calculation can be simplified to:

$$\alpha(x^{(n-1)}, x^\star) = \min\left\{1,\ \frac{f(x^*)}{f(x^{(n-1)})}\right\}.$$

To apply the MH algorithm and obtain the Bayesian posterior samples, our target function is the Bayesian posterior PDF:

$$p(\theta|\mathbf{X}) \propto \pi(\theta)\cdot L(\theta|\mathbf{X}),$$

Usually, we don't know the normalizing constant value c, such that $p(\theta|\mathbf{X}) = c^{-1}\pi(\theta)\cdot L(\theta|\mathbf{X})$ is a valid PDF. However, this will not be a problem, as the PDF only appears in the ratio when we calculate the $\alpha(x^{(n-1)}, x^\star)$ where the constant c will be canceled.

1.6 Screening data format

A general format of the screening data is introduced here. A mass screening trial is usually composed of a sequence of screening exams. There were a different number of exams and different time intervals between the two consecutive exams. For example, the *Minnesota Colon Cancer Control Study (MCCCS)* randomized approximately 46,000 subjects to receive either five annual *fecal occult blood test (FOBT)* screenings, or three biennial FOBT screenings, or no screening between 1976 and 1982 (Church et al [10], Wu et al 2009a [65]). In the *Mayo Lung Project* between 1971 and 1983, male heavy smokers took a screening exam every 4 months, with 19 exams altogether (Fontana et al 1975[16], Wu et al[67]).

Consider a group of initially asymptomatic individuals scheduled with K ordered screening exams at $t_0 < t_1 < \cdots < t_{K-1}$, where t_{i-1} represents a person's age at the i-th screen, $i = 1, \ldots, K$. In a periodic screening program,

TABLE 1.1
A sample of mass cancer screening data.

t_0	n_1	s_1	r_1	n_2	s_2	r_2	$\cdots$	n_K	s_K	r_K
...	...		...							
60	2100	2	1	2045	3	2	$\cdots$	1677	0	0
...	...		...							
65	1420	3	0	1368	0	0	$\cdots$	1038	1	0
...	...		...							

$\Delta = t_i - t_{i-1}, i = 1, \ldots, K-1$, is the time duration between any two consecutive exams, so $t_i = t_0 + i \cdot \Delta, i = 0, \ldots, K-1$. The mass screening data usually consists of three pieces of information in the i-th *screening interval* (t_{i-1}, t_i):

- n_i is the total number of individuals examined at the i-th screening.
- s_i denotes the number of individuals diagnosed by the i-th exam, that is, the number of *screen-detected cases.*
- r_i is the number of individuals found in the clinical state S_c within the i-th screening interval (t_{i-1}, t_i), that is, the number of *interval cases.*

Table 1.1 shows the data format for a mass screening program with K scheduled exams, where t_0 is the age at the first exam, and the triplets (n_i, s_i, r_i) stratified by the initial age are the data we use. We have collected a few screening datasets, including breast cancer, lung cancer, colorectal cancer, and ovarian cancer. These datasets were organized in a similar format as in Table 1.1, and we will introduce some datasets in the next few sections. Two full datasets were provided, and readers can use them in the study.

1.7 The Minnesota Colorectal Cancer Study

Colorectal cancer (CRC) is the third most common form of cancer and the second leading cause of death for both genders in the United States. CRC is most often found in people 50 years and older. The age-specific colorectal cancer risk rises continuously with advancing age (SEER Fast Stats Results).

Between 1976 and 1982 the *Minnesota Colon Cancer Control Study (MCCCS)* randomized approximately 46,000 subjects to receive either five annual FOBT screenings, three biennial FOBT screenings, or no screening. Each screening cycle consisted of six hemoccult slides (Hemoccult®, Beckman Coulter, Palo Alto, California), about 83% of slides were re-hydrated. If any of the slides were positive, then the screen was considered positive and a definitive workup exam was done, including a colonoscopy. Due to a lower-than-expected death rate among the controls, the investigators resumed screening between 1986 and 1992. We restricted the analysis to the original 5 annual screening groups. The initial screening age for males is between 28 and 90 inclusive, and it is between 36 and 93 for females. The MCCCS data were summarized in Tables 1.2 and 1.3, and were published in Wu et al 2009 [65].

1.8 The Mayo Lung Project

Lung cancer is the most common cancer in terms of both incidence and mortality with 1.35 million new cases per year and 1.18 million deaths, with the highest rates in Europe and North America. The most common cause of lung cancer is long-term exposure to tobacco usage. There are two major types of lung cancer: small cell or non-small cell. Non-small cell lung cancer grows and spreads less aggressively, and it often can be treated more successfully with treatments.

There were several major randomized controlled lung cancer screening studies carried out in North America: the Mayo Lung Project, the Johns Hopkins Lung Project (JHLP), the Lung Cancer Screening Program at the Memorial Sloan Kettering Cancer Center (MSKC-LCSP), the Early Lung Cancer Action Project, the Prostate, Lung, Colorectal and Ovarian Cancer Screening Trial (PLCO), and the National Lung Screening Trial (NLST). The lung cancer screening techniques are chest X-ray, sputum cytology, and low-dose computed tomography. Many people do not have symptoms or have only vague symptoms until the disease has progressed significantly. As a result, only 15% of lung cancers are discovered in the early stages, when the possibility of curative treatment is the greatest.

The Mayo Lung Project was started in August 1971, with the purpose to determine whether the death rate from bronchogenic carcinoma can be significantly reduced by vigorous application of modern detecting techniques and aggressive treatment (Fontana et al 1975 [16]). Between 1971 and 1983, 9309 candidates for the Mayo Lung Project had been enrolled in the study. They were male heavy smokers. As a group, 85% were smoking between 1 and 2.5 packs of cigarettes per day. More than 97% had smoked for at least 20 years. More than 90% of the participants were still smoking regardless of the warnings that they received. Each participant took a screening test every 4 months, with 19 tests altogether. Each screening test includes a chest X-ray and a three-day pooled sputum cytology study. If any of the tests were positive, then the screen was considered positive and a definitive workup exam, such as a biopsy, was done. The age at entry ranges from 44 to 76 years old in the Mayo Lung Project. However, we only used the data from age 45 to 69, because the other age groups have too few participants, and may cause large variations in the estimation. Table 1.4 summarizes the Mayo Lung Project screening data.

TABLE 1.2
The MCCCS males annual screening data.

t_0	n_1	s_1	r_1	n_2	s_2	r_2	n_3	s_3	r_3	n_4	s_4	r_4	n_5	s_5	r_5
28	1	0	0	1	0	0	0	0	0	0	0	0	0	0	0
35	1	0	0	1	0	0	0	0	0	0	0	0	0	0	0
37	1	0	0	1	0	0	1	0	0	1	0	0	1	0	0
41	2	0	0	1	0	0	1	0	0	1	0	0	1	0	0
42	1	0	0	1	0	0	1	0	0	1	0	0	1	0	0
43	1	0	0	1	0	0	0	0	0	0	0	0	1	0	0
44	1	0	0	1	0	0	1	0	0	1	0	0	1	0	0
45	1	0	0	1	0	0	0	0	0	0	0	0	0	0	0
46	3	0	0	3	0	0	2	0	0	2	0	0	2	0	0
47	9	0	0	8	0	0	9	0	0	7	0	0	8	0	0
48	8	0	0	8	0	0	7	0	0	6	0	0	6	0	0
49	47	0	0	47	0	0	39	0	0	40	0	0	42	0	1
50	200	0	0	178	0	0	165	0	0	162	1	0	165	0	0
51	263	0	0	235	0	0	214	0	0	228	0	0	227	0	0
52	275	0	0	243	0	0	234	0	0	231	0	0	230	0	0
53	247	0	0	225	0	0	211	1	0	217	0	0	208	0	0
54	270	0	0	251	1	0	236	0	0	244	0	0	237	0	0
55	262	1	0	234	0	0	214	1	0	223	0	0	224	0	0
56	257	0	0	239	1	0	232	0	0	229	0	0	228	0	0
57	279	1	0	255	0	1	248	1	0	248	0	0	248	0	0
58	255	0	0	235	0	0	225	0	0	227	0	0	223	1	0
59	271	0	0	247	0	0	247	1	0	243	1	0	236	0	0
60	275	0	2	244	0	0	235	0	0	230	0	0	224	0	0
61	275	1	0	252	0	0	242	0	0	232	0	0	234	0	0
62	277	1	0	245	0	0	237	1	0	225	1	0	229	2	0
63	268	2	0	243	0	0	229	1	0	225	0	0	222	1	0
64	276	1	0	253	0	0	237	1	0	226	1	0	226	1	0
65	250	1	0	225	1	0	212	0	0	199	0	0	192	0	0
66	251	2	0	224	1	0	211	0	0	202	1	0	197	1	0
67	249	0	0	230	0	0	210	0	0	198	0	0	199	0	0
68	205	1	1	188	1	0	181	0	0	174	0	0	172	0	0
69	188	0	0	178	0	0	162	0	0	149	0	0	151	0	0
70	175	0	0	153	0	0	142	0	0	134	0	0	123	0	0
71	137	0	0	127	1	0	117	0	0	106	0	0	102	0	0
72	135	0	0	117	0	0	107	0	0	100	0	0	98	0	1
73	106	0	0	87	1	0	82	1	0	76	0	0	75	0	0
74	111	0	0	97	0	0	89	1	1	77	0	0	69	0	0
75	82	0	0	74	0	0	68	0	0	57	0	0	55	0	0
76	77	0	0	59	0	0	49	1	0	48	0	0	46	0	0
77	52	0	0	43	0	0	38	0	0	42	0	0	34	0	0
78	37	1	0	37	0	0	32	0	0	26	0	0	28	0	0
79	38	0	0	33	0	0	35	0	0	27	0	0	26	0	0
80	22	0	0	15	0	0	14	0	0	13	0	0	14	1	0
81	16	0	0	12	0	0	10	0	0	9	0	0	6	0	0
82	12	0	0	11	0	0	7	0	0	4	0	0	5	0	0
83	5	0	0	4	0	0	3	0	0	1	0	0	2	0	0
84	4	0	0	2	0	0	2	0	0	1	0	0	1	0	0
85	1	0	0	1	0	0	0	0	0	0	0	0	0	0	0
86	2	0	0	1	0	0	1	0	0	0	0	0	0	0	0
87	1	0	0	1	0	0	1	0	0	1	0	0	1	0	0
90	1	0	0	1	0	0	0	0	0	1	0	0	0	0	0

Adapted from Table 1 in Wu et al 2009 [65].

TABLE 1.3
The MCCCS females annual screening data.

t_0	n_1	s_1	r_1	n_2	s_2	r_2	n_3	s_3	r_3	n_4	s_4	r_4	n_5	s_5	r_5
36	1	0	0	1	0	0	1	0	0	0	0	0	0	0	0
38	1	0	0	1	0	0	1	0	0	0	0	0	1	0	0
40	2	0	0	2	0	0	2	0	0	2	0	0	2	0	0
42	2	0	0	2	0	0	2	0	0	1	0	0	2	0	0
43	1	0	0	1	0	0	1	0	0	1	0	0	1	0	0
44	3	0	0	3	0	0	3	0	0	2	0	0	2	0	0
45	2	0	0	3	0	0	2	0	0	2	0	0	2	0	0
46	4	0	0	4	0	0	4	0	0	5	0	0	5	0	0
47	6	0	0	6	0	0	6	0	0	6	0	0	6	0	0
48	16	0	0	14	0	0	13	0	0	12	0	0	13	0	0
49	67	0	0	59	0	0	50	0	0	55	0	0	52	0	0
50	194	0	0	178	0	0	168	0	0	171	1	0	162	0	0
51	223	0	0	207	0	0	195	0	0	197	1	0	189	1	0
52	237	0	0	222	0	0	202	0	0	204	0	0	202	0	0
53	248	0	0	230	0	1	222	0	0	206	0	0	215	0	0
54	251	0	0	226	0	0	215	0	0	217	1	0	214	0	0
55	261	0	0	239	0	0	216	0	0	215	0	0	225	0	0
56	282	0	0	254	1	0	253	0	0	250	0	0	253	0	0
57	311	0	0	285	0	0	269	0	0	279	0	0	266	0	0
58	333	0	0	316	0	0	297	0	0	299	1	0	299	1	0
59	283	1	0	255	0	0	246	0	0	243	0	0	246	0	0
60	339	0	0	314	0	0	303	0	0	293	1	0	301	0	0
61	320	1	0	303	0	0	291	1	0	274	0	0	282	0	1
62	341	0	0	313	0	0	312	1	0	282	1	0	293	0	0
63	350	0	0	333	0	0	314	1	0	298	0	0	306	0	0
64	308	1	0	283	0	0	265	0	0	245	0	0	253	1	0
65	316	0	0	289	0	0	288	0	0	270	0	0	276	0	0
66	308	0	0	283	0	0	278	2	0	264	0	0	260	0	0
67	289	1	0	269	1	0	250	0	0	245	2	0	240	1	0
68	266	1	0	241	1	0	229	0	0	212	1	0	213	0	0
69	199	1	0	186	1	0	183	0	0	170	0	0	167	0	0
70	201	1	0	184	1	0	175	0	0	163	0	0	160	2	0
71	197	3	0	175	0	0	173	0	0	167	2	0	160	1	0
72	150	0	1	135	1	0	128	0	0	117	1	0	118	0	0
73	143	1	0	133	0	0	132	0	0	119	0	0	116	0	0
74	102	0	0	90	0	0	92	0	0	84	0	0	77	0	0
75	92	1	0	82	0	0	81	0	0	67	0	0	69	0	0
76	84	0	0	77	0	0	72	0	0	67	1	0	66	0	0
77	82	0	0	74	0	0	65	0	0	58	1	0	60	0	0
78	47	0	0	42	0	0	39	0	0	34	0	0	34	1	0
79	35	0	0	29	0	0	29	0	0	21	0	0	18	0	0
80	33	0	0	28	0	0	27	0	0	22	0	0	19	0	0
81	16	0	0	9	0	0	10	0	0	7	0	0	7	0	0
82	11	0	0	9	0	0	7	0	0	7	0	0	7	0	0
83	9	0	0	7	0	0	7	0	0	3	0	0	4	0	0
84	5	0	0	4	0	0	3	0	0	3	0	0	3	0	0
85	3	0	0	2	0	0	1	0	0	1	0	0	1	0	0
87	1	0	0	1	0	0	0	0	0	0	0	0	0	0	0
88	2	0	0	2	0	0	2	0	0	2	0	0	1	0	0
93	1	0	0	0	0	0	0	0	0	0	0	0	0	0	0

Adapted from Table 2 in Wu et al 2009 [65].

TABLE 1.4

MAYO: 19 screenings at four months apart, censoring all interval cancers at four months after the last exam.

44	1 0 0	0 0 0	0 0 0	0 0 0	0 0 0	0 0 0	0 0 0	0 0 0	0 0 0	0 0 0	0 0 0	0 0 0	0 0 0	0 0 0	0 0 0	0 0 0	0 0 0	0 0 0	0 0 0
45	491 1 0	215 0 0	199 0 0	190 0 0	186 0 0	179 0 0	175 0 0	171 0 0	168 0 0	166 0 0	162 0 0	159 0 0	154 0 0	153 0 0	151 0 0	147 0 0	146 0 0	139 0 0	121 0 1
46	442 0 0	223 0 0	214 0 0	207 0 0	201 0 0	193 0 0	190 0 0	186 0 0	180 0 0	175 0 0	170 0 0	165 0 0	162 0 0	156 0 0	152 0 0	150 0 0	148 0 0	145 1 0	126 0 0
47	461 0 0	224 0 0	211 0 0	204 1 0	194 0 0	190 0 0	182 0 0	179 0 0	175 0 0	171 0 0	170 0 0	167 0 0	162 0 0	159 0 0	153 0 0	150 0 0	142 0 0	140 0 0	125 0 0
48	444 1 0	184 0 0	177 0 0	171 0 0	165 0 0	161 0 0	160 0 0	156 0 0	152 1 0	149 0 0	145 0 0	143 0 0	137 0 0	135 0 0	133 0 0	129 0 0	123 0 0	119 1 0	99 0 0
49	478 1 0	221 0 0	212 0 0	201 0 0	191 0 0	183 0 0	178 0 0	177 0 0	177 0 0	172 0 0	170 1 0	167 0 0	166 0 0	162 0 0	158 1 0	155 0 0	152 0 0	142 0 0	128 1 0
50	461 2 0	221 0 0	211 0 1	202 0 0	194 0 0	191 0 0	190 0 0	184 0 0	182 0 0	177 0 0	175 1 0	170 0 0	167 0 0	163 0 0	158 0 0	156 0 0	150 0 0	148 0 0	135 0 0
51	458 3 0	201 0 0	196 0 0	193 0 0	186 0 0	183 0 0	179 1 1	171 0 0	169 1 0	166 0 0	163 0 0	162 0 0	156 0 0	152 0 0	151 0 0	148 0 0	145 0 0	139 1 0	118 0 0
52	467 5 0	222 0 0	216 0 0	211 0 0	206 0 0	204 0 0	203 2 0	197 0 0	195 0 0	188 0 0	185 0 0	181 0 0	180 1 0	178 0 0	174 0 1	167 0 0	166 0 0	153 0 0	134 0 0
53	431 4 0	191 0 0	184 0 0	181 0 0	178 0 0	173 0 0	170 0 0	168 0 0	165 0 1	160 0 0	157 1 0	151 0 0	146 0 0	141 0 0	138 1 0	134 0 0	127 0 0	121 0 0	104 0 0
54	439 4 0	194 0 0	190 0 0	181 0 0	174 0 0	171 1 0	167 0 0	162 0 0	159 0 0	157 0 0	153 0 0	152 1 0	149 0 0	149 0 0	147 0 0	143 0 0	140 0 0	137 0 0	123 0 0
55	427 5 0	206 1 0	197 1 0	188 0 0	183 0 0	180 0 0	177 1 0	172 0 0	171 2 0	167 1 0	162 0 0	160 0 0	157 1 0	151 0 0	147 0 1	142 0 0	136 1 0	130 0 0	121 0 0
56	434 5 0	212 0 0	208 0 0	201 0 0	197 0 0	195 0 0	192 0 0	190 1 0	187 0 0	185 0 0	179 0 0	172 1 0	166 0 0	160 1 0	158 0 0	153 1 0	145 0 0	135 1 0	124 0 0
57	436 3 1	193 1 0	183 0 0	179 0 0	174 0 0	168 0 0	163 1 0	160 0 0	159 0 0	156 0 1	154 0 0	148 1 0	146 1 0	144 0 0	140 0 0	137 0 0	137 0 0	133 1 0	121 1 1
58	386 6 0	194 0 0	185 0 0	177 0 0	174 0 0	168 0 0	162 0 0	160 0 0	159 0 0	156 0 0	152 0 0	149 0 0	146 0 0	142 0 0	139 0 0	135 0 0	131 0 0	129 0 0	121 0 0
59	402 4 0	183 0 0	175 1 0	171 0 0	169 0 0	166 0 0	163 0 0	157 0 0	155 0 0	152 0 0	151 0 0	151 0 0	145 0 0	143 1 0	140 1 0	136 0 0	132 1 1	124 0 0	119 1 0
60	371 4 0	172 0 0	168 0 0	163 1 0	158 0 0	155 0 0	153 1 0	147 0 0	145 0 0	142 0 0	137 0 0	133 0 0	132 0 0	127 0 0	124 1 0	121 0 1	114 1 0	109 0 0	104 0 0
61	342 6 0	170 1 0	166 0 0	156 0 0	152 0 0	150 1 0	148 0 0	147 1 0	142 0 0	140 0 0	134 1 0	130 1 0	126 0 0	125 0 1	123 0 1	121 0 1	118 0 0	116 0 0	106 0 0
62	347 5 0	155 0 0	151 0 0	143 0 0	140 0 0	136 0 0	130 0 0	128 1 0	126 0 0	124 0 0	121 0 0	119 1 0	116 0 0	112 1 0	110 1 0	105 0 1	102 0 0	98 0 0	90 0 0
63	278 5 0	143 0 0	139 0 0	137 0 0	132 0 2	126 1 0	123 0 0	123 0 0	122 0 0	120 0 1	119 0 0	115 1 0	111 0 0	110 0 0	108 1 0	105 1 1	99 1 1	94 0 0	85 0 0
64	285 6 0	125 1 0	118 1 0	116 0 0	113 1 0	109 0 0	105 0 0	103 0 0	102 0 0	101 0 0	101 0 0	97 0 0	94 0 0	90 0 0	88 1 0	87 0 0	85 2 0	82 0 0	74 1 0
65	259 3 0	120 1 0	112 0 0	109 0 0	109 0 0	106 0 0	102 1 0	101 0 0	99 0 0	93 0 0	90 0 0	87 0 0	83 0 0	82 0 0	81 0 0	76 0 0	75 0 0	72 0 0	66 1 0
66	188 5 0	86 0 0	81 0 0	79 0 0	78 1 0	71 2 0	66 0 0	66 0 0	64 2 0	60 0 0	60 0 0	60 0 0	58 0 0	54 0 0	52 0 0	51 1 0	50 0 0	48 0 0	42 0 0
67	207 4 0	104 1 1	97 0 0	92 0 1	86 0 0	85 1 0	82 1 0	79 1 0	76 0 0	73 0 0	70 0 0	68 0 0	67 0 0	66 0 0	64 0 0	60 0 0	58 1 0	55 0 0	51 0 0
68	177 5 0	72 1 1	68 0 0	66 0 0	63 0 0	62 0 0	60 0 0	58 0 0	58 0 0	57 1 0	53 0 0	52 0 0	52 1 0	48 1 0	46 0 1	43 1 0	42 0 0	39 0 0	35 0 0
69	144 3 0	69 0 0	64 0 0	59 2 0	55 0 0	54 1 0	52 0 0	52 0 0	49 0 0	47 0 0	46 0 0	45 0 0	45 0 0	44 0 2	42 2 0	39 0 0	38 0 0	38 0 0	34 0 0
70	14 0 0	6 0 0	6 0 0	6 0 0	6 0 0	6 0 0	5 0 0	5 0 0	4 0 0	4 0 0	4 0 0	4 0 0	3 0 0	3 0 0	3 0 0	3 0 0	3 0 0	3 0 0	3 0 0
71	14 0 0	5 0 0	5 0 0	5 0 0	4 0 0	4 0 0	4 0 0	4 0 0	4 0 0	4 0 0	4 0 0	4 0 0	4 0 0	4 0 0	4 0 0	3 0 0	3 0 0	3 0 0	3 0 0
72	9 0 0	4 0 0	4 0 0	4 0 0	4 0 0	4 0 0	4 0 0	4 0 0	4 0 0	4 0 0	4 0 0	4 0 0	4 0 0	3 0 0	3 0 0	1 0 0	1 0 0	1 0 0	1 0 0
73	10 0 1	3 0 0	3 0 0	3 0 0	3 0 0	3 0 0	3 0 0	3 0 0	3 0 0	3 0 0	3 0 0	3 0 0	3 0 0	3 0 0	3 0 0	3 0 0	3 0 0	3 0 0	3 0 0
74	2 0 0	1 0 0	1 0 0	1 0 0	1 0 0	1 0 0	1 0 0	1 0 0	1 0 0	1 0 0	1 0 0	1 0 0	1 0 0	1 0 0	1 0 0	1 0 0	1 0 0	1 0 0	1 0 0
75	3 0 0	2 0 0	2 0 0	2 0 0	2 0 0	2 0 0	2 0 0	2 0 0	2 0 0	2 0 0	2 0 0	2 0 0	2 0 0	2 0 0	2 0 0	2 0 0	2 0 0	2 0 0	2 0 0
76	1 0 0	0 0 0	0 0 0	0 0 0	0 0 0	0 0 0	0 0 0	0 0 0	0 0 0	0 0 0	0 0 0	0 0 0	0 0 0	0 0 0	0 0 0	0 0 0	0 0 0	0 0 0	0 0 0

1.9 The Health Insurance Plan (HIP) of Greater New York

The Health Insurance Plan of Greater New York (HIP) study, began at the end of 1963 (Shapiro et al 1988 [47]). It was the first randomized mass clinical trial that use *mammograms* and *clinical breast exams* as diagnostic screening tests for breast cancer. The study randomized initially *asymptomatic* women aged 40 to 64 years without a history of breast cancer into two groups: the study and the control group. Each group consisted of about 31,000 women. The study group was composed of four annual breast cancer screening exams, with each exam including both a mammogram and a clinical breast exam. The control group only received the usual care. After 15 years of follow-up, more than 1100 (1171 vs. 1154) breast cancer cases were diagnosed in the study and the control group correspondingly, with about 300 cases within the first 5 years of follow-up. In the study group, 132 cases were detected by scheduled screening exams. Shapiro et al wrote a book on the HIP study, with many data summary tables [47].

1.10 The National Lung Screening Trial (NLST) study

The National Lung Screening Trial (NLST) is a recently finished mass screening study on lung cancer. The purpose of the project was to compare two different screening modalities for early detection: low-dose helical computed tomography (or spiral CT) versus standard chest X-rays for heavy smokers [53]. The spiral CT uses X-rays to obtain a multiple-image scan of the entire chest, while a standard chest X-ray produces a single image of the whole chest. Participants were either current or former heavy smokers but were without signs, symptoms, or history of lung cancer, i.e., asymptomatic heavy smokers. There were 54,000 male or female heavy smokers enrolled in the study, with initial screening ages between 55 and 74 in 33 centers across the United States. The study was carried out between August 2002 and April 2004. All participants were evenly randomized to one of two arms: chest X-ray arm or the low-dose CT arm. Three annual screening exams were provided to each participant in each arm. Although 5-year survival rates approach 70% with surgical resection of stage IA lung cancer (i.e., non-small cell lung cancer (NSCLC) that is 3 cm across or smaller), more than 75% of patients with locally advanced or metastatic lung cancer have a 5-year survival of less than 5%. The primary endpoint of the NLST is lung cancer mortality. Since March 2021, the United States Preventive Services Task Force (USPSTF) recommends "annual screening for lung cancer with low-dose computed tomography (LDCT)

TABLE 1.5
Overview of the NLST data.

Group within Study	[a]Total subj.	[b]Screen-diag. No.	[c]Interval No.
	The NLST: Chest X-ray		
Overall	26226	279	177
male smokers	15500	165	107
female smokers	10726	114	70
	The NLST: Spiral CT		
Overall	26452	649	60
male smokers	15621	384	44
female smokers	10831	265	16

[a]Total number of people who ever received lung cancer screens.
[b]Total number of subjects diagnosed by regular screening.
[c]Total number of clinical incident cases between two regular screenings.

in adults aged 50 to 80 years who have a 20 pack-year smoking history and currently smoke or have quit within the past 15 years. Screening should be discontinued once a person has not smoked for 15 years or develops a health problem that substantially limits life expectancy or the ability or willingness to have curative lung surgery"[18]. For more information, see the USPSTF website: *https://www.uspreventiveservicestaskforce.org/uspstf/*.

The NLST screening data were summarized in Table 1.5. It is obvious that more tumors were diagnosed in the low-dose CT arm than in the chest X-ray arm, which implies that the sensitivity of spiral CT may be higher than that of chest X-rays. Two cohorts from the CT arms (male vs. female heavy smokers) will be used as examples. The NLST data cannot be released here due to the contract with NCI, although we will use it in many examples.

The presented dataset in the previous sections can be used for learning purposes and for understanding the modeling in this book. Readers are encouraged to find their own dataset. It is straightforward to generate pseudo-screening data using the method in section 2.4 of Chapter 2.

2

Estimating the Three Key Parameters

CONTENTS

The first mass cancer screening was carried out in the 1960s in the United States targeting breast cancer, i.e., the Health Insurance Plan of Greater New York (HIP) study. Since then, several major randomized controlled cancer screening trials for other cancer sites have been carried out in the Western world. For lung cancer, there were at least six large-scale mass screenings using pooled sputum cytology, chest X-ray, or low-dose computed tomography, including the Mayo Lung Project, the Johns Hopkins Study, the Memorial Sloan Kettering study, the Early Lung Cancer Action Project, the Prostate, Lung, Colorectal, and Ovarian (PLCO) Cancer Screening Trial, and the most recent National Lung Screening Trial (NLST). For colon cancer, there was the Minnesota colorectal cancer study using the fecal occult blood test (FOBT).

However, after six decades, more controversy rather than solutions appeared in the practice. Is cancer screening beneficial? Is it harmful? What is the chance of overdiagnosis? Should people take part in screening regularly?

DOI: 10.1201/9781003404125-2

When should we start screening, and how frequently should one be screened? To address these problems, observational studies are not enough, while probability modeling may provide more accurate information.

In this chapter, we start by introducing concepts in cancer screening modeling, and deriving the probability of various cases, including screen-detected, clinical incidence, lifetime risk, etc. It is important to understand the probability calculation, as we will use these and a similar derivation procedure to estimate the probability of other terms, such as the *lead time* (i.e., the diagnosis time advanced by screening), the *overdiagnosis* (i.e., the diagnosis of tumor that would not have caused any symptoms in one's lifetime), etc. Then we focus on the estimation of the three key parameters: the *sensitivity* of screening modality, the *sojourn time* in the preclinical state, and the *transition density* which is the probability density of the time in the disease-free state.

The three key parameters are important because all other terms are functions of the three key parameters. Therefore, accurate estimation of the three key parameters is critical. We will use two different models to estimate the three key parameters: one assumes that the sensitivity is a function of age, and the other assumes that sensitivity is a function of time spent in the preclinical state and the sojourn time. In both models, we use the maximum likelihood estimate (MLE) and Bayesian posterior estimation to make inferences for the three key model parameters. The Bayesian method provides more information, such as the posterior density curves, the measures of uncertainty, the predictive distribution, etc.

2.1 Introduction

The purpose of screening is to detect tumors early before clinical symptoms would appear, so that patients may have a better prognosis and more available treatments, and hence increase the chance for complete healing and survival. There are different kinds of screening modalities targeting different kinds of cancer, for example, mammograms, digital mammograms, and clinical breast exams (CBE) for breast cancer, chest X-ray or computed tomography (CT) for lung cancer, fecal occult blood test (FOBT) for colon cancer, and prostate-specific antigen (PSA) test for prostate cancer.

Using breast cancer screening as an example, we introduce concepts and parameters used in cancer screening. The *disease progressive model* was first proposed by Zelen and Feinleib 1969 shortly after the screening program of the Health Insurance Plan of Greater New York (HIP) study was completed [87]. It is assumed that clinical disease progresses through three states, denoted by $S_0 \to S_p \to S_c$. See Figure 2.1, where S_0 is the *disease-free state* or the

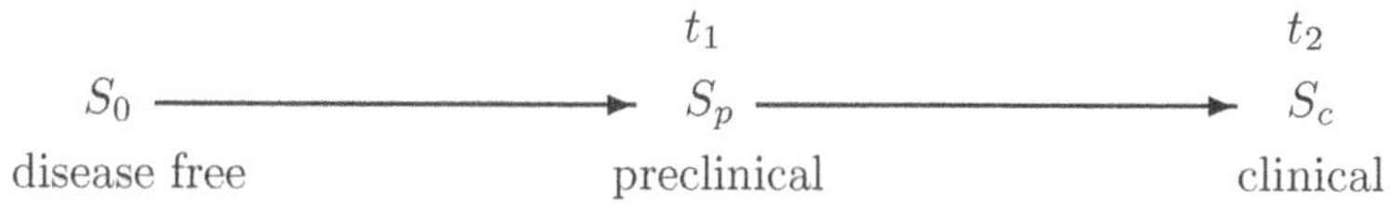

$$S_0 \xrightarrow{} \overset{t_1}{S_p} \xrightarrow{} \overset{t_2}{S_c}$$

disease free — preclinical — clinical

FIGURE 2.1
Disease development model.

state in which the disease cannot be detected by any technology; S_p refers to the *preclinical state* , in which an asymptomatic individual unknowingly has the disease that a screening exam can detect; and S_c is the *clinical state* at which the disease manifests itself in clinical symptoms. In fact, each state is a period of time, not a single time point; therefore, Figure 2.2 is a better description of the three states: S_0 is the time period from birth to age t_1, S_p refers the time period from t_1 to t_2, and S_c starts at age t_2, the onset of clinical symptoms. The progressive disease model describes the natural history of tumor development. The goal of screening programs is to detect the tumor in the preclinical state S_p before any clinical symptom appears.

2.2 The three key parameters and other terminology

Zelen and Feinleib 1969 provided a simple probability model in cancer screening when an individual was examined only once [87]. However, it defined some concepts in cancer screening that are widely used today: screening sensitivity, transition probability density from the disease-free state to the preclinical state, and sojourn time distribution in the preclinical state. We will introduce them and other important parameters as well.

The *sensitivity* is the probability that a screening exam result is positive, given that an individual is in the preclinical state S_p. We let D represent the

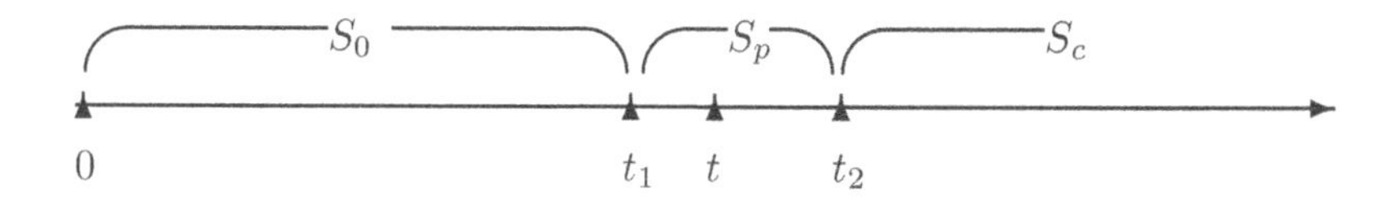

FIGURE 2.2
Disease development and the lead time.

true disease status of an individual:

$$D = \begin{cases} 1, & \text{if an individual has the disease.} \\ 0, & \text{if an individual doesn't have the disease.} \end{cases}$$

And we let X represent the test result of a screening exam:

$$X = \begin{cases} 1, & \text{if a test is positive.} \\ 0, & \text{if a test is negative.} \end{cases}$$

The sensitivity β is the probability of correctly identifying those who have the disease: $\beta = P(X = 1|D = 1)$.

Specificity is the probability of correctly identifying those who do *not* have the disease, that is, $\alpha = P(X = 0|D = 0)$. Ideally, we wish to have a test with both sensitivity and specificity equal to 100%, but in reality, this is unachievable. In fact, both sensitivity and specificity cannot be estimated directly from data summary in mass screening. Here is the reason: Suppose there are n people taking part in one screening exam, according to their true disease status and the screening results, the data can be separated into 4 groups as in Table 2.1.

From Table 2.1, we can see that the sensitivity $\beta = P(X = 1|D = 1) = n_{11}/(n_{11} + n_{21})$, and the specificity $\alpha = P(X = 0|D = 0) = n_{22}/(n_{12} + n_{22})$. However, in a mass screening program, only n_{11} and n_{12} can be obtained by a follow-up exam, such as a biopsy after a positive screening result to confirm whether it is cancerous or not. The other two numbers n_{21} and n_{22} are usually unknown. Because confirmation of the true disease status is not cost-effective, nor ethical for those screened negative individuals (who are the majority in mass screening). Therefore, we cannot directly obtain the β and the α from data collection, but we can use a probability model to estimate the sensitivity (Wu et al 2005 [79]). Another important concept is *false-positive rate* , which is defined as the ratio of the number of false positives (n_{12}), and the total number of disease-free cases. That is, the false-positive rate equals to $n_{12}/(n_{12} + n_{22}) = 1 - \alpha$ in Table 2.1.

The *sojourn time* is the time duration in the preclinical state; that is, the time from when the disease first develops (onset of S_p at t_1) to the manifestation of clinical symptoms (onset of S_c at t_2); it is $(t_2 - t_1)$ in Figure 2.2. The nature of disease development prevents the observation of the onset of S_p; that

TABLE 2.1
True disease status and test result in one mass screening.

		Disease Status	
		Diseased: $D = 1$	*Not diseased:* $D = 0$
Test	+	True positive (n_{11})	False positive (n_{12})
Result	−	False negative (n_{21})	True negative (n_{22})

is, we cannot observe when the preclinical state starts. And data collection in a screening program makes it impossible to observe the onset of S_c if cancer was detected at a screening exam. Therefore, estimation of the sojourn time is difficult. However, this information can be obtained under model assumptions, and different kinds of cancer usually have different lengths of sojourn time. For example, the preclinical phase of breast cancer may last from 1 to 5 years (Wu et al 2005 [79], Shen and Zelen 1999 [49], Walter and Day 1983 [54]), and it may last longer for colorectal cancer (Wu et al 2009a [65]), and the sojourn time of lung cancer may cover a wide range, depending on whether it is small cell lung cancer or non-small cell lung cancer. For those with a long sojourn time, it is relatively easier to catch cancer in its preclinical stage.

The *transition probability density* was defined in Zelen and Feinleib (1969) as making a transition from the disease-free state (S_0) to the preclinical state (S_p). It is in fact a probability density function (PDF) of the time duration in the disease-free state S_0. Since some people may stay in a disease-free state all their lifetime and never make a transition to the preclinical state S_p, this PDF is in fact a sub-PDF. This means the whole area under the transition density curve is less than 1 (Wu et al 2005 [79]), and it is difficult to estimate its distribution without proper probability modeling.

The *lead time* is the length of time that the diagnosis is advanced by screening. The effectiveness of the screening program is directly related to the lead time. In Figure 2.2, one enters the preclinical state S_p at age t_1, and enters the clinical state S_c at age t_2 if there is no screening intervention, so $(t_2 - t_1)$ is the sojourn time. However, if she is offered a screening exam at the time t within the time interval (t_1, t_2), and cancer is diagnosed, then the length of the time $(t_2 - t)$ is the lead time. An individual with a longer lead time usually has a better prognosis than those with a shorter one. For a particular case detected by the screening, the lead time is unobservable. When evaluating the effectiveness of a screening program, we must consider the fact that age at diagnosis is advanced if the disease is detected by screening rather than by the onset of clinical symptoms. Even in the absence of effective therapy, screening may appear to lengthen one's *survival time*, the time from diagnosis until death. If we do not account for the lead time when analyzing the benefit of screening, then our inference is subject to *lead time bias*; that is, the survival time appears longer because of earlier diagnosis. Fortunately, probability modeling makes it possible to accurately estimate the distribution of lead time. It is a function of the three key parameters: sensitivity, sojourn time distribution, and transition probability density.

The *overdiagnosis* is another important concept in cancer screening. It refers to people who were confirmed with cancer (not false positive); however, if the cancer were left untreated, no symptom would have come up before they die of other causes. Overdiagnosis has caused hot debates for some time, estimates based on the observation studies vary greatly, from 7% [46] to 52% [29]. To address this issue, we will separate all screening participants into 4 mutually exclusive groups: symptom-free-life, no-early-detection, true-early-detection, and overdiagnosis. The probability of each outcome with or without a screening history for asymptomatic individuals could be derived, and it is also a function of the three key parameters. The probability of overdiagnosis among those screen-detected can be obtained by conditional probability; and this is the number that causes much attention and concern from the general public.

In summary, it is very important to have an accurate estimation of the three key parameters, since all other terms are functions of the three. Once these three key parameters are determined, the whole process is well-defined.

2.3 Probability calculation

The probability of different events lays the foundation for the methods in this book. We will provide detailed probability calculations for a few cases in this section, and mastering probability calculation is very important in understanding the rest of the book. Throughout this chapter, the time t usually represents a participating individual's age.

2.3.1 Probability of incidence and lifetime risk

For an individual who has clinical cancer without any screening, we let T_1 be the time duration in S_0, and T_2 be the time duration in S_p, i.e., the sojourn time; see Figure 2.2. We usually cannot observe T_1 and T_2, though sometimes we can observe the incidence time, or the value $(T_1 + T_2)$ if the cancer is a clinical incident case.

We assume that T_1 and T_2 are independent random variables, and let $T_1 \sim w(t)$, and $T_2 \sim q(x)$, where $w(t)$ and $q(x)$ are the corresponding probability density functions (PDF). In fact, $w(t)$ is a sub-PDF, because some people may never have cancer in their lifetime, which means, the lifetime risk for a specific cancer is less than 1, i.e., $\int w(t)dt < 1$. We let $Q(z) = \int_z^\infty q(x)dx$ be the survival function of the sojourn time in the preclinical state S_p.

We let $Y = T_1 + T_2$ be the clinical incidence time, that is, the time when clinical symptoms present. When there is no screening involved, the probability density function (PDF) of Y can be obtained by applying equation (1.11):

$$I_Y(y) = \int_0^y w(x)q(y-x)dx. \tag{2.1}$$

We can derive the probability of having clinical symptoms during one's lifetime for an individual at the current age t_0. First, we derive the formula when one's lifetime $T(> t_0)$ is fixed, then we allow T to be random. When lifetime

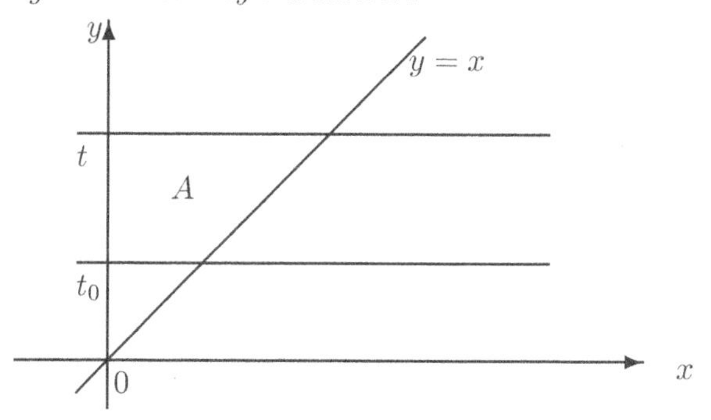

FIGURE 2.3
The area A defined by $\{t_0 < y < t, 0 < x < y\}$.

$T = t(> t_0)$ is fixed, the probability of incidence in (t_0, t) is

$$\begin{aligned}
&P(t_0 < Y < T|T = t) = P(t_0 < Y < t) \\
&= \int_{t_0}^{t} I_Y(y)dy = \int_{t_0}^{t}\int_{0}^{y} w(x)q(y-x)dxdy \quad \text{(switch } dx \text{ and } dy\text{)} \\
&= \int_{0}^{t_0}\int_{t_0}^{t} w(x)q(y-x)dydx + \int_{t_0}^{t}\int_{x}^{t} w(x)q(y-x)dydx \\
&= \int_{0}^{t_0} w(x)\left\{\int_{t_0}^{t} q(y-x)dy\right\}dx + \int_{t_0}^{t} w(x)\left\{\int_{x}^{t} q(y-x)dy\right\}dx \\
&= \int_{0}^{t_0} w(x)[Q(t_0-x) - Q(t-x)]dx + \int_{t_0}^{t} w(x)[1 - Q(t-x)]dx.
\end{aligned} \tag{2.2}$$

See Figure 2.3 to understand switching the order of dx and dy in the (2.2).

When the lifetime T is random, the probability of having clinical symptoms after age t_0 and before one's death is

$$\begin{aligned}
&P(t_0 < Y < T|T > t_0) = \int_{t_0}^{\infty} P(t_0 < Y < T|T = t)f_T(t|T > t_0)dt \\
&= \int_{t_0}^{\infty} P(t_0 < Y < t)f_T(t|T > t_0)dt.
\end{aligned} \tag{2.3}$$

Where the conditional PDF of the lifetime

$$f_T(t|T > t_0) = \begin{cases} \frac{f_T(t)}{P(T>t_0)} = \frac{f_T(t)}{1-F_T(t_0)}, & \text{if } t > t_0; \\ 0, & \text{otherwise.} \end{cases} \tag{2.4}$$

The $f_T(t)$ can be obtained by transforming the actuarial life table from the US Social Security Administration[1]. We will provide more details on how to obtain the $f_T(t)$ in section 4.3.2 of Chapter 4.

[1] http://www.ssa.gov/OACT/STATS/table4c6.html, last access 11/19/2022.

Exercise 2.1.
For an individual currently at age 60, numerically calculate the lifetime risk of certain cancer if his lifetime T is 85, i.e., calculate $P(60 < Y < 85)$, under the following scenarios:

(a) $w(t) = 0.003, Q(x) = e^{-x}$.

(b)

$$
\begin{aligned}
w(t) &= \frac{0.2}{\sqrt{2\pi}\sigma t} \exp\left\{-(\log t - \mu)^2/(2\sigma^2)\right\}, \quad \mu = 4.4,\ \sigma^2 = 0.15; \\
Q(x) &= \frac{1}{1 + (x\rho)^\kappa}, \quad \kappa = 2.5,\ \rho = 0.8.
\end{aligned}
$$

(c)

$$
\begin{aligned}
w(t) &= \frac{0.3}{\sqrt{2\pi}\sigma t} \exp\left\{-(\log t - \mu)^2/(2\sigma^2)\right\}, \quad \mu = 4.3, \&\sigma^2 = 0.1; \\
Q(x) &= \exp(-\lambda x^\alpha), \quad \lambda = 0.2,\ \alpha = 2.5.
\end{aligned}
$$

(d) Prove that

$$
\int_0^\infty I_Y(y)dy = \int_0^\infty w(t)dt.
$$

For numerical calculation in (a) to (c), readers can pick 0.1 as the step length in the integral approximation, and answers are provided at the end of this chapter.

2.3.2 Probability of screen-detected cases

Consider an asymptomatic woman at age t_0, who will go through a sequence of K screening exams, happening at her age $t_0 < t_1 < \cdots < t_{K-1}$. We let the sensitivity $\beta_i = \beta(t_i)$ at her age t_i. $T_1 \sim w(t)$ is her time in the S_0, $T_2 \sim q(x)$ is her sojourn time in the S_p, and $Q(z) = \int_z^\infty q(x)dx$ is the survival function of the sojourn time. We assume that T_1 and T_2 are independent and that β_i doesn't depend on T_1 nor T_2. How to calculate the probability that one is in the preclinical state S_p and will be detected at the i–th exam t_{i-1} for the first time? and how to calculate the probability of clinical incidence between any two screening exams? We start by defining two events:

$$
\begin{aligned}
D_i &= \{\text{She is in the preclinical state and is detected at } t_{i-1}\}. \\
I_i &= \{\text{She is a clinical incidence case in } (t_{i-1}, t_i)\}.
\end{aligned}
$$

We use female breast cancer as an example, and start with the simplest case of one or two screenings, and then we move on to the general situation.

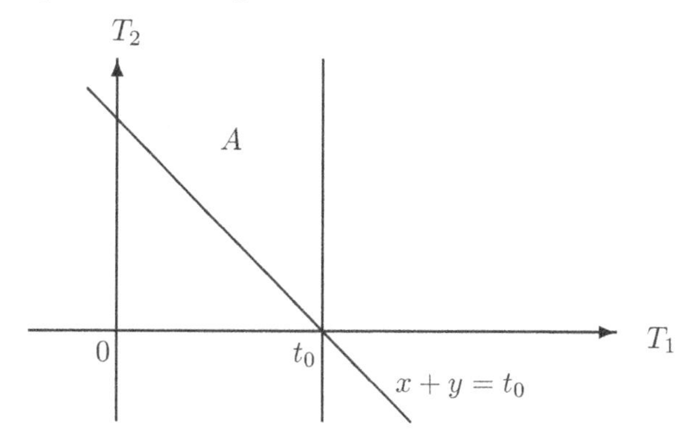

FIGURE 2.4
The area A defined by $\{T_1 < t_0, T_1 + T_2 > t_0\}$.

To calculate $P(D_1)$, the probability of diagnosis at the first exam at her age t_0, she must have entered the preclinical state S_p before t_0, and has remained in the preclinical state at t_0. Then

$$\begin{aligned} P(D_1) &= \beta_0 P(\text{onset age of } S_p < t_0, \text{onset age of } S_c > t_0) \\ &= \beta_0 P(T_1 < t_0, T_1 + T_2 > t_0), \end{aligned} \tag{2.5}$$

Let A be the area defined by $\{T_1 < t_0, T_1 + T_2 > t_0\}$; see Figure 2.4. Since we know the distribution of T_1, T_2 and they are independent, we can calculate the joint probability of two random variables:

$$\begin{aligned} P(D_1) =& \beta_0 P(T_1 < t_0, T_1 + T_2 > t_0) \\ =& \beta_0 \int_A f_{T_1,T_2}(x,y)dxdy = \beta_0 \int_0^{t_0} \int_{t_0-x}^{\infty} f_{T_1,T_2}(x,y)dydx \\ =& \beta_0 \int_0^{t_0} f_{T_1}(x) \int_{t_0-x}^{\infty} f_{T_2}(y)dydx \\ =& \beta_0 \int_0^{t_0} w(x) \int_{t_0-x}^{\infty} q(y)dydx \\ =& \beta_0 \int_0^{t_0} w(x)Q(t_0 - x)dx. \end{aligned} \tag{2.6}$$

In fact, there is another way to calculate this using the conditional distribution and reach the same answer:

$$\begin{aligned} P(D_1) =& \beta_0 P(T_1 < t_0, T_1 + T_2 > t_0) \\ =& \beta_0 \int_0^{t_0} f_{T_1}(x) P(T_1 + T_2 > t_0 | T_1 = x)dx \\ =& \beta_0 \int_0^{t_0} w(x) P(T_2 > t_0 - x | T_1 = x)dx, \ T_1, T_2 \text{ are independent} \\ =& \beta_0 \int_0^{t_0} w(x) P(T_2 > t_0 - x)dx = \beta_0 \int_0^{t_0} w(x)Q(t_0 - x)dx. \end{aligned}$$

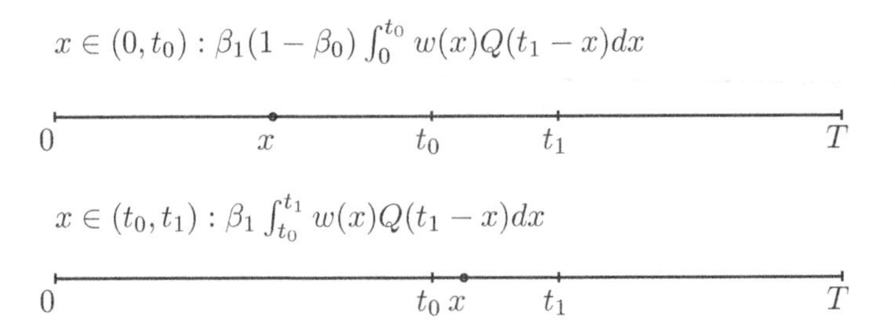

FIGURE 2.5
Two possible onset cases of the S_p in D_2.

Now to calculate $P(D_2)$, there are two possible cases depending on when she enters the preclinical state S_p. See Figure 2.5, where x is the onset age of the preclinical state S_p. In both cases, the sojourn time is longer than $(t_1 - x)$.

$$
\begin{aligned}
P(D_2) &= \beta_1(1-\beta_0) \int_0^{t_0} w(x)Q(t_1 - x)dx \\
&\quad + \beta_1 \int_{t_0}^{t_1} w(x)Q(t_1 - x)dx
\end{aligned}
$$

Exercise 2.2.

(a) Derive $P(D_3)$, the probability of being detected at the 3rd exam at t_2.

(b) Derive $P(D_4)$, the probability of being detected at the 4th exam at t_3.

In general, people who will develop clinical cancer can be classified by *generation* depending on when she enters the preclinical state. This classification will separate people into mutually exclusive groups, and make it easy to calculate probabilities for different events. Let (t_{i-1}, t_i) be the i-th screening interval, $i = 1, 2, \cdots, K-1$. The i-th generation of individuals are those women who enter S_p during the i-th screening interval (t_{i-1}, t_i). The 0-th generation consists of women who entered S_p before the first exam t_0. We let $t_{-1} = 0$. The concept of *generation* was given in Zelen 1993 [88].

For an individual who was detected at the k-th screening exam at her age t_{k-1}, she could belong to the 0-th, or the 1st, 2nd, $\ldots$, or the $(k-1)$-th generation, depending on when she entered the state S_p. If she belongs to the i-th generation $(i < k-1)$, she must have passed her previous $(k-i-1)$ exams undetected and had a sojourn time of at least $(t_{k-1} - x)$, where $x \in (t_{i-1}, t_i)$ is her age entering the state S_p (i.e., onset age). If she belongs to the $(k-1)$-th generation, then she must have entered the S_p in the age interval (t_{k-2}, t_{k-1}). We simply add all these possibilities and obtain[79]:

$$\begin{aligned} P(D_k) =& \beta_{k-1} \left\{ \sum_{i=0}^{k-2} [1-\beta_i] \cdots [1-\beta_{k-2}] \int_{t_{i-1}}^{t_i} w(x) Q(t_{k-1}-x) dx \right. \\ & \left. + \int_{t_{k-2}}^{t_{k-1}} w(x) Q(t_{k-1}-x) dx \right\}, \quad \text{for all } k = 2, \cdots, K, \end{aligned} \tag{2.7}$$

where β_i is the sensitivity at the i-th screening exam.

2.3.3 Probability of interval incidence cases

We will use the distribution of T_1 (time duration in S_0) and T_2 (sojourn time in S_p) to calculate the probability of being a clinical incidence case between the first two exams (t_0, t_1). We notice that for an incident case in (t_0, t_1), there are only two mutually exclusive cases: either she has entered the preclinical state before t_0, or she has entered the S_p in (t_0, t_1). These two events are represented by areas A and B in Figure 2.6.

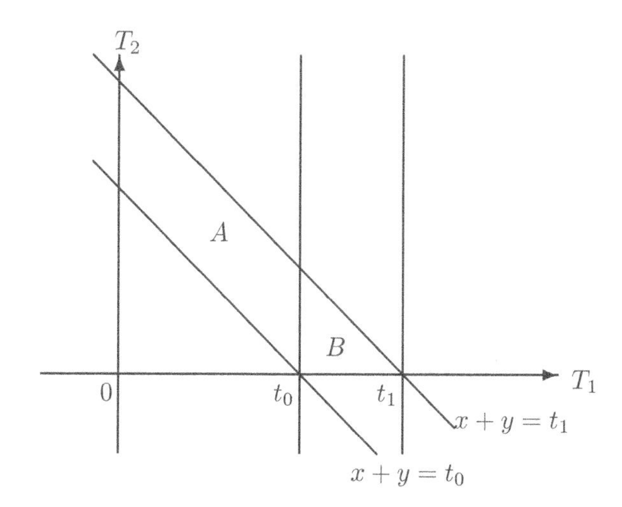

FIGURE 2.6
The areas A = $\{T_1 < t_0 < T_1 + T_2 < t_1\}$ and B = $\{t_0 < T_1 < T_1 + T_2 < t_1\}$ in $P(I_1)$.

Therefore,

$$
\begin{aligned}
P(I_1) &= P(\text{One is an incident case in } (t_0, t_1)) \\
&= (1-\beta_0)P(T_1 < t_0 < T_1 + T_2 < t_1) + P(t_0 < T_1 < T_1 + T_2 < t_1) \\
&= (1-\beta_0)\int_0^{t_0}\int_{t_0-x}^{t_1-x} f_{T_1,T_2}(x,y)dydx + \int_{t_0}^{t_1}\int_0^{t_1-x} f_{T_1,T_2}(x,y)dydx \\
&= (1-\beta_0)\int_0^{t_0}\int_{t_0-x}^{t_1-x} w(x)q(y)dydx + \int_{t_0}^{t_1}\int_0^{t_1-x} w(x)q(y)dydx \\
&= (1-\beta_0)\int_0^{t_0} w(x)[Q(t_0-x) - Q(t_1-x)]dx \qquad (2.8) \\
&\quad + \int_{t_0}^{t_1} w(x)[1-Q(t_1-x)]dx.
\end{aligned}
$$

We will get the same answer using the conditional distribution of T_2 given T_1 as follows:

$$
\begin{aligned}
P(I_1) &= (1-\beta_0)P(T_1 < t_0 < T_1 + T_2 < t_1) + P(t_0 < T_1 < T_1 + T_2 < t_1) \\
&= (1-\beta_0)\int_0^{t_0} f_{T_1}(x)P(t_0 < T_1 + T_2 < t_1 | T_1 = x)dx \\
&\quad + \int_{t_0}^{t_1} f_{T_1}(x)P(T_1 < T_1 + T_2 < t_1 | T_1 = x)dx \\
&= (1-\beta_0)\int_0^{t_0} w(x)P(t_0 - x < T_2 < t_1 - x | T_1 = x)dx \\
&\quad + \int_{t_0}^{t_1} w(x)P(0 < T_2 < t_1 - x | T_1 = x)dx \\
&= (1-\beta_0)\int_0^{t_0} w(x)P(t_0 - x < T_2 < t_1 - x)dx \\
&\quad + \int_{t_0}^{t_1} w(x)P(0 < T_2 < t_1 - x)dx \\
&= (1-\beta_0)\int_0^{t_0} w(x)[Q(t_0-x) - Q(t_1-x)]dx \\
&\quad + \int_{t_0}^{t_1} w(x)[1-Q(t_1-x)]dx.
\end{aligned}
$$

Now to get $P(I_2)$, the probability of incidence in (t_1, t_2), there are three mutually exclusive events depending on the onset age of the S_p (see Figure 2.7), where x is the onset age of the S_p. And we simply add the three probabilities

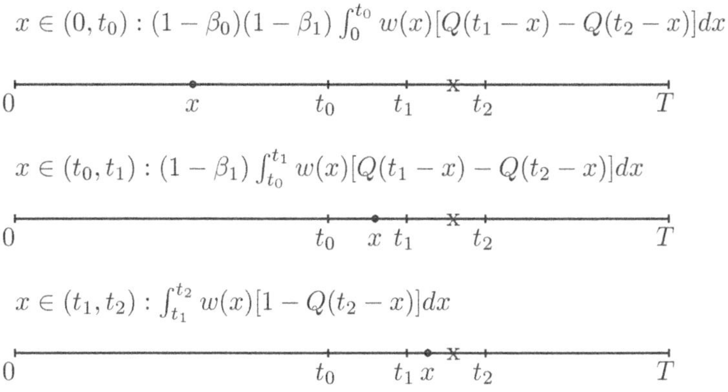

$x \in (0, t_0) : (1-\beta_0)(1-\beta_1) \int_0^{t_0} w(x)[Q(t_1 - x) - Q(t_2 - x)]dx$

0 x t_0 t_1 t_2 T

$x \in (t_0, t_1) : (1-\beta_1) \int_{t_0}^{t_1} w(x)[Q(t_1 - x) - Q(t_2 - x)]dx$

0 t_0 x t_1 t_2 T

$x \in (t_1, t_2) : \int_{t_1}^{t_2} w(x)[1 - Q(t_2 - x)]dx$

0 t_0 t_1 x t_2 T

FIGURE 2.7
Three mutually exclusive events in I_2.

to obtain

$$\begin{aligned} P(I_2) =& (1-\beta_0)(1-\beta_1) \int_0^{t_0} w(x)[Q(t_1 - x) - Q(t_2 - x)]dx \\ &+ (1-\beta_1) \int_{t_0}^{t_1} w(x)[Q(t_1 - x) - Q(t_2 - x)]dx \\ &+ \int_{t_1}^{t_2} w(x)[1 - Q(t_2 - x)]dx. \end{aligned} \tag{2.9}$$

Exercise 2.3.

(a) Derive $P(I_3)$, the probability of an interval case in (t_2, t_3).

(b) Derive $P(I_4)$, the probability of an interval case in (t_3, t_4).

In general, to calculate the probability of incidence in (t_{k-1}, t_k), we let $I_k(t)dt$ be the probability that an individual enters the state S_c at age interval $(t, t+dt)$, where $t \in (t_{k-1}, t_k)$. If this woman belonged to the i-th $(i < k)$ generation, then she must have gone through her previous $(k-i)$ screening exams undetected, and have a sojourn time $(t-x)$, where x is her onset age of the preclinical state S_p; or, she may have entered S_p after the k-th exam and developed the clinical disease at time t. Hence,

$$\begin{aligned} I_k(t) =& \sum_{i=0}^{k-1} [1-\beta_i] \cdots [1-\beta_{k-1}] \int_{t_{i-1}}^{t_i} w(x) q(t-x) dx \\ &+ \int_{t_{k-1}}^{t} w(x) q(t-x) dx, \quad \text{for } \forall t \in (t_{k-1}, t_k). \end{aligned} \tag{2.10}$$

The probability of an incident case in the k-th screening interval (t_{k-1}, t_k) is

$$
\begin{aligned}
P(I_k) &= \int_{t_{k-1}}^{t_k} I_k(t)dt \quad \text{(switching the order of } dx, dt) \\
&= \sum_{i=0}^{k-1} [1-\beta_i]\cdots[1-\beta_{k-1}] \int_{t_{i-1}}^{t_i} w(x)[Q(t_{k-1}-x) - Q(t_k - x)]dx \\
&+ \int_{t_{k-1}}^{t_k} w(x)[1 - Q(t_k - x)]dx, \quad \text{for all } k = 1, \cdots, K. \qquad (2.11)
\end{aligned}
$$

The next exercise will help us know the values of $P(D_k)$ and $P(I_k)$.

Exercise 2.4. If a woman took a screening exam at her age 50, 51, 52, 53, 54, numerically calculate the $P(D_k), P(I_k), k = 1, 2, 3, 4$ using R/S-PLUS or any software, in the following scenario:

(a) $\beta_i = 0.8, w(t) = 0.002, Q(x) = \exp(-\lambda x),\ \lambda = 0.5.$

(b) $\beta_i = 0.9, w(t) = 0.004, Q(x) = \frac{1}{1+(x\rho)^\kappa}$, where $\kappa = 2.5, \rho = 0.8.$

(c) The sensitivity is changing with one's age

$$
\begin{aligned}
\beta_i &= \{1 + \exp(-b_0 - b_1 * (t_i - m))\}^{-1}, \quad m = 55, b_0 = 1.2, b_1 = 0.1; \\
w(t) &= \frac{0.2}{\sqrt{2\pi}\sigma t} \exp\left\{-(\log t - \mu)^2/(2\sigma^2)\right\}, \quad \mu = 4.4, \sigma^2 = 0.15; \\
Q(x) &= \frac{1}{1+(x\rho)^\kappa}, \quad \kappa = 2.3, \rho = 0.8.
\end{aligned}
$$

(d) The sensitivity is changing with one's age

$$
\begin{aligned}
\beta_i &= \{1 + \exp(-b_0 - b_1 * (t_i - m))\}^{-1}, \quad m = 60, b_0 = 1.0, b_1 = 0.05; \\
w(t) &= \frac{0.3}{\sqrt{2\pi}\sigma t} \exp\left\{-(\log t - \mu)^2/(2\sigma^2)\right\}, \quad \mu = 4.3, \sigma^2 = 0.1; \\
Q(x) &= \exp(-\lambda x^\alpha), \quad \lambda = 0.2, \alpha = 2.5.
\end{aligned}
$$

In the next section, we will use these probabilities to build up the likelihood function and estimate the three key parameters.

2.4 Sensitivity as a function of age

Some studies have suggested that a woman's age may affect the sensitivity, the sojourn time distribution, and the transition density into the preclinical state of breast cancer (Eddy 1980[15]; Lee and Zelen 1998 [30]; Shen and Zelen 1999 [49]; Walter and Day 1983 [54]). For example, breast cancer is rare for people under 40 years old, but more common in the older age groups, which means, the $w(t)$ is close to zero for younger females and is larger for older females for breast cancer. The sensitivity also depends on many factors, such as tumor size, or how long one has stayed in the preclinical state. Wu, Rosner, and Broemeling 2005 modeled such relationships and explored quantitatively the changing pattern of these parameters across different age groups [79]. Link functions were used to connect one's age with screening sensitivity, and the transition probability density.

2.4.1 Probability formulation and the likelihood

Consider a cohort of initially asymptomatic women who enroll in a screening program. The sensitivity is denoted by $\beta(t)$, where t is an individual's age at the exam. We let $w(t)$ be the probability density function (PDF) of time duration in the disease-free state S_0. We let $q(x)$ be the PDF of the sojourn time in S_p; and we let $Q(z) = \int_z^\infty q(x)dx$ be the survival function of the sojourn time.

Assume that the study design calls for K ordered screening examinations that occur for a specific individual at ages $t_0 < t_1 < \cdots < t_{K-1}$. If the exams are equally spaced with a time interval Δ, then $t_i = t_0 + i \times \Delta, i = 0, 1, \ldots, (K-1)$. We call $(t_{i-1}, t_i), i = 1, 2, \cdots, K-1$ the i-th screening interval. The i-th generation of individuals is that who enter the S_p in the i-th screening interval (t_{i-1}, t_i). The 0-th generation consists of all those who enter the S_p before the first exam at t_0. We let $t_{-1} = 0$.

We have derived the probability of screen-detected cases and the probability of interval cases in section 2.3. To simplify notation, we use $D_{k,t_0} = P(D_k)$ to represent the probability of a diagnosis at the k-th scheduled exam at age t_{k-1}, and we use $I_{k,t_0} = P(I_k)$ to represent the probability of being an incident case in the k-th screening interval $(t_{k-1}, t_k), k = 1, \ldots, K$. We added t_0 in the subscription to emphasize that the probability depends on the initial screening age t_0. And we summarize the results here

$$D_{1,t_0} = \beta(t_0) \int_0^{t_0} w(x)Q(t_0 - x)dx; \tag{2.12}$$

$$\begin{aligned} D_{k,t_0} &= \beta(t_{k-1}) \left\{ \sum_{i=0}^{k-2} [1 - \beta(t_i)] \cdots [1 - \beta(t_{k-2})] \int_{t_{i-1}}^{t_i} w(x)Q(t_{k-1} - x)dx \right. \\ &\quad \left. + \int_{t_{k-2}}^{t_{k-1}} w(x)Q(t_{k-1} - x)dx \right\}, \quad \text{for } k = 2, \cdots, K. \end{aligned} \tag{2.13}$$

This is the same probability $P(D_k)$ in the equation (2.7). And

$$
\begin{aligned}
I_{k,t_0} & \\
&= \sum_{i=0}^{k-1}[1-\beta(t_i)]\cdots[1-\beta(t_{k-1})]\int_{t_{i-1}}^{t_i} w(x)[Q(t_{k-1}-x)-Q(t_k-x)]dx \\
&+ \int_{t_{k-1}}^{t_k} w(x)[1-Q(t_k-x)]dx, \qquad \text{for } k=1,\cdots,K. \qquad (2.14)
\end{aligned}
$$

This is the same probability $P(I_k)$ in the equation (2.11).

We let n_{i,t_0} be the total number of individuals examined at the i-th screening; s_{i,t_0} is the number of cases diagnosed (confirmed cancer cases, not including false positives) at the i-th screening exam; and r_{i,t_0} is the number of cases diagnosed in the clinical state S_c in the interval (t_{i-1}, t_i), these are called interval cases. The likelihood for women aged t_0 at the first exam is proportional to:

$$
L(\cdot|t_0) = \prod_{k=1}^{K} D_{k,t_0}^{s_{k,t_0}} I_{k,t_0}^{r_{k,t_0}} (1 - D_{k,t_0} - I_{k,t_0})^{n_{k,t_0}-s_{k,t_0}-r_{k,t_0}} . \qquad (2.15)
$$

The likelihood function for the whole study group is the product of the age-specific contributions across all ages,

$$
L = \prod_{t_0} L(\cdot|t_0) = \prod_{t_0}\prod_{k=1}^{K} D_{k,t_0}^{s_{k,t_0}} I_{k,t_0}^{r_{k,t_0}} (1 - D_{k,t_0} - I_{k,t_0})^{n_{k,t_0}-s_{k,t_0}-r_{k,t_0}} . \qquad (2.16)
$$

We usually use the log-likelihood function to find the MLE and to carry out the MCMC simulation to obtain posterior samples.

Exercise 2.5. Suppose that we have collected data from an initially asymptomatic age group $t_0 = 60$, with four biennial screening exams at 60, 62, 64, and 66, as the following:

$$
(n_1, s_1, r_1, \ldots, n_4, s_4, r_4) = (944, 3, 2, 939, 1, 2, 936, 3, 0, 933, 3, 2).
$$

Assume the last screening interval data r_4 is collected from age 66 to 68. Using the following link functions

$$
\begin{aligned}
\beta(t_i) &= \{1 + \exp(-b_0 - b_1 * (t_i - m))\}^{-1}, \quad m = 54, b_0 = 1.0, b_1 = 0.05; \\
w(t) &= \frac{0.2}{\sqrt{2\pi}\sigma t} \exp\left\{-(\log t - \mu)^2/(2\sigma^2)\right\}, \quad \mu = 4.3, \sigma^2 = 0.1; \\
Q(x) &= \exp(-\lambda x^\alpha), \quad \lambda = 0.25, \alpha = 3.0.
\end{aligned}
$$

Calculate the value of the log-likelihood using (2.15).

2.4.2 Simulation: Checking model reliability

We want to check whether the likelihood function can provide unbiased estimates of the parameters due to the complicated model. So we have done simulations to verify this for different parametric link functions. Here we will present one type of parametric functions that we have used for breast cancer screening.

The sensitivity is a probability limited to (0,1), and it is assumed to increase with age. A mathematically convenient model for associating sensitivity β with age t is the logistic model:

$$\beta(t) = \{1 + \exp(-b_0 - b_1 * (t - m))\}^{-1}, \tag{2.17}$$

where m is the average age at the first exam in the screening group. If $b_1 > 0$, $\beta(t)$ will be a monotone increasing function of age t.

The transition density function $w(t)$ measures time duration in the disease-free state S_0, and $w(t)dt$ is the probability of making a transition from the S_0 to the S_p in the age interval $(t, t + dt)$. The integral $\int_0^\infty w(t)dt$ represents the lifetime risk of entering the preclinical state. According to the NCI's SEER database (Ries et al 2002[44]), a woman's lifetime risk of being diagnosed with breast cancer (invasive and *in situ*) is 15.7%, which is (slightly) less than or equal to a woman's lifetime risk of entering the preclinical disease state. Therefore, we choose 20% as a reasonable upper bound for breast cancer. The $w(t)$ was estimated by Lee and Zelen 1998 using the age-specific breast cancer incidence rates from the Surveillance, Epidemiology, and End Results (SEER) program of the National Cancer Institute [30], where the $w(t)$ were summarized in age intervals of 5 years as a step function. We plotted the step function based on their estimates, and it was right-skewed and could fit well by a lognormal distribution. Therefore, we chose

$$w(t|\mu, \sigma^2) = \frac{0.2}{\sqrt{2\pi}\sigma t} \exp\left\{-(\log t - \mu)^2/(2\sigma^2)\right\}, \quad t > 0, \tag{2.18}$$

which is the PDF of the lognormal (μ, σ^2) multiplied by 20%.

The sojourn time in the preclinical state was modeled to follow an exponential distribution [30, 49, 54]. However, the exponential distribution has only one parameter and methods based on it are rather sensitive to modest departures in the tail. We picked the log-logistic distribution for the sojourn time for mathematical convenience. This distribution has analytical forms for the density function $q(x)$, the survival function $Q(x)$, and the hazard function $h(x)$ as follows (Cox and Oakes 1984 [11]):

$$q(x) = \frac{\kappa x^{\kappa-1}\rho^\kappa}{[1 + (x\rho)^\kappa]^2}, \qquad Q(x) = \frac{1}{1 + (x\rho)^\kappa}, \qquad h(x) = \frac{\kappa x^{\kappa-1}\rho^\kappa}{1 + (x\rho)^\kappa}, \tag{2.19}$$

where $x > 0$ is the sojourn time in the preclinical state S_p, $\kappa > 0, \rho > 0$ are parameters to be estimated. This density is right-skewed. An advantage of this family over others is the relatively simple form of $Q(x)$ and $h(x)$. The first moment is $E(X) = \frac{\pi}{\rho\kappa}\csc(\frac{\pi}{\kappa})$. And for the rth moment to exist, $\kappa > r$ is needed. We assumed that the time duration in the disease-free state and the sojourn time in the preclinical state are independent.

The purpose of the simulation is to check the reliability of the likelihood function as screening sensitivity and transition density are both age-independent. There are six unknown parameters $\theta = (b_0, b_1, \mu, \sigma^2, \kappa, \rho)$ in the model. The simulation is composed of two major steps: (1). We generate pseudo-screening data using a fixed input vector θ_0 and the total screening number $K = 4$, the initial number of people at age 0 is 100,000 for each age group, and the age group at the first exam is from age 40 to 64, inclusive, the same as in the HIP study. The generated screening data is saved in a data matrix as in Table 1.1. (2). We estimate the parameter θ using the generated screening data and the likelihood function, the result was saved in $\hat{\theta}$. The two-step procedure was repeated 1000 times, the mean and standard error of the estimated $\hat{\theta}_j$ was calculated and summarized in Table 2.2. See Wu et al 2005b for more details [84].

For step (1) to generate the screening data: for each age group with the initial screening exam at age t_0, we assume there were $M = 100,000$ individuals at age 0. Since someone may have clinical symptoms before the age t_0, the number of individuals who would take the first exam at t_0 would be less than M, that is, $n_1 < M$. Their time spent in the disease-free state S_0 and in the preclinical state S_p can be generated by the probability density functions $w(t)$ and $q(x)$ correspondingly. And we generated 25 age groups independently, with the initial screening age t_0 between 40 and 64, inclusive. At each screening exam, generate a Bernoulli random variable (using the sensitivity as the probability of success p) to decide who would be detected for those in the preclinical state.

Exercise 2.6. Generate (pseudo) screening data using the input parameters $\theta_0 = (b_0, b_1, \mu, \sigma^2, \kappa, \rho) = (0.8, 0.1, 4.3, 0.09, 3.0, 0.7)$, and the $\beta(t), w(t), q(x)$ defined in this subsection, assuming $m = 52$, for age 40 to 64 years old age groups, with $M = 1,000$ and four annual screenings ($K = 4, \Delta = 1$ year), and put the generated screening data into a data matrix as in Table 1.1.

For step (2) to calculate the MLE using the generated screening data: one major issue is calculating the log-likelihood as fast as possible; and we implemented this part in C/C++, then, taking the *negative* value of the log-likelihood and calling the S-PLUS routine "nlminb" to provide a local minimum. This local minimum corresponds to a local maximum in the log-likelihood. The built-in function "nlminb" needs a starting value of θ, an interval for each parameter to be estimated, and the evaluating function (the log-likelihood in this case) as input. However, since all computer software can only find a local minimum (maximum) and the found minimum value depends on the starting point, so it has trouble finding the global minimum (maximum) for a general function. To overcome this problem, the starting value of θ was

TABLE 2.2
Simulation results for the six parameters, with bias = $\bar{\hat{\theta}} - \theta_0$.

	b_0	b_1	μ	σ^2	κ	ρ
θ_0	2.07	-0.05	4.05	0.80	4.54	0.70
$\bar{\hat{\theta}}$	2.073	-0.051	4.053	0.799	4.525	0.698
bias	0.003	-0.001	0.003	-0.001	-0.015	-0.002
S.E.	0.112	0.006	0.042	0.018	0.245	0.016
θ_0	0.91	-0.07	4.24	0.51	3.01	0.74
$\bar{\hat{\theta}}$	0.879	-0.069	4.242	0.510	3.046	0.730
bias	-0.031	0.001	0.002	0	0.036	-0.01
S.E.	0.093	0.004	0.019	0.015	0.150	0.029
θ_0	2.72	-0.12	3.65	0.55	3.73	0.65
$\bar{\hat{\theta}}$	2.714	-0.120	3.652	0.551	3.750	0.647
bias	-0.006	0	0.002	0.001	0.02	-0.003
S.E.	0.157	0.011	0.021	0.018	0.133	0.012
θ_0	3.14	0.12	4.42	0.86	1.16	1.23
$\bar{\hat{\theta}}$	3.169	0.123	4.420	0.861	1.161	1.223
bias	0.029	0.003	0	0.001	0.001	-0.007
S.E.	0.308	0.029	0.024	0.034	0.015	0.025
θ_0	0.47	-0.17	3.59	0.15	1.67	0.76
$\bar{\hat{\theta}}$	0.475	-0.170	3.591	0.150	1.667	0.752
bias	0.005	0	0.001	0	-0.003	-0.008
S.E.	0.053	0.004	0.005	0.004	0.023	0.018
θ_0	1.64	0.02	3.93	0.08	2.37	1.05
$\bar{\hat{\theta}}$	1.612	0.022	3.930	0.080	2.377	1.037
bias	-0.028	0.002	0	0	0.007	-0.013
S.E.	0.150	0.004	0.003	0.001	0.054	0.037
θ_0	2.81	0.19	4.03	0.67	3.07	0.82
$\bar{\hat{\theta}}$	2.710	0.181	4.029	0.670	3.094	0.812
bias	-0.1	-0.09	-0.01	0	0.024	-0.008
S.E.	0.137	0.013	0.033	0.014	0.083	0.012
θ_0	3.74	-0.04	4.36	0.72	2.74	0.81
$\bar{\hat{\theta}}$	3.650	-0.039	4.361	0.721	2.762	0.801
bias	-0.09	-0.001	0.001	0.001	0.022	-0.009
S.E.	0.538	0.030	0.024	0.027	0.075	0.021

Adapted from Table 1 in Wu et al 2005b [84].

chosen randomly and the procedure was repeated five times for each generated screening data to (hopefully) find the global maximum. Although the procedure (of five replacements) cannot guarantee that the true MLE was found, it at least provides a better estimation, equal or close to the MLE. Eight simulation results are listed in Table 2.2. For each input value of θ_0, the sample mean and sample standard error (S.E.) of the MLE $\hat{\theta}_j, j = 1, 2, \ldots, 1000$ from 1000 simulations are listed. The consistency between the sample mean of the MLE and the input parameters is clearly shown.

Theoretically, the parameters have a domain of either $(-\infty, \infty)$ or $(0, \infty)$. The practical meaning of these parameters will limit them to a finite range. The range for each parameter was identified as: $0.50 < b_0 < 5, -0.2 < b_1 <$

$0.2, 3.5 < \mu < 4.5, 0 < \sigma^2 < 1, 0.1 < \rho < 2.0$, and $1 < \kappa < 5$. For justifications of these ranges, see Wu et al 2005 [79]. For the input values of θ, all six values were randomly chosen from the valid range above. One issue with the simulation is that we have to assume a large number of people in each group. However, in reality, participants in the screening program are much fewer than 100,000 in the simulation. There are some problems with the current likelihood, and we will discuss that in section 2.6.

2.4.3 Application: The HIP for breast cancer

We applied our method to the Health Insurance Plan for Greater New York (HIP) data (Shapiro 1988 [47]). Wu, Rosner and Broemeling 2005 [79] estimated the age-dependent sensitivity $\beta(t)$, the transition density $w(t)$, and the sojourn time distribution $q(x)$ using the HIP study group data. The sensitivity $\beta(t)$ was a function of age t using a logistic link function,

$$\beta(t) = \{1 + \exp[-b_0 - b_1(t - \bar{t})]\}^{-1} ,$$

where $\bar{t}$ is the average age at the initial exam in the study group. The transition density function was

$$w(t|\mu, \sigma^2) = \frac{0.2}{\sqrt{2\pi}\sigma t} \exp\left\{-(\log t - \mu)^2/(2\sigma^2)\right\}, \quad \sigma > 0,$$

which is the pdf of a $lognormal(\mu, \sigma^2)$ multiplied by 20% (the upper limit corresponding to a lifetime risk). The log-logistic distribution was adopted as the distribution for the sojourn time in the preclinical state, so that the survivor function and the hazard function are, respectively,

$$Q(x) = \frac{1}{1 + (x\rho)^\kappa} \quad \text{and} \quad h(x) = \frac{\kappa x^{\kappa-1}\rho^\kappa}{1 + (x\rho)^\kappa}, \qquad \kappa > 0, \quad \rho > 0,$$

where x is the sojourn time in the state of S_p. The density is $q(x) = h(x)Q(x)$.

The unknown parameters in the model are $\theta = (b_0, b_1, \mu, \sigma^2, \kappa, \rho)$. Let H represent the HIP data. The posterior distribution is

$$f(\theta|H) \propto L(\theta|H)\pi(\theta). \tag{2.20}$$

We used the likelihood function in equation (2.16) to find the maximum likelihood estimate (MLE). And we use equation (2.20) to find Bayesian posterior samples of θ, and then make inferences for the model parameters θ.

We used Markov Chain Monte Carlo (MCMC) to generate random samples from the joint posterior distribution of the parameters for Bayesian inference. We partitioned the posterior simulation into four subchains, sampling the posterior for (b_0, b_1), μ, σ^2, and (κ, ρ) separately. A noninformative bivariate normal prior for (b_0, b_1) (i.e., mean vector $(0, 0)$ and variance equal to 10^{10} times the identity matrix) was adopted. A noninformative normal prior of

TABLE 2.3
The MLE and Bayesian posterior estimates using the HIP data.

Parameters	MLE (s.e.)	Bayesian Posterior Estimate		
		median	mean	s.e.
b_0	1.122 (0.733)	1.581	1.676	1.338
b_1	0.081 (0.042)	0.084	0.085	0.078
μ	4.331 (0.048)	4.329	4.340	0.076
σ^2	0.145 (0.046)	0.172	0.190	0.076
κ	2.205 (0.732)	2.275	2.509	0.927
ρ	0.808 (0.181)	0.917	0.886	0.287

Adapted from Table 1 in Wu et al 2005 [79].

$\mu \sim N(0, 10^{10})$ was chosen. And the prior for σ^2 was uniform (0, 1). The prior for κ was uniform (1, 5), and it was uniform (0, 2) for ρ. Numerical approximation using the trapezoidal rule was used to evaluate the two integrals $\int_a^b w(x)dx$ and $\int_a^b w(x)Q(t-x)dx$ in the likelihood calculation.

We ran the MCMC for 30,000 steps, with a burn-in of 10,000 iterations. After the burn-in steps, we sampled the posterior every 20 steps to obtain 1000 posterior samples for the vector θ. We ran two parallel chains, with overdispersed starting values. Bayesian output analysis showed convergence. We combined the saved posterior samples from both chains for the analysis, with the posterior sample size $n = 2000$. The Bayesian method provides more information, such as posterior density curves, measures of uncertainty, predictive distributions, etc. Simulation results of the MLE and Bayesian posterior estimates are summarized in Table 2.3.

The sensitivity seems to increase with age. The trend is shown in Figure 2.8, which shows age-specific posterior quantiles based on the posterior samples of the parameters. From ages 40 to 65, the posterior mean sensitivity increased from 0.603 to 0.875 and the posterior standard error dropped from 0.236 to 0.144. The posterior error of sensitivity was largest for women 40 years old, as one might expect since the sensitivity was closest to 0.5 for this age group. At the average age of 51.6 years, the posterior mean sensitivity was 0.779, with a posterior standard error of 0.186. For comparison, the estimated sensitivity for the HIP study by Shapiro et al 1988 was 0.737, defined as the ratio of the screen-detected cases (132) divided by the total number of cancer cases (screen-detected and interval cases 132 + 47) during the first 5 years of follow-up. This result is close to the posterior mean sensitivity we estimated when we fit a model without an age effect on sensitivity: posterior mean = 0.74 and 90% credible interval (0.43, 0.97). We computed the posterior probability of a positive slope: $P(b_1 > 0|\text{HIP data}) = 0.904$. A likelihood ratio test for the slope gives a p-value of 0.092, where the p-value was calculated by $P(\chi_1^2 > -2\log(LR))$, with

$$-2\log(LR) = 2\left[\log L(\hat{b}_0, \hat{b}_1, \hat{\mu}, \hat{\sigma}^2, \hat{\kappa}, \hat{\rho}) - \log L(\tilde{b}_0, \tilde{\mu}, \tilde{\sigma}^2, \tilde{\kappa}, \tilde{\rho})\right].$$

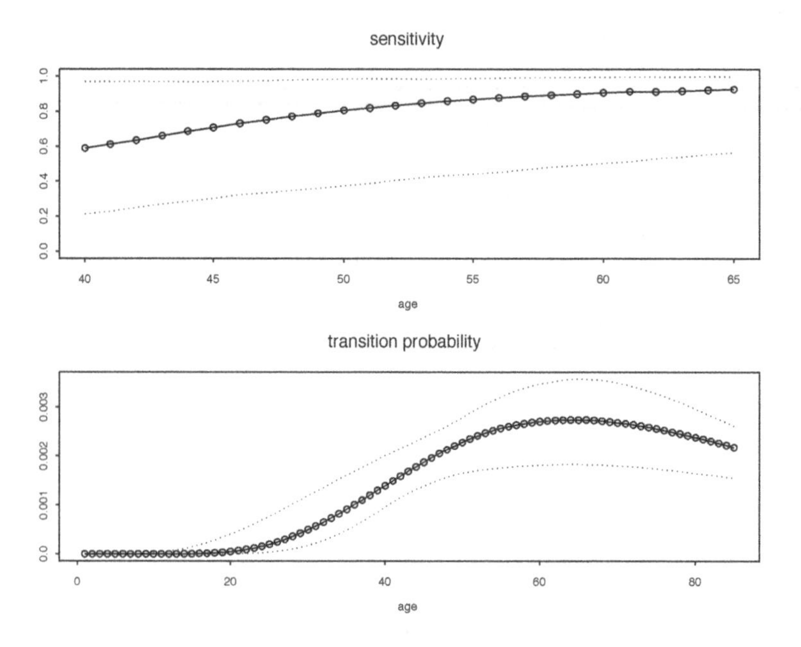

FIGURE 2.8
The posterior median and 90% credible intervals (5%, 95%) of sensitivity and transition density using the HIP data. Adapted from Figure 1 in Wu et al 2005 [79].

Thus, there is some evidence of an age effect on sensitivity in the HIP data.

The posterior median of the age-dependent transition probabilities from S_0 to S_p are also shown in Figure 2.8. The transition probabilities do not appear monotone with age; the function appears to peak around age 60. The posterior mean sojourn time was 1.88 years, and the posterior median was 1.51 years. The posterior standard deviation of the sojourn time was large, 1.65 years. The MLE for the mean sojourn time was 1.78 years.

2.4.4 Application: The Minnesota Colorectal Cancer study

The Minnesota colorectal cancer study was introduced in Chapter 1. We applied the age-dependent sensitivity model to males and females separately using this data. The only modeling difference is in the $w(t)$, where the upper limit of the log-normal density was changed from 0.2 to 0.1, that is,

$$w(t|\mu, \sigma^2) = \frac{0.1}{\sqrt{2\pi}\sigma t} \exp\left\{-(\log t - \mu)^2/(2\sigma^2)\right\} \quad t > 0.$$

TABLE 2.4
Bayesian posterior estimates for the annual screening groups in MCCCS.

Parameters	MALE			FEMALE		
	Median	Mean	S.E.	Median	Mean	S.E.
b_0	0.816	0.983	1.638	0.686	0.801	1.443
b_1	0.128	0.140	0.156	0.188	0.206	0.142
μ	4.365	4.368	0.091	4.427	4.432	0.052
σ^2	0.091	0.119	0.081	0.058	0.065	0.037
κ	3.019	3.055	1.015	3.607	3.543	0.899
ρ	0.791	0.749	0.278	0.633	0.626	0.194

Adapted from Table 3 in Wu et al 2009 [65].

According to the NCI's "SEER Fast Fact Stats" database, the lifetime risk of being diagnosed with colorectal cancer is about 5.3% for females and 5.9% for males. Therefore, we picked 10% as a reasonable upper limit for the $w(t)$.

There are six unknown parameters $\theta = (b_0, b_1, \mu, \sigma^2, \kappa, \rho)$ as before. The MCMC was run for 20,000 steps, with a burn-in of 15,000 iterations. After the burn-in time, the posteriors were sampled every 20 steps, giving 250 posterior samples for the parameter vector. Four parallel chains were simulated, with dispersed starting values with respect to the target distribution. The 250 posterior samples from each of the four chains were pooled for the analysis, giving a total of 1,000 posterior samples for each gender. We plotted the estimated sensitivity and transition density in Figures 2.9 and 2.10. Table 2.4 summarized the MCMC simulation results.

The sensitivity appears to increase with age for both genders. However, the posterior mean sensitivity is not monotonic with age for males; it has a small bump around age 74. The standard errors of the sensitivity are not monotone either; there is a minimum at age 69 for males and at age 78 for females. The age-dependent transition probability is not a monotone function of age; it has a single maximum at age 72 for males and a single maximum at age 75 for females. Age dependency seems more dramatic for females than for males. The posterior mean sojourn time is 4.08 years for males and 2.41 years for females, with a posterior median of 1.66 years for males and 1.88 years for females. The 95% Highest Posterior Density (HPD) interval for sojourn time is (0.97, 20.28) years for males and (1.15, 5.96) years for females, which are very large ranges, especially for males. It seems that males take a longer time to develop colorectal cancer symptoms than females. However, this estimate may not be so accurate, due to the fact that there were fewer men than women in the MCCCS annual screening program.

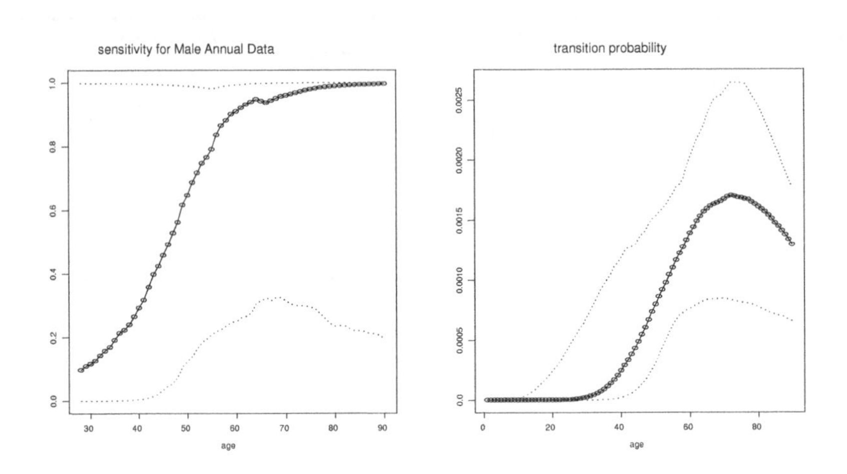

FIGURE 2.9
Estimates of sensitivity and transition density using posterior quantiles (5%, 50%, 95%) for males in the MCCCS. Adapted from Figure 1 in Wu et al 2009 [65].

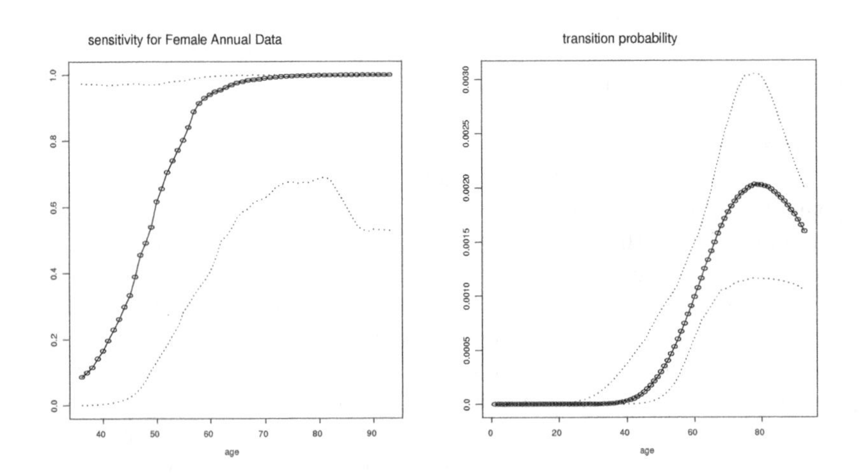

FIGURE 2.10
Estimates of sensitivity and transition density using posterior quantiles (5%, 50%, 95%) for females in the MCCCS. Adapted from Figure 2 in Wu et al 2009 [65].

TABLE 2.5
Bayesian posterior estimates for the five parameters in Mayo Lung Project.

Parameters	Median	Mean	S.E.
b_0	2.357	2.395	0.845
μ	4.252	4.252	0.017
σ^2	0.034	0.035	0.005
κ	1.531	1.545	0.043
ρ	1.040	1.054	0.189

Adapted from Table 1 in Wu et al 2011 [64].

2.4.5 Application: The Mayo Lung Project

We applied the method to the Mayo Lung Project data. The age at entry was from 44 to 76 years old in the study. We only used the data from age 45 to age 69, because the other age groups have too few participants and may cause large variations in the estimation. The original method was designed for breast cancer screening, where the sensitivity was a logistic function of age ([79]). After consulting with lung cancer radiologists and oncologists, there seems no obvious age effect connected with sensitivity in practice in lung cancer screening. Hence in this study, the sensitivity is simplified as $\beta(t) = \beta$. According to the NCI's "SEER Fast Fact Stats" database, the lifetime risk of being diagnosed with lung and bronchus cancer is about 6.94% for both genders in the general population. However, according to Wikipedia, the lifetime risk for male smokers is 17.2%. Since the Mayo Lung Project participants were male heavy smokers, the risk should be much higher than that. Therefore, we picked 30% as a reasonable upper limit for the log-normal density used in $w(t)$.

Markov Chain Monte Carlo (MCMC) simulation was run for 30,000 steps, with a burn-in of 5000 steps. After the burn-in, the posteriors were sampled every 100 steps, giving 250 posterior samples for the parameter vector θ. Four chains were simulated, each with different starting values that are over-dispersed with respect to the target distribution. The 250 posterior samples from each of the 4 chains were pooled for the analysis, giving a total of 1000 posterior samples. The posterior estimates for the parameters and the standard errors are listed in Table 2.5.

The posterior sensitivity is skewed to the left, see Figure 2.11. The posterior mean sensitivity is 0.894, and its posterior median is 0.914, the 95% highest posterior density (HPD) interval for the sensitivity is (0.718, 0.981). The posterior mean sojourn time is 2.24 years, with a posterior median of 2.20 years for male heavy smokers; the 95% HPD interval for the mean sojourn time is (1.57, 3.35) years. The age-dependent transition probability is not a monotone function of age; it has a single maximum at age 68, see Figure 2.12.

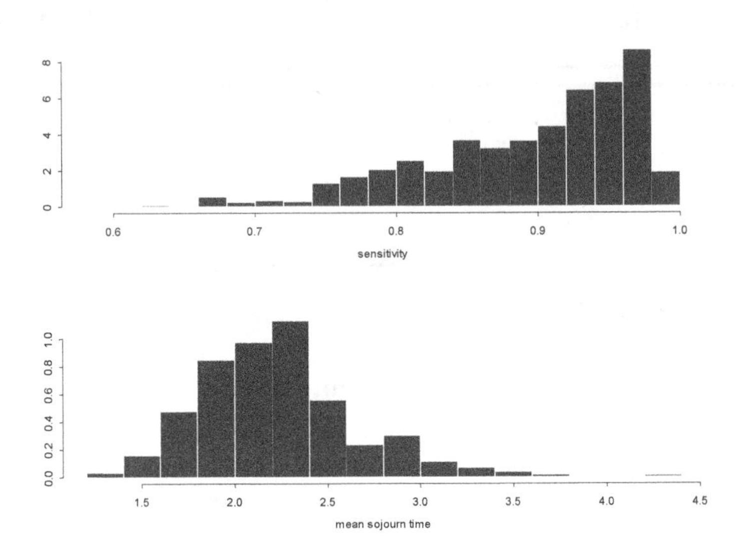

FIGURE 2.11
Histogram of the estimated sensitivity and the sojourn time in the Mayo study. Adapted from Figure 2 in Wu et al 2011 [64].

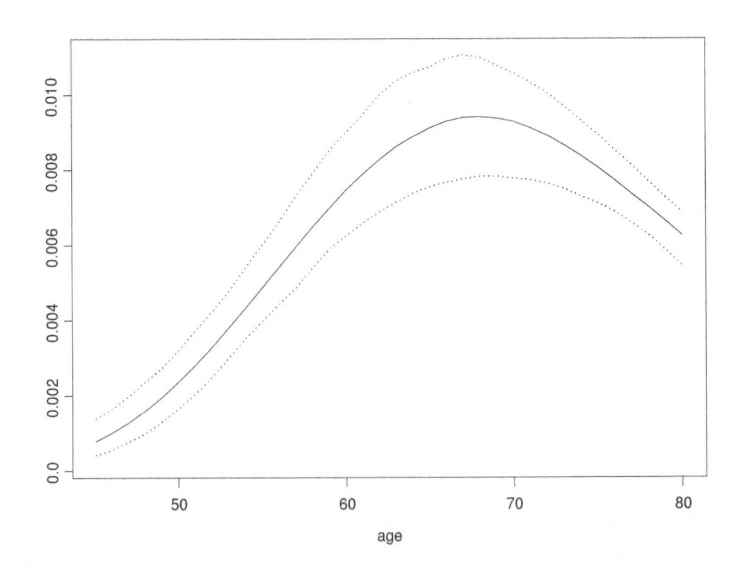

FIGURE 2.12
Estimated transition density for male heavy smokers in the Mayo study. Adapted from Figure 3 in Wu et al 2011 [64].

TABLE 2.6
Bayesian posterior estimates for the six parameters in NLST CT arm.

	Mean	S.E.	2.5%	50%	97.5%
			CT Overall		
b_0	3.263	0.503	2.154	3.339	3.963
b_1	0.002	0.053	-0.094	0.005	0.094
μ	4.271	0.008	4.255	4.270	4.288
σ^2	0.022	0.002	0.018	0.022	0.027
λ	0.270	0.053	0.163	0.275	0.370
α	2.703	0.496	1.899	2.643	3.822
			CT Male		
b_0	2.923	0.622	1.705	2.950	3.939
b_1	0.002	0.058	-0.095	0.003	0.096
μ	4.268	0.010	4.249	4.268	4.288
σ^2	0.021	0.003	0.016	0.020	0.026
λ	0.306	0.079	0.140	0.312	0.452
α	2.713	0.601	1.715	2.672	3.903
			CT Female		
b_0	3.247	0.516	2.182	3.330	3.968
b_1	0.017	0.054	-0.091	0.026	0.096
μ	4.276	0.014	4.248	4.275	4.303
σ^2	0.026	0.004	0.019	0.026	0.034
λ	0.194	0.059	0.090	0.189	0.330
α	2.983	0.562	1.945	2.948	3.934

Adapted from Table 1 in Liu et al 2015 [32].

2.4.6 Application: The National Lung Screening Trial

We applied the method to the NLST low-dose CT screening data for three groups: males, females, and combined. The parametric functions were:

$$\begin{aligned} \beta(t) &= \{1+\exp(-b_0 - b_1 * (t-m))\}^{-1}, \\ w(t|\mu,\sigma^2) &= \frac{0.3}{\sqrt{2\pi}\sigma t}\exp\left\{-(\log t - \mu)^2/(2\sigma^2)\right\}, \\ Q(x) &= \exp(-\lambda x^\alpha), \alpha > 0, \lambda > 0, \end{aligned} \tag{2.21}$$

where $m = 64.5$ is the average age at the first exam. The six unknown parameters were $\theta = (b_0, b_1, \mu, \sigma^2, \lambda, \alpha)$. MCMC was used to draw posterior samples with non-informative Uniform priors. Two parallel chains were running for each group, and after the burn-in and thinning steps, 1000 posterior samples from two chains were collected. The results are summarized in Table 2.6.

The estimated sensitivity and transition density based on the posterior θ at different ages are summarized in Table 2.7. The posterior quantiles of

TABLE 2.7
Bayesian posterior estimates of $\beta(t)$ and $w(t)$ at different ages using the NLST CT data.

Age	Sensitivity β			Transition density $w(t)$		
	Median	Mean	S.E.	Median	Mean	S.E.
			CT Overall			
55	0.9642	0.9551	0.0306	0.0030	0.0030	3.07×10-4
60	0.9657	0.9581	0.0238	0.0066	0.0066	3.86×10-4
65	0.9642	0.9587	0.0220	0.0101	0.0100	5.63×10-4
70	0.9616	0.9570	0.0256	0.0114	0.0114	6.01×10-4
75	0.9613	0.9529	0.0343	0.0102	0.0102	3.96×10-4
			CT Male			
55	0.9484	0.9360	0.0461	0.0029	0.0029	4.01×10-4
60	0.9496	0.9398	0.0369	0.0067	0.0067	4.95×10-4
65	0.9497	0.9396	0.0385	0.0104	0.0104	7.16×10-4
70	0.9495	0.9355	0.0497	0.0118	0.0118	7.74×10-4
75	0.9506	0.9274	0.0678	0.0105	0.0105	5.07×10-4
			CT Female			
55	0.9601	0.9499	0.0337	0.0034	0.0034	4.98×10-4
60	0.9641	0.9563	0.0255	0.0065	0.0065	5.76×10-4
65	0.9665	0.9599	0.0228	0.0094	0.0094	7.75×10-4
70	0.9666	0.9610	0.0256	0.0104	0.0104	8.31×10-4
75	0.9710	0.9596	0.0332	0.0096	0.0095	6.00×10-4

Adapted from Table 2 in Liu et al 2015 [32]

sensitivity and transition density curve were plotted in Figure 2.13. One interesting finding is that sensitivity is not changing with one's age using CT. The posterior probability $P(b_1 > 0|NLST) = 0.532$ for the overall group, and similar probability for each gender group. So we would think sensitivity for lung cancer screening using CT is independent of one's age.

The posterior mean sojourn time is 1.48 years for the combined group, and it is 1.44 (1.62) years for male (female) heavy smokers respectively, with a posterior median of 1.47 years for the combined group, 1.41 (1.58) years for the male (female) group respectively. The 95% highest posterior density (HPD) interval is (1.22, 1.77) years for the combined group, (1.11, 1.78) years for males, and (1.21, 2.04) years for females. For detailed results, see Liu et al 2015 [32].

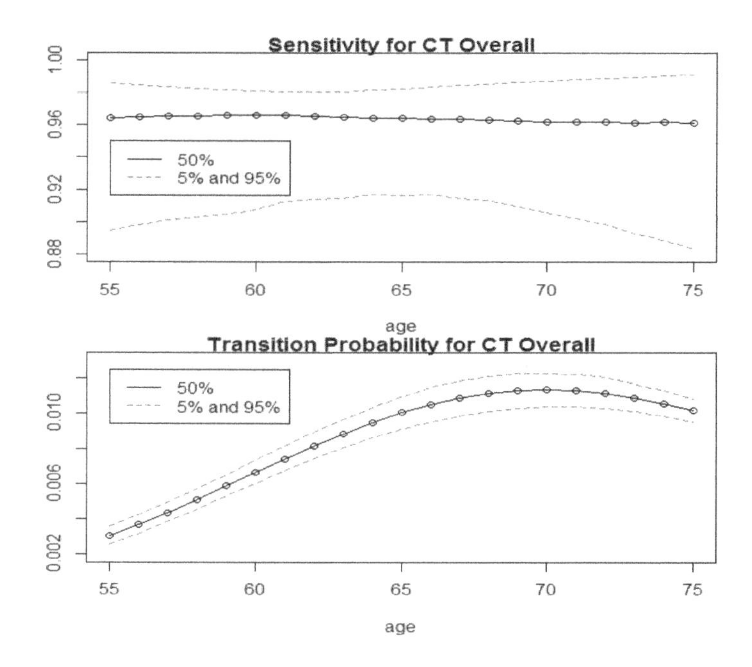

FIGURE 2.13
Posterior quantiles (5%, 50%, 95%) of sensitivity and transition density for the CT overall group. Adapted from Figure 6 in Liu et al 2015 [32].

2.5 Sensitivity as a function of time in the S_p and sojourn time

The sensitivity was assumed to be related to age in the previous sections. One problem is that under this assumption, the estimated sensitivity and sojourn time are negatively correlated: when the sensitivity is over-estimated, the sojourn time will be under-estimated, and vice versa. Intuitively, when the tumor cell is just formed, the sensitivity is fairly small; while at the late stage, when a patient is at the end of the preclinical state S_p and the clinical stage S_c will soon start, the sensitivity might be very close to one. Hence the sensitivity not only depends on the age at diagnosis but also depends on the time that an individual spent in the preclinical state relative to the total sojourn time. For lung cancer, there is evidence to show that sensitivity doesn't depend on age. Therefore, we will model the sensitivity as a function of the ratio of time in the preclinical state and the sojourn time.

2.5.1 Probability formulation and likelihood

We will model the sensitivity as a function of the time spent in the preclinical state and the sojourn time. This may provide better modeling and more accurate statistical inference for the key parameters.

We consider an asymptomatic individual who will go through a sequence of screening exams at the ages $t_0 < t_1 < \cdots < t_{K-1}$. We let $\beta(x|Y), 0 \leq x \leq Y$ be the sensitivity, where x is the length of time that she has stayed in the preclinical state S_p, and Y represents the sojourn time in the S_p, which is a random variable. Intuitively, β will increase as x increases and will decrease as Y increases. We let $w(t)$ and $q(x)$ be the probability density function of the time duration in the S_0 and the S_p respectively. We let $Q(z) = \int_z^{\infty} q(x)dx$ be the survival function of the sojourn time Y.

We let D_{k,t_0} be the probability that an individual is diagnosed with cancer at the k-th exam, given that she is already in the preclinical state. The probability that an individual in the S_p is detected at the first exam at her age t_0 is

$$D_{1,t_0} = \int_0^{t_0} w(x) \int_{t_0-x}^{\infty} q(t)\beta(t_0 - x|t)dtdx. \tag{2.22}$$

Because she must have entered the preclinical state S_p at some point $x \in (0, t_0)$, and she would have remained in this state until t_0 or after. So her time spent in the preclinical state is $(t_0 - x)$ at the exam, and her sojourn time t is larger than $(t_0 - x)$; hence; the double integral appears. We can use a similar way to calculate the probability of the screen-detected cases and the interval cases:

$$\begin{aligned} D_{k,t_0} =& \sum_{i=0}^{k-2} \int_{t_{i-1}}^{t_i} w(x) \int_{t_{k-1}-x}^{\infty} q(t) \left\{ \prod_{j=i}^{k-2} [1 - \beta(t_j - x|t)] \right\} \beta(t_{k-1} - x|t)dtdx \\ &+ \int_{t_{k-2}}^{t_{k-1}} w(x) \int_{t_{k-1}-x}^{\infty} q(t)\beta(t_{k-1} - x|t)dtdx, \text{ for } k = 2, \cdots, K. \end{aligned} \tag{2.23}$$

$$\begin{aligned} I_{k,t_0} =& \sum_{i=0}^{k-1} \int_{t_{i-1}}^{t_i} w(x) \int_{t_{k-1}-x}^{t_k-x} q(t) \left\{ \prod_{j=i}^{k-1} [1 - \beta(t_j - x|t)] \right\} dtdx \\ &+ \int_{t_{k-1}}^{t_k} w(x)[1 - Q(t_k - x)]dx, \quad \text{for } k = 1, \cdots, K. \end{aligned} \tag{2.24}$$

Notice that if the sensitivity doesn't depend on the sojourn time t in the above formula, the probabilities will be the same as in section 2.4. Finally, the likelihood function of each age group t_0 is proportional to the multinomial probability:

$$L(\cdot|t_0) = \prod_{k=1}^{K} D_{k,t_0}^{s_{k,t_0}} I_{k,t_0}^{r_{k,t_0}} (1 - D_{k,t_0} - I_{k,t_0})^{n_{k,t_0} - s_{k,t_0} - r_{k,t_0}}$$

And the total likelihood is proportional to:

$$
\begin{aligned}
L &= \prod_{t_0} L(\cdot|t_0) \\
&= \prod_{t_0} \prod_{k=1}^{K} D_{k,t_0}^{s_{k,t_0}} I_{k,t_0}^{r_{k,t_0}} (1 - D_{k,t_0} - I_{k,t_0})^{n_{k,t_0} - s_{k,t_0} - r_{k,t_0}}
\end{aligned}
$$

We would use this likelihood to find the maximum likelihood estimate (MLE) of the parameters and to generate Bayesian posterior samples using the Markov Chain Monte Carlo (MCMC) simulations. Then we make inferences using both the MLE and the MCMC posterior samples.

2.5.2 Application: The NLST-CT for heavy smokers

We applied the method with the sensitivity as a function of the sojourn time to the NLST low-dose CT data for male and female heavy smokers separately. See section 1.10 for a description of the NLST-CT data.

We use the ratio x/Y to measure the tumor growth, where x represents the time that one has stayed in the preclinical state S_p, and Y represents the total sojourn time in the S_p. Given the sojourn time Y, the sensitivity is defined as

$$\beta(x|Y) = [1 + \exp(-b_0 - b_1 \times \frac{x}{Y})]^{-1}, \ 0 \leq x \leq Y, b_0 \geq 0, b_1 \geq 0.$$

For the transition probability $w(t)$ and the sojourn time distribution $q(x)$, we will use the parametric functions [12, 32]

$$
\begin{aligned}
w(t) &= \frac{0.3}{\sqrt{2\pi}\sigma t} \exp\{-(\log t - \mu)^2/(2\sigma^2)\}, \ \sigma > 0. \\
Q(x) &= \exp(-\lambda x^{\alpha}), \quad q(x) = \lambda \alpha x^{\alpha-1} Q(x), \ \lambda > 0, \alpha > 0.
\end{aligned}
$$

There were six parameters $\theta = (b_0, b_1, \mu, \sigma^2, \lambda, \alpha)$ in the model. For male and female heavy smokers, we found the maximum likelihood estimate (MLE) numerically, and also ran Markov Chain Monte Carlo simulations to obtain the posterior samples of θ.

We used the Gibbs sampler combined with the Metropolis-Hasting (MH) algorithm to generate posterior samples using the likelihood and non-informative (flat) priors. For each gender group, eight chains have run 6000 steps with overdispersed initial values, with a burn-in of 1000 steps, then thinning the chain every 50 steps, which provides 100 posterior samples from each chain. We combined the posterior samples to get 800 posterior samples for each gender. See Wu et al 2022 for more details and results [12]. Table 2.8 summarized the MLE and Bayesian posterior estimates.

It was clear from Table 2.8 that the MLE of (μ, σ^2) and the posterior mean (or median) were close to each other for each gender, implying that the

TABLE 2.8
MLE and Bayesian posterior estimates using the NLST-CT data.

	Female heavy smokers				Male heavy smokers			
		Bayesian estimate				Bayesian estimate		
θ	MLE	Mean	Median	S.E.	MLE	Mean	Median	S.E.
b_0	3.139	2.972	2.992	1.242	4.084	2.636	2.577	1.339
b_1	1.860	1.223	0.875	1.107	0	1.285	0.936	1.112
μ	4.266	4.254	4.253	0.014	4.262	4.253	4.253	0.010
σ^2	0.023	0.021	0.021	0.004	0.019	0.017	0.017	0.002
λ	0.214	0.194	0.190	0.089	0.354	0.294	0.305	0.109
α	2.803	4.238	3.512	2.173	2.288	3.168	2.614	1.662

Adapted from Table 1 in Wu et al 2022 [12].

transition density curves using the MLE or using the posterior mean/median should be close for each gender. However, the MLE of (b_0, b_1) was very different from the posterior mean estimates for both genders; specifically, the MLE of b_1 was zero for male heavy smokers, suggesting that the sensitivity was the same at the beginning and at the end of the preclinical state, which seems incompatible with clinical observations. Similarly, the MLE of (λ, α) was also different from that of the posterior mean estimates for each gender. In general, we prefer Bayesian estimates since the posterior samples provide the distribution for each parameter, not just a single value; hence, it is easier to make inferences on the variation and the credible interval.

Figure 2.14 shows the estimated density of the six parameters in the $\theta = (b_0, b_1, \mu, \sigma^2, \lambda, \alpha)$ using the posterior samples for both genders: the solid and the dotted line represent the estimated density for the female and male heavy smokers respectively. The posterior distribution of the b_1 is close for both genders, implying that screening sensitivity increased at about the same rate for both genders as one's time in the preclinical state increases. However, the distribution of b_0 for female smokers was shifting to the right of their male counterparts, implying that the sensitivity for female smokers was higher at the onset of S_p.

We can calculate the sensitivity at the onset and at the end of the S_p using either the MLE of (b_0, b_1), or the mean value of the posterior samples. However, a better inference is to use all 800 posterior samples (b_0^*, b_1^*). The sensitivity at the onset of S_p is $\beta_0^* = 1/(1 + \exp(-b_0^*))$, and at the end of S_p is $\beta_1^* = 1/(1 + \exp(-b_0^* - b_1^*))$; that gives 800 posterior samples of β_0^* and β_1^*. Then we take the average and calculate the 95% highest posterior density (HPD) interval. We summarized the result using all three approaches in Table 2.9.

Figure 2.15 helps to visualize the result: there are 4 curves in each panel; the pointwise mean sensitivity at each point $x/Y \in [0, 1]$ (the solid line),

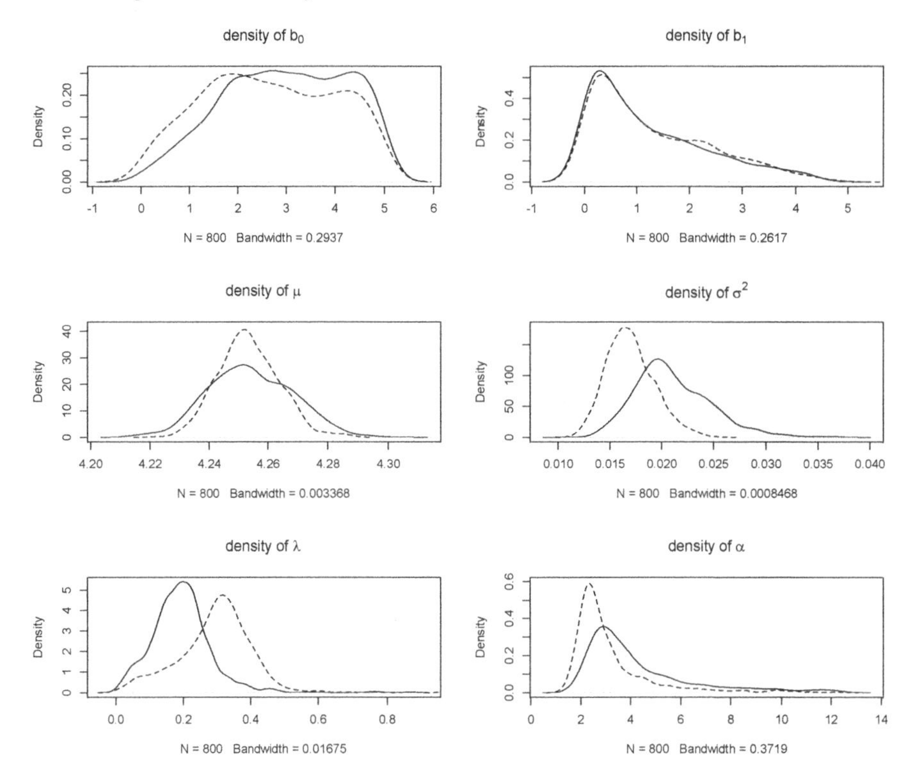

FIGURE 2.14
Estimated density of parameters using the posterior samples: The solid line is for female heavy smokers; the dotted line is for the male counterparts. Adapted from Figure 2 in Wu et al 2022 [12].

the corresponding point-wise 95% highest posterior density (HPD) intervals (the two dotted lines), and the sensitivity curve using the posterior mean (the broken line).

TABLE 2.9
Estimate of sensitivity at onset and end of the S_p using the NLST-CT data.

	Female heavy smokers				Male heavy smokers			
		Bayesian posterior				Bayesian posterior		
β	MLE	^{a}Mean	^{b}All	95% HPD	MLE	^{a}Mean	^{b}All	95% HPD
onset	0.958	0.951	0.915	(0.700, 0.993)	0.983	0.933	0.884	(0.613, 0.993)
end	0.993	0.985	0.981	(0.952, 0.993)	0.983	0.980	0.972	(0.906, 0.993)

^{a} use the mean of the 800 posterior samples.
^{b} use all 800 posterior samples.

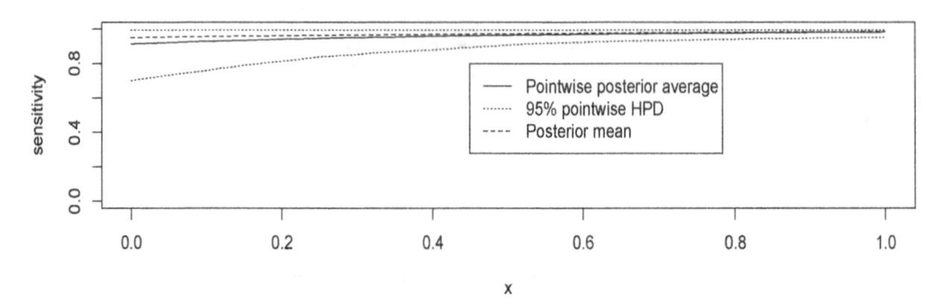

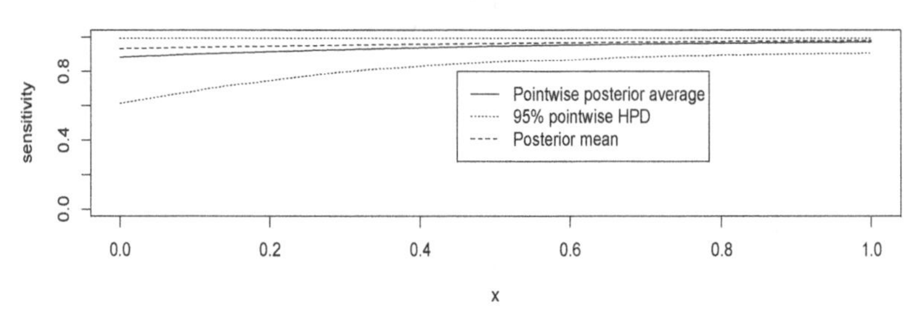

FIGURE 2.15
Plots of estimated sensitivity for male and female heavy smokers. Adapted from Figure 3 in Wu et al 2022 [12].

Similarly, we can use all posterior samples to estimate the transition age from the disease-free state S_0 to the preclinical state S_p and the sojourn time. We summarized the mean, median, and mode with the corresponding 95% HPD intervals (in years) in Table 2.10. The first row under the column

TABLE 2.10
Transition age and sojourn time with corresponding 95% HPD credible intervals (in years) based on the posterior samples.

	Female heavy smokers		
	Mean	Median	Mode
Transition age	71.15 (69.25,73.28)	70.40(68.55, 72.31)	68.93(67.26,70.65)
Sojourn time	1.49 (1.02, 1.92)	1.47(1.06, 1.89)	1.46 (1.10, 1.80)
	Male heavy smokers		
	Mean	Median	Mode
Transition age	70.94(69.40,72.32)	70.34(68.96,71.66)	69.16 (68.03, 70.38)
Sojourn time	1.43(1.05,1.83)	1.39(1.09,1.73)	1.30 (1.01, 1.64)

Adapted from Table 2 in Wu et al 2022 [12].

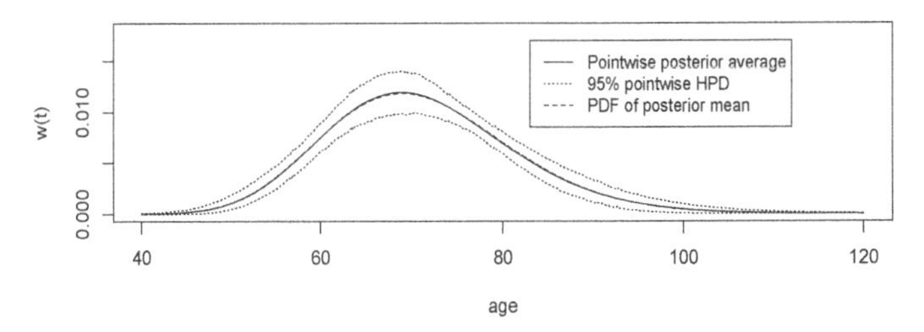

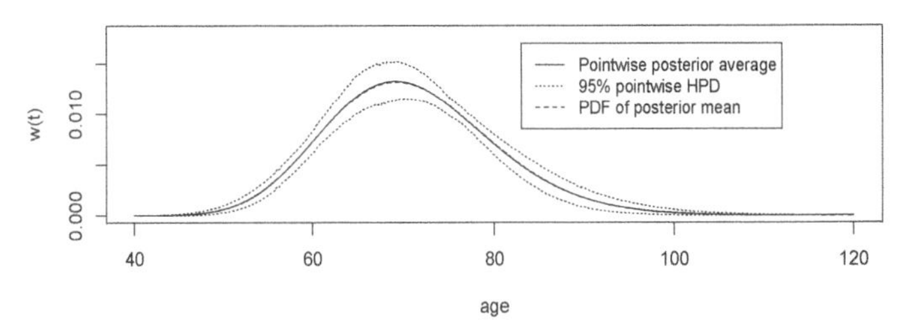

FIGURE 2.16
Plots of estimated transition density for heavy smokers. Adapted from Figure 4 in Wu et al 2022 [12].

"Mean" showed that the average mean transition age into the preclinical state for female heavy smokers was 71.15 years, with a 95% HPD interval of (69.25, 73.28) years. See Wu et al 2022 for more details [12].

Figure 2.16 showed the transition density curve and the pointwise 95% HPD intervals. The density curve plotted using the posterior mean (the broken line) was almost the same as the pointwise posterior average (the solid line). Figure 2.17 showed the density curve of the sojourn time and the pointwise 95% HPD intervals. For comparison, the density curve using the posterior sample mean of (λ^*, α^*) was also plotted in the same graph, using the broken line.

2.6 An open problem

A careful study of the likelihood function shows that some individuals' screening data was used more than once. It may be used multiple times depending on the situation. For example, for a person who was diagnosed at the second exam t_1, the likelihood contribution from this individual should be D_2, but in

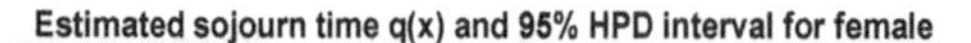

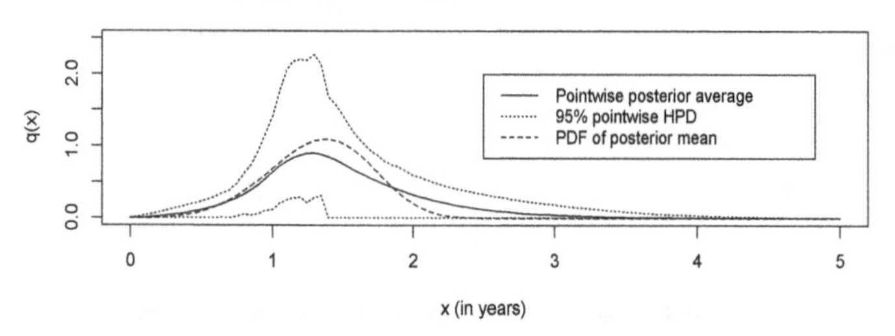

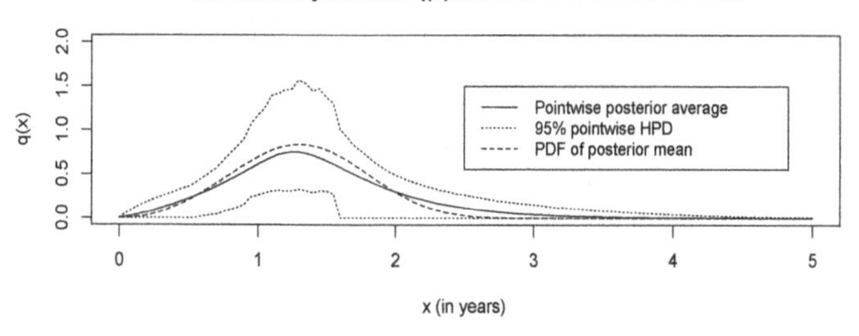

FIGURE 2.17
Plots of estimated sojourn time density for heavy smokers. Adapted from Figure 5 in Wu et al 2022 [12].

the existing likelihood function, it is $(1 - D_1 - I_1) \times D_2$. Because this person was included in the number $(n_1 - s_1 - r_1)$ at the first screening, and then it was counted again in the number s_2 at the second screening. And for an individual who was an interval incident case in (t_2, t_3), her contribution to the likelihood should be I_3, but in the existing likelihood, it is $(1-D_1-I_1)\times(1-D_2-I_2)\times I_3$, as it was counted in the two previous screening groups.

A better way is to avoid double or multiple counting, but use each person's data exactly once in the likelihood. For the individual who was diagnosed at the i-th screening, the contribution to the likelihood should be D_i, and for individuals who experienced the interval case, the contribution to the likelihood should be I_i, there is no doubt about this. However, for those who went through a sequence of exams and not being detected and not being an interval case, the contribution to the likelihood should be based on the probability that this person reached the last time in the sequence of screening. We leave this as an open problem for researchers to explore for a better likelihood.

2.7 Bibliographic notes

There are many publications to estimate the sensitivity, the sojourn time distribution, and the transition probability from the disease-free to the preclinical state in a screening program [54, 14, 51, 30, 49]. Some good review articles in this area are Liu et al 2017[31], Wu and Rosner [77] and Wu and Perez 2012 [75].

Shen and Zelen 1999 was the first paper to use a likelihood function to estimate the screening sensitivity and the mean sojourn time under the assumptions of a stable and a nonstable disease model [49]. The stable model assumed that the transition density $w(t) = w$ was a constant for all ages. Their non-stable model considered $w(t)$ to be a step-function of age t, with $w(t)$ to be a constant in every 5-year age group (40-44, 45-49, etc.). In both models, the screening sensitivity was assumed to be a constant across all exams, and the sojourn time was assumed to follow an exponential distribution, i.e., $Q(x) = \exp(-x/\mu)$. The estimated parameters are the sensitivity β, the mean sojourn time μ and the transition parameter w. The non-stable disease model requires more assumptions, however. For example, a person's age at the initial and the last screening exams should fall into the same age group. The innovative part of their paper was that they used a likelihood function to estimate these parameters.

We have built up on the previous models and introduced parametric link functions for the sensitivity, the transition density, and the sojourn time. A major contribution is to clearly derive the probability formula for different events under different assumptions. Two different modeling assumptions were introduced in this chapter: (i) the sensitivity as a function of age, or (ii) the sensitivity depends on the ratio of time in the preclinical state and the total sojourn time. Major methodologies presented in this chapter are in Wu et al 2005 [79] and Wu et al 2022 [76]. Wu et al 2005b [84] provides the simulation procedure to generate pseudo-screening data and check modal reliability.

The methods were applied to a few different cancer screening data. Wu et al 2009a estimated the three key parameters for FOBT screening in colorectal cancer [65]. Chen et al 2010 [7] applied the method to the Canadian National Breast Screening Study Data [36, 37]. Wu et al 2011 applied the method to the Mayo Lung Project (MLP) data, to make Bayesian inferences for the three key parameters for male heavy smokers [67]. Jang et al 2013 applied the method to the Johns Hopkins Lung Project (JHLP) data, where a chest X-ray exam was carried out annually for eight consecutive years for male heavy smokers in the Baltimore metropolitan area between 1973 and 1978 [21]. Chen et al 2014 applied the method to the lung cancer screening program data at the Memorial Sloan Kettering Cancer Center (MSKC-LCSP), which was carried out in the New York City area since 1974 for male heavy smokers, using data from the annual chest X-ray group [8]. In all three lung cancer screening data analyses above, the sensitivity was treated as a constant across all age groups and they were all for male heavy smokers. Liu et al 2015 applied the method to the NLST CT data for three groups: male, and female heavy smokers, and combined, with three annual low-dose CT exams [32]. Wang et al 2017 used the likelihood method to the lung cancer data from the Prostate, Lung, Colorectal, and Ovarian Cancer Screening Trial [55]. Rahman and Wu 2021 applied the method to the NLST chest X-ray data [43]. Wu and Kim 2022 adopted the model that sensitivity is a function of the ratio of time in the preclinical stage and the sojourn time, and applied it to the HIP data [83].

There are other publications on methodologies that we didn't cover in this chapter. Wu et al 2008 modeled sensitivity as a function of an individual's age and the time spent in the preclinical state, and applied it to the HIP data [63]. Kim et al 2015 used a nonlinear mixed-effects approach to generalize the probability model for sensitivity to depend on age at diagnosis, time spent in the preclinical state and sojourn time, and applied the method to the HIP data and the Johns Hopkins Lung Project data [26]. Kim and Wu 2016 proposed a family of link functions to model the sensitivity as a function of time spent in the preclinical state and the sojourn time, and used simulations to check model reliability, then applied it to the Johns Hopkins Lung Project data [27]. Finally, Wu and Kim 2020 is an editorial article discussing the problems in the MLE calculation when the screening number is too few [82].

2.8 Solution for some exercises

Exercise 2.1:

(a) 0.075

(b) 0.0657059

(c) 0.12636

(d) Proof:

$$
\begin{aligned}
&\int_0^\infty I_Y(y)dy \\
&= \int_0^\infty \int_0^y w(x)q(y-x)dxdy, \text{ switch } dx\ dy \\
&= \int_0^\infty \int_x^\infty w(x)q(y-x)dydx \\
&= \int_0^\infty w(x)\int_x^\infty q(y-x)dydx = \int_0^\infty w(x)[-Q(y-x)|_x^\infty]dx \\
&= \int_0^\infty w(x)[Q(x-x)-Q(\infty-x)]dx, Q(0)=1, Q(\infty)=0 \\
&= \int_0^\infty w(x)dx.
\end{aligned}
$$

Exercise 2.4:

	k	$P(D_k)$	$P(I_k)$
(a)			
	1	0.00320067	0.000740636
	2	0.00164762	0.000587867
	3	0.00145923	0.000569335
	4	0.00143638	0.000567087
(b)			
	1	0.00593402	0.000849272
	2	0.00342906	0.000703596
	3	0.00330967	0.000697972
	4	0.00330279	0.000697711
(c)			
	1	0.00195818	0.000754722
	2	0.00146423	0.000608541
	3	0.00144659	0.000587825
	4	0.00150831	0.000581912
(d)			
	1	0.00352923	0.00137412
	2	0.00281184	0.000974177
	3	0.00291437	0.000950634
	4	0.00309053	0.000963696

Exercise 2.5: The log-likelihood $\approx$ -116.37.

Exercise 2.6: Due to randomness in simulation, the answer varies. However, three samples are provided here using the input parameters, and your generated data matrix should be similar to these.

Sample 1:

t_0	n_1	s_1	r_1	n_2	s_2	r_2	n_3	s_3	r_3	n_4	s_4	r_4
40	991	1	0	990	0	0	990	1	1	988	2	0
41	989	2	1	986	1	0	985	1	1	983	0	2
42	982	0	2	980	0	0	980	2	0	978	1	2
43	986	0	0	986	1	0	985	2	2	981	0	1
44	979	2	0	977	2	4	971	1	0	970	3	2
45	981	1	1	979	3	0	976	2	0	974	0	1
46	974	4	2	968	0	2	966	2	1	963	2	1
47	980	1	2	977	2	0	975	1	1	973	1	0
48	969	4	0	965	2	1	962	3	3	956	3	1
49	972	4	0	968	0	0	968	3	1	964	2	0
50	972	3	1	968	3	2	963	0	0	963	1	0
51	972	1	1	970	2	2	966	5	0	961	1	3
52	960	1	0	959	1	0	958	2	0	956	6	0
53	966	6	1	959	2	0	957	2	0	955	0	0
54	946	5	0	941	1	0	940	2	0	938	1	1
55	945	3	0	942	3	2	937	1	0	936	5	0
56	955	6	2	947	5	1	941	4	0	937	5	1
57	949	6	0	943	3	0	940	3	1	936	1	0
58	937	4	1	932	1	1	930	0	1	929	2	1
59	935	8	1	926	2	0	924	3	0	921	0	0
60	938	4	1	933	4	0	929	3	0	926	5	1
61	931	4	1	926	5	0	921	2	0	919	3	0
62	945	1	2	942	2	0	940	0	1	939	1	0
63	935	4	0	931	2	0	929	1	0	928	4	0
64	922	8	0	914	3	2	909	2	0	907	3	0

Sample 2:

t_0	n_1	s_1	r_1	n_2	s_2	r_2	n_3	s_3	r_3	n_4	s_4	r_4
40	983	1	0	982	0	0	982	2	0	980	3	0
41	978	0	1	977	0	1	976	3	0	973	0	0
42	985	2	1	982	0	0	982	0	0	982	1	1
43	980	3	1	976	2	1	973	0	1	972	2	0
44	976	1	2	973	0	0	973	0	1	972	3	0
45	984	2	1	981	3	0	978	1	0	977	4	1
46	975	5	1	969	3	0	966	1	1	964	4	0
47	978	2	4	972	2	1	969	1	2	966	2	2
48	973	3	0	970	1	1	968	1	1	966	0	0
49	966	4	1	961	2	0	959	3	0	956	3	1
50	961	2	0	959	1	0	958	2	1	955	2	0
51	967	1	1	965	0	1	964	0	2	962	0	0
52	955	4	0	951	3	1	947	2	1	944	1	0
53	956	1	0	955	3	0	952	4	1	947	4	2
54	960	5	1	954	2	1	951	1	0	950	3	0
55	945	1	2	942	1	1	940	3	1	936	2	0
56	937	2	0	935	1	1	933	3	1	929	6	2
57	941	6	1	934	2	0	932	2	1	929	3	1
58	944	4	0	940	3	0	937	0	0	937	0	0
59	928	6	6	916	2	1	913	2	0	911	1	1
60	933	5	1	927	2	2	923	3	0	920	2	0
61	952	6	0	946	2	0	944	1	1	942	0	0
62	939	4	1	934	2	0	932	2	0	930	3	1
63	920	5	2	913	2	0	911	5	0	906	7	0
64	922	3	0	919	5	0	914	0	1	913	1	0

Sample 3:

t_0	n_1	s_1	r_1	n_2	s_2	r_2	n_3	s_3	r_3	n_4	s_4	r_4
40	982	3	1	978	1	1	976	1	0	975	0	1
41	984	2	1	981	0	0	981	2	2	977	1	1
42	985	0	0	985	0	0	985	2	1	982	2	0
43	980	2	1	977	3	0	974	0	0	974	1	1
44	973	2	2	969	1	1	967	1	0	966	2	0
45	973	2	1	970	1	0	969	0	1	968	1	2
46	980	2	0	978	1	1	976	1	1	974	0	0
47	967	1	1	965	1	1	963	0	0	963	4	0
48	959	3	3	953	1	3	949	0	0	949	1	0
49	964	2	0	962	1	1	960	1	0	959	2	1
50	974	4	2	968	1	0	967	2	0	965	3	0
51	967	0	0	967	3	4	960	2	2	956	1	0
52	972	1	2	969	2	0	967	2	1	964	2	0
53	959	4	1	954	1	1	952	2	1	949	2	1
54	948	4	2	942	1	1	940	1	0	939	1	1
55	937	4	0	933	0	1	932	3	0	929	2	0
56	951	9	0	942	4	0	938	2	0	936	0	0
57	957	8	0	949	1	1	947	5	0	942	10	1
58	941	3	1	937	2	0	935	2	1	932	2	0
59	949	6	2	941	3	1	937	0	1	936	1	0
60	944	5	1	938	3	0	935	4	0	931	0	0
61	929	6	0	923	0	1	922	1	2	919	2	0
62	951	3	0	948	0	0	948	3	0	945	2	0
63	930	4	0	926	2	0	924	2	1	921	2	1
64	918	5	0	913	3	0	910	0	0	910	4	0

3

Testing Dependency of Two Screening Modalities

CONTENTS

There were a few screening programs using two diagnostic procedures, with binary outcomes. If one of the two tests results in a positive finding, a more definitive diagnostic procedure, such as a biopsy, will be carried out to establish the presence or absence of disease. The use of both tests may considerably improve the overall screening sensitivity if the two tests are independent or negatively correlated, compared to employing two tests that are positively correlated. A likelihood ratio test was developed for testing the independence of the two diagnostic procedures. The motivation comes from the need to investigate the independence of mammograms and clinical breast exams in the HIP study. And it was later used to investigate the independence of chest X-rays and sputum cytology for lung cancer in the Johns Hopkins Lung Project. Since most screening programs use only one screening modality, you can safely skip this chapter without much loss.

3.1 Introduction

Some cancer screening programs adopted two diagnostic modalities with the purpose of increasing the overall sensitivity and assessing test reliability. We

DOI: 10.1201/9781003404125-3

will investigate the *correlation* between two testing techniques or modalities in this chapter. We will investigate the independent use of both a clinical breast examination and a mammogram to screen for breast cancer in the Health Insurance Plan of Greater New York (HIP) study and the independent use of chest X-rays and the sputum cytology for lung cancer in the Johns Hopkins Lung Project. The motivation for using two screening procedures is the expectation that the different natures of the procedures may lead to increased overall sensitivity. For example, in diagnosing lung cancer, the size, shape, and location of a lesion are important indicators for a chest X-ray radiologist, whereas in sputum cytology, a sample of mucus is viewed under the microscope to identify possible cancer cells. Usually, sputum cytology is more useful in diagnosing squamous cell lung cancers, a type of non-small cell carcinoma, which starts in the central airways, and it may not be effective in identifying other types of lung cancer. Similarly, for breast cancer, a clinical breast exam may find one kind of breast cancer easily while mammograms may find another kind. Even if some breast cancer screening trials have been designed to conduct two screening tests independently (Shapiro et al, 1988 [47]), it is likely that some factors related to patients may influence the detectability of the screening procedures, therefore resulting in dependency on the tests. As some investigators reasoned, early diagnosis by mammogram and clinical breast exam may be based on some similar biological features, so that certain breast cancer lesions are easily detected by both procedures, while others are unlikely to be found by either procedure (Walter and Day 1983 [54]). So, if there is a strong positive correlation among two screening procedures, using only the one with the higher sensitivity will be more cost-effective than utilizing both. On the other hand, if two screening procedures are independent, the use of both screening procedures will substantially increase the overall screening sensitivity. The knowledge of the dependence structure between two diagnostics tests will provide a basis to guide health policymakers in designing cost-effective screening programs.

In this chapter, we use the likelihood function and hypothesis testing to address this problem. We present the general data format when two exams are carried out at each screening. First, we introduce the likelihood function for testing the dependence under the stable disease model when the sensitivity and the transition density are constants (Shen et al 2001 [48]). Then we expand to the case when the transition density $w(t)$ is age-dependent (Kim et al 2012 [28]).

3.2 Data format for two screening modalities

The data format is similar to that in Chapter 1, section 1.6. For the i-th screening interval $[t_{i-1}, t_i)$, for $i = 1, 2, \cdots, k-1$, we use the following

TABLE 3.1
A sample of mass cancer screening data.

t_0	n_1	$s_{10}^{(1)}$	$s_{01}^{(1)}$	$s_{11}^{(1)}$	r_1	n_2	$s_{10}^{(2)}$	$s_{01}^{(2)}$	$s_{11}^{(2)}$	r_2	$\cdots$
$\cdots$	$\cdots$		$\cdots$								
55	1800	2	1	1	1	1645	1	3	2	2	$\cdots$
$\cdots$	$\cdots$		$\cdots$								
65	1520	1	2	2	0	1368	0	1	1	0	$\cdots$
$\cdots$	$\cdots$		$\cdots$								

notation: n_i is the total number of individuals examined at t_{i-1}; s_i is the number of cases detected and confirmed (excluding false-positive cases) at the exam given at t_{i-1}; and r_i is the number of clinical cases that appeared within the interval (t_{i-1}, t_i). Let $s_{10}^{(i)}$ represents the number of positive cases diagnosed by screening modality 1 only, but not by modality 2; and $s_{01}^{(i)}$ refers to the number of positive cases diagnosed by screening modality 2 only, but not by modality 1; and $s_{11}^{(i)}$ refers to the number of cases detected by both modalities. It is obvious that $s_i = s_{10}^{(i)} + s_{01}^{(i)} + s_{11}^{(i)}$. Table 3.1 shows the data format. The only difference is to replace the s_i in Table 1.1, with three columns $s_{10}^{(i)}, s_{01}^{(i)}, s_{11}^{(i)}$.

3.3 Testing dependency under the stable disease model

We will start with the stable disease model [48] and expand it to the more complicated one.

3.3.1 The likelihood function

We consider an early detection trial with two screening procedures independently applied to each individual during a study (e.g., clinical breast exam and mammography in breast cancer screening). There are three situations for a tumor to be detected: the case diagnosed by procedure 1 only, diagnosed by procedure 2 only, and detected by both procedures. We let X_i be a binary random variable that denotes the outcome of procedure i $(i = 1, 2)$ with one denoting a positive finding and zero denoting a negative or normal finding. We let D be a binary random variable that gives the true disease status of an individual. That is, $D = 1$ means that the individual has the disease and $D = 0$ means that the individual does not have the disease. We are interested in the situation of $D = 1$ for detection purposes, and let

$$\alpha_{ij} = P\{X_1 = i, X_2 = j | D = 1\}, \quad i, j \in \{0, 1\}. \tag{3.1}$$

Then the overall sensitivity is

$$\beta = P\{\max(X_1, X_2) = 1 | D = 1\} = \alpha_{10} + \alpha_{01} + \alpha_{11}. \tag{3.2}$$

The individual sensitivities of the two tests are

$$\begin{aligned} \beta_1 &= P\{X_1 = 1 | D = 1\} = \alpha_{10} + \alpha_{11}, & (3.3) \\ \beta_2 &= P\{X_2 = 1 | D = 1\} = \alpha_{01} + \alpha_{11}. & (3.4) \end{aligned}$$

If X_1 and X_2 are independent given that $D = 1$, then

$$\begin{aligned} \alpha_{11} &= P\{X_1 = 1, X_2 = 1 | D = 1\} = P\{X_1 = 1 | D = 1\} P\{X_2 = 1 | D = 1\} \\ &= \beta_1 \beta_2. \end{aligned}$$

Similarly, if X_1 and X_2 are independent given that $D = 1$, then

$$\begin{aligned} \alpha_{00} &= (1 - \beta_1)(1 - \beta_2), \\ \alpha_{10} &= \beta_1 (1 - \beta_2), \\ \alpha_{01} &= (1 - \beta_1) \beta_2. \end{aligned}$$

These are the necessary and sufficient conditions for the independence of X_1 and X_2 given that $D = 1$.

We let ρ be the *correlation coefficient* between X_1 and X_2 conditional on $D = 1$. Since the conditional distribution of X_i given $D = 1$ are Bernoulli random variables with success rate β_i, for $i = 1, 2$,

$$\begin{aligned} \rho &= corr(X_1, X_2 | D = 1) = \frac{Cov(X_1, X_2 | D = 1)}{\sqrt{Var(X_1 | D = 1) Var(X_2 | D = 1)}} \\ &= \frac{Pr(X_1 = 1, X_2 = 1 | D = 1) - Pr(X_1 = 1 | D = 1) Pr(X_2 = 1 | D = 1)}{\sqrt{\beta_1 (1 - \beta_1) \beta_2 (1 - \beta_2)}} \\ &= \frac{\alpha_{11} - \beta_1 \beta_2}{\sqrt{\beta_1 \beta_2 (1 - \beta_1)(1 - \beta_2)}}. \end{aligned} \tag{3.5}$$

From this equation, we know that

$$\alpha_{11} = \beta_1 \beta_2 + \rho \sqrt{\beta_1 \beta_2 (1 - \beta_1)(1 - \beta_2)}\,. \tag{3.6}$$

And we can express α_{10}, α_{01} in terms of β_1, β_2 and ρ in the general case

$$\begin{aligned} \alpha_{10} = \beta_1 - \alpha_{11} = \beta_1 - \beta_1 \beta_2 - \rho \sqrt{\beta_1 \beta_2 (1 - \beta_1)(1 - \beta_2)}\,; \\ \alpha_{01} = \beta_2 - \alpha_{11} = \beta_2 - \beta_1 \beta_2 - \rho \sqrt{\beta_1 \beta_2 (1 - \beta_1)(1 - \beta_2)}\,. \end{aligned} \tag{3.7}$$

The overall sensitivity, $\beta = \beta_1 + \beta_2 - \alpha_{11}$, can be expressed as

$$\beta = \beta_1 + \beta_2 - \beta_1\beta_2 - \rho\sqrt{\beta_1\beta_2(1-\beta_1)(1-\beta_2)}\,. \tag{3.8}$$

It is clear that a positive correlation ρ reduces the overall sensitivity and a negative correlation increases the overall sensitivity. A test of independence of two screening modalities is to test

$$H_0 : \rho = 0, \quad vs. \quad H_1 : \rho \neq 0.$$

Equivalently, it is to test

$$H_0 : \alpha_{11} = \beta_1\beta_2, \quad vs. \quad H_1 : \alpha_{11} \neq \beta_1\beta_2.$$

Or equivalently, to test

$$H_0 : \beta = \beta_1 + \beta_2 - \beta_1\beta_2, \quad vs. \quad H_1 : \beta \neq \beta_1 + \beta_2 - \beta_1\beta_2.$$

Let $t_0 < t_1 < \cdots < t_{K-1}$ represent K ordered screening exam ages/times. Consider the i-th screening interval $[t_{i-1}, t_i)$. Let $D_i(\beta)$ be the probability of an individual diagnosed at the i-th scheduled exam given at t_{i-1}, and let $I_i(\beta)$ be the probability of an interval case occurring in the i-th interval (t_{i-1}, t_i). The contribution to the likelihood from the i-th screening interval would be [48]:

$$L_i(\beta, \beta_1, \beta_2 | D = 1) = L_{1i}(\beta | D = 1) L_{2i}(\beta_1, \beta_2 | \beta, D = 1), \tag{3.9}$$

where

$$\begin{aligned} L_{1i}(\beta | D = 1) &= D_i(\beta)^{s_i} I_i(\beta)^{r_i} [1 - D_i(\beta) - I_i(\beta)]^{n_i - s_i - r_i}\,, \\ L_{2i}(\beta_1, \beta_2 | \beta, D = 1) &= \alpha_{10}^{s_{10}^{(i)}} \alpha_{01}^{s_{01}^{(i)}} \alpha_{11}^{s_{11}^{(i)}} / \beta^{s_i}\,. \end{aligned} \tag{3.10}$$

And for K screening intervals, the full likelihood is

$$L = L_1(\beta | D = 1) L_2(\beta_1, \beta_2 | \beta, D = 1), \tag{3.11}$$

with

$$\begin{aligned} L_1(\beta | D = 1) &= \prod_{i=1}^{K} D_i(\beta)^{s_i} I_i(\beta)^{r_i} [1 - D_i(\beta) - I_i(\beta)]^{n_i - s_i - r_i}\,, \\ L_2(\beta_1, \beta_2 | D = 1) &= \prod_{i=1}^{K} \alpha_{10}^{s_{10}^{(i)}} \alpha_{01}^{s_{01}^{(i)}} \alpha_{11}^{s_{11}^{(i)}} / \beta^{s_i}\,. \end{aligned} \tag{3.12}$$

The $L_1(\beta | D = 1)$ depends only on β, and it does not involves β_1 and β_2. The $L_2(\beta_1, \beta_2 | D = 1)$ involves all three β_1, β_2 and β. And the total screen-detected number at the i-th screening is $s_i = s_{10}^{(i)} + s_{01}^{(i)} + s_{11}^{(i)}$. A simplified likelihood that replaces the first part of (3.10) was called the conditional likelihood in Shen et al 2001:

$$L_{1i}(\beta|D=1) = \frac{D_i(\beta)^{s_i} I_i(\beta)^{r_i}}{[D_i(\beta)+I_i(\beta)]^{s_i+r_i}}. \tag{3.13}$$

The $D_i(\beta)$ and $I_i(\beta)$ were first derived by Zelen 1993 when the sensitivity $\beta(t_i)=\beta$ was the same at all exams [88]. However, the derivation procedure using the concept of forward/backward recurrence time was complicated and difficult to follow. In fact, their formula of $D_i(\beta)$ and $I_i(\beta)$ is just the same as in the equations (2.12), (2.13), and (2.14) with the sensitivity $\beta(t_i)=\beta$. Hence,

$$D_1(\beta) = \beta\int_0^{t_0} w(x)Q(t_0-x)dx; \tag{3.14}$$

$$\begin{aligned} D_i(\beta) &= \beta\left\{\sum_{j=0}^{i-2}(1-\beta)^{i-j-1}\int_{t_{j-1}}^{t_j} w(x)Q(t_{i-1}-x)dx \right. \\ &\left. + \int_{t_{i-2}}^{t_{i-1}} w(x)Q(t_{i-1}-x)dx\right\}, \text{ for } i=2,\cdots,K. \end{aligned} \tag{3.15}$$

$$\begin{aligned} I_i(\beta) &= \sum_{j=0}^{i-1}(1-\beta)^{i-j}\int_{t_{j-1}}^{t_j} w(x)[Q(t_{i-1}-x)-Q(t_i-x)]dx \\ &+ \int_{t_{i-1}}^{t_i} w(x)[1-Q(t_i-x)]dx, \text{ for } i=1,\cdots,K. \end{aligned} \tag{3.16}$$

The above probabilities can be simplified under the stable disease model, that is, $w(t)=w$. If the sojourn time is assumed to follow the exponential distribution with mean μ,

$$q(x) = \frac{1}{\mu}e^{-x/\mu}, \quad Q(x)=e^{-x/\mu}, \ x>0, \mu>0.$$

And $w(t)=w$ is a constant, then the $D_i(\beta)$ and $I_i(\beta)$ are greatly simplified to [48]:

$$D_i(\beta) = \begin{cases} \beta P\left[1-\beta\sum_{j=1}^{i-1}(1-\beta)^{i-j-1}Q_0(t_{i-1}-t_{j-1})\right] & \text{if } i>1 \\ \beta P & \text{if } i=1, \end{cases} \tag{3.17}$$

$$I_i(\beta) = P\left[\frac{\Delta_i}{\mu} - \beta\sum_{j=0}^{i-1}(1-\beta)^{i-j-1}\{Q_0(t_{i-1}-t_j)-Q_0(t_i-t_j)\}\right]. \tag{3.18}$$

where $\Delta_i = t_i - t_{i-1}$ is the screening time interval, and

$$Q_0(t) = \mu^{-1} \int_t^{\infty} Q(t)dt = e^{-t/\mu}, \quad t > 0.$$

and

$$P = \int_0^{t_0} wQ(t_0 - x)dx = w\mu(1 - e^{-t_0/\mu}) \approx \mu w,$$

the last approximation comes from the fact that when t_0 is larger, $e^{-t_0/\mu}$ is almost zero. As most screening programs were designed with equal screening intervals; i.e., $\Delta_i = \Delta$, the above formula can be further simplified as

$$D_i(\beta) = \begin{cases} \mu w \beta \left(1 - \beta \sum_{j=1}^{i-1} (1-\beta)^{i-j-1} e^{-(t_{i-1}-t_{j-1})/\mu}\right) & \text{if } i > 1 \\ \mu w \beta & \text{if } i = 1, \end{cases} \quad (3.19)$$

$$I_i(\beta) = \mu w \left[\frac{\Delta}{\mu} - \beta \sum_{j=0}^{i-1} (1-\beta)^{i-j-1} \left\{ e^{-(t_{i-1}-t_j)/\mu} - e^{-(t_i - t_j)/\mu} \right\} \right]. \quad (3.20)$$

There are three parameters (β, w, μ) in the stable disease model, and in the HIP study $\Delta = 1$ year.

To test the independence of the two procedures $H_0 : \rho = 0$, we can use the *Wald test* by finding the maximum likelihood estimate (MLE) of ρ and using the normal approximation when the sample size is large,

$$\hat{\rho}/\sqrt{var(\hat{\rho})} \sim N(0, 1).$$

Another way is to use the *likelihood ratio test* $-2log(LR)$, which is asymptotically distributed as a chi-square random variable with one degree of freedom. Specifically, the log-likelihood function $log(L) = l(\beta_1, \beta_2, \rho, \mu)$, is reduced to the log-likelihood $l(\beta_1, \beta_2, \mu)$ under the null hypothesis H_0. Under some standard regularity conditions, the log-likelihood ratio test statistic for testing H_0 is

$$-2log(LR) = 2\left\{ l(\hat{\beta}_1, \hat{\beta}_2, \hat{\rho}, \hat{\mu}) - l(\tilde{\beta}_1, \tilde{\beta}_2, \tilde{\mu}) \right\} \sim \chi_1^2$$

where the estimators $(\hat{\beta}_1, \hat{\beta}_2, \hat{\rho}, \hat{\mu})$ and $(\tilde{\beta}_1, \tilde{\beta}_2, \tilde{\mu})$ are the MLEs under H_1 and H_0 correspondingly.

Simulation studies were performed to evaluate the reliability of both likelihood functions and the proposed estimation. It seems that the MLE obtained from the likelihood in (3.10) is slightly more accurate than using the conditional likelihood in (3.13), and with a smaller variance. For more details, see Shen et al 2001 [48].

TABLE 3.2
The HIP screening data using two modalities.

scr.	n_i	$s_{10}^{(1)}$	$s_{01}^{(1)}$	$s_{11}^{(1)}$	r_i
1	20166	24	21	10	13
2	15936	15	9	8	8
3	13679	8	5	5	10
4	11971	12	9	6	10

n_i is the total number of people being screened at the i-th exam, $i = 1, 2, 3, 4$. $s_{10}^{(1)}$ is the number of people diagnosed by clinical breast exam (i.e., physical exam) only. $s_{01}^{(1)}$ is the number of people diagnosed by mammogram only. $s_{11}^{(1)}$ is the number of people diagnosed by both modalities.

3.3.2 Application: Mammogram and clinical breast exam in the HIP study

The method was applied to estimate the correlation coefficient and test the dependence between the two screening modalities (clinical breast examination and mammography) in the HIP study. There were four annual screenings, each one composed of a clinical breast exam and a mammogram. Data are available for the total number of screening-detected cases at each screening exam, the total number of interval cases between two consecutive screening exams, and the total number of screening-detected cases by mammography only, or by clinical breast exam only, or by both procedures. The HIP data used for this application is presented in Table 3.2.

The MLE using the conditional likelihood was obtained and presented in Table 3.3. The original likelihood could not be used as the maximum likelihood estimates did not converge to the interior of the parameter space.

Table 3.3 summarizes the estimates for overall screening sensitivity (β), the screening sensitivities for mammography (β_1), clinical breast exam (β_2), the correlation coefficient ρ and the other two parameters. The standard

TABLE 3.3
The MLE using the conditional likelihood and the HIP data.

Parameter	β	β_1	β_2	ρ	α_{10}	α_{01}
MLE	0.703	0.389	0.469	-0.114	0.234	0.314
[a]S.E.	0.158	0.097	0.108	0.192	0.066	0.081

[a]S.E. is the standard error obtained by the bootstrapping method.
Adapted from Table 5 in Shen et al 2001 [48]

deviations were estimated based on 300 bootstrap simulations. In the HIP study, the estimated correlation is -0.114, with a standard deviation of 0.192. The p-value is 0.553 from the Wald statistic for testing the null hypothesis $H_0 : \rho = 0$. Using the likelihood ratio test, the conditional likelihood ratio test yielded a chi-square test statistic of 0.137 with one degree of freedom, and the p-value is 0.711. Therefore we failed to reject the null hypothesis $H_0 : \rho = 0$. That is, there is no significant evidence to show that the two screening procedures are dependent [48].

3.4 Testing dependency under the non-stable disease model

The method can be extended to the general disease progressive model when the transition density $w(t)$ and the sensitivity were both age-dependent. We will present the extended method and then apply it to lung cancer screening using the Johns Hopkins Lung Project data.

3.4.1 The likelihood function

The transition density $w(t)$ is not a constant in reality, as younger people usually have a much lower incidence. It is a sub-probability density function, that is, $\int w(t)dt < 1$, as most people may not enter the preclinical state in their lifetime. We assume that the screening sensitivity is age-dependent, to simplify the situation, we also assume that the correlation coefficient ρ between the two screening modalities is not changing with one's age. And we want to test $H_0 : \rho = 0$.

Assume a group of people with initial age t_0 went through a sequence of exams at $t_0 < t_1 < \cdots < t_{K-1}$, and there were two screening modalities at each exam. Using the result in Chapter 2, the probability of an individual being diagnosed at the k-th exam at the age t_{k-1} is

$$D_{1,t_0} = \beta_0 \int_0^{t_0} w(x)Q(t_0 - x)dx. \tag{3.21}$$

$$\begin{aligned} D_{k,t_0} &= \beta_{k-1}\left\{\sum_{i=0}^{k-2}[1-\beta_i]\cdots[1-\beta_{k-2}]\int_{t_{i-1}}^{t_i} w(x)Q(t_{k-1}-x)dx \right. \\ &+ \left. \int_{t_{k-2}}^{t_{k-1}} w(x)Q(t_{k-1}-x)dx\right\}, \quad \text{for } k = 2, \cdots, K. \end{aligned} \tag{3.22}$$

And the probability of incidence in the interval (t_{k-1}, t_k) is

$$
\begin{aligned}
& I_{k,t_0} \\
= & \sum_{i=0}^{k-1} [1-\beta_i]\cdots[1-\beta_{k-1}] \int_{t_{i-1}}^{t_i} w(x)[Q(t_{k-1}-x) - Q(t_k - x)]dx \\
& + \int_{t_{k-1}}^{t_k} w(x)[1 - Q(t_k - x)]dx, \qquad \text{for } k = 1, \cdots, K, \qquad (3.23)
\end{aligned}
$$

where $\beta_i = \beta(t_i)$ is the overall sensitivity of both modalities at t_i, and we know from the previous section that

$$\beta_i = \beta_{i1} + \beta_{i2} - \beta_{i1}\beta_{i2} - \rho\sqrt{\beta_{i1}\beta_{i2}(1-\beta_{i1})(1-\beta_{i2})}$$

where $\beta_{i1} = \beta_1(t_i), \beta_{i2} = \beta_2(t_i)$ are the corresponding sensitivity of modalities 1 and 2 at the age t_i.

A natural extension of the likelihood function for the age group t_0 would be

$$L(\theta|t_0) = \prod_{i=1}^{K} D_{i,t_0}^{s_{i,t_0}} I_{i,t_0}^{r_{i,t_0}} [1 - D_{i,t_0} - I_{i,t_0}]^{n_{i,t_0} - s_{i,t_0} - r_{i,t_0}} \frac{\alpha_{10}^{s_{10}^{(i)}} \alpha_{01}^{s_{01}^{(i)}} \alpha_{11}^{s_{11}^{(i)}}}{\beta_i^{s_i}}.$$

And the likelihood function including all age groups would be

$$L(\theta) = \prod_{t_0} L(\theta|t_0).$$

To test $H_0 : \rho = 0$, under some regular conditions, the log-likelihood ratio test follows a chi-square distribution with one degree of freedom. That is,

$$
\begin{aligned}
-2\log(LR) &= 2\Big\{\log L(\hat{\beta}_{0,1}, \hat{\beta}_{0,2}, \ldots, \hat{\beta}_{K-1,1}, \hat{\beta}_{K-1,2}, \hat{\rho}) \\
&\quad - \log L(\tilde{\beta}_{0,1}, \tilde{\beta}_{0,2}, \ldots, \tilde{\beta}_{K-1,1}, \tilde{\beta}_{K-1,2})\Big\} \sim \chi_1^2.
\end{aligned}
$$

where $(\hat{\beta}_{0,1}, \hat{\beta}_{0,2}, \ldots, \hat{\beta}_{K-1,1}, \hat{\beta}_{K-1,2}, \hat{\rho})$ and $(\tilde{\beta}_{0,1}, \tilde{\beta}_{0,2}, \ldots, \tilde{\beta}_{K-1,1}, \tilde{\beta}_{K-1,2})$ are the corresponding MLE of θ under the hypothesis H_1 and H_0.

3.4.2 Application: Chest X-ray and sputum cytology in the Johns Hopkins Lung Project

Kim et al 2012 tested the dependency of chest X-ray and sputum cytology using the Johns Hopkins Lung Project (JHLP) data when the transition density $w(t)$ is age-dependent[28].

The JHLP enrolled 10,386 male smokers in the Baltimore metropolitan area between 1973 and 1978. They were at least 45 years old and smoked at least one pack of cigarettes per day, or had smoked this much within one year of enrollment, and they had no prior history of respiratory tract cancer. All participants were randomized to either chest X-ray only or a dual screen (chest X-ray and sputum cytology) group, resulting in 5160 to the chest X-ray-only arm and 5226 to the dual-screen arm. Participants in the chest X-ray group received chest X-ray screening tests annually, for eight consecutive years. Participants in the dual-screen group took chest X-rays annually and received sputum cytology every 4 months, for 8 consecutive years, with a total of 22 screening time points altogether. Out of the 22 screenings, only 8 annual screenings include both chest X-ray and sputum cytology procedures. If any of the tests were positive, then the test was considered positive and a definitive workup exam, such as a biopsy, was done. The data that we used includes the total number of participants in each screening exam, the number of detected and confirmed cancer cases in each screening exam, and the number of interval cases. These data were stratified by age at entry. The age at entry ranges from 45 to 88 years old in the study. However, we only used the data from age 45 to 67 because the other age groups have too few participants, and may cause large deviations in the estimation.

In this application, the transition probability density is the PDF of a log-normal distribution multiplied by 20% (i.e., a sub-PDF),

$$w(t) = \frac{0.2}{\sqrt{2\pi}\sigma t} \exp\left\{-\frac{(\log t - \mu)^2}{2\sigma^2}\right\}.$$

The sojourn time in the preclinical state follows the log-logistic distribution,

$$q(x) = \frac{\kappa x^{\kappa-1}\rho^\kappa}{[1+(x\rho)^\kappa]^2}, \qquad Q(x) = \frac{1}{1+(x\rho)^\kappa} \qquad \kappa > 0, \rho > 0.$$

The sensitivity for each screening modality and the overall sensitivity were assumed to be the same across the screening period, that is, $\beta_i = \beta$, and $\beta_{i1} = \beta_1, \beta_{i2} = \beta_2$. We let r be the correlation coefficient, and since

$$\alpha_{11} = \beta_1 + \beta_2 - \beta,$$

we can write the expression (3.5) as

$$r = \frac{\beta_1 + \beta_2 - \beta - \beta_1\beta_2}{\sqrt{\beta_1\beta_2(1-\beta_1)(1-\beta_2)}}.$$

The JHLP data have annual chest X-rays and 4-monthly sputum cytology with different screening intervals. Therefore, there were two screens each year with only cytology. In other words, there was one dual-screening (X-ray and cytology) and two single-screening (cytology only) exams each year. To correct two missing x-ray screenings on cytology a year, we used the following likelihood:

$$
\begin{aligned}
&L(\theta|t_0)\\
&= \left\{ \prod_{i=1}^{K_d} D(\beta)_{i,t_0}^{s_{i,t_0}} I(\beta)_{i,t_0}^{r_{i,t_0}} [1 - D(\beta)_{i,t_0} - I(\beta)_{i,t_0}]^{n_{i,t_0} - s_{i,t_0} - r_{i,t_0}} \right.\\
&\quad \left. \times \frac{\alpha_{10}^{s_{10}^{(i,t_0)}} \alpha_{01}^{s_{01}^{(i,t_0)}} \alpha_{11}^{s_{11}^{(i,t_0)}}}{\beta^{s_{i,t_0}}} \right\}\\
&\quad \times \left\{ \prod_{j=1}^{K_s} D(\beta_2)_{j,t_0}^{s_{j,t_0}} I(\beta_2)_{j,t_0}^{r_{j,t_0}} [1 - D(\beta_2)_{j,t_0} - I(\beta_2)_{j,t_0}]^{n_{j,t_0} - s_{j,t_0} - r_{j,t_0}} \right\}
\end{aligned}
$$

where K_d is the number of dual screenings and K_s is the number of single-screenings (i.e., cytology only), with $K = K_d + K_s$. Note that the probabilities of being diagnosed and incident for the single-screenings only depend on the sensitivity of cytology; i.e., only β_2 is considered.

We used the likelihood ratio test (LRT) to test the hypothesis $H_0 : r = 0$ versus $H_1 : r \neq 0$:

$$2\left[\log L(\hat{\beta}_1, \hat{\beta}_2, \hat{r}, \hat{\mu}, \hat{\sigma}^2, \hat{\kappa}, \hat{\rho}) - \log L(\tilde{\beta}_1, \tilde{\beta}_2, \tilde{\mu}, \tilde{\sigma}^2, \tilde{\kappa}, \tilde{\rho})\right] \sim \chi_1^2.$$

The result is summarized in Table 3.4.

The estimated sensitivity of the dual screening (β) is 0.8534 and 0.8550 under H_0 and H_1, respectively. The LRT was performed, and the resulting p-value is 0.5903. Therefore, there is no strong evidence to support that the correlation coefficient is different from zero. The sensitivity is 79.93% for X-ray and 26.98% for cytology, and the overall sensitivity β is 85.34%. It seems that the dual screening improves the overall sensitivity up to about 5%.

TABLE 3.4
Parameter estimates under the two hypotheses.

Model	β_1	β_2	r	μ	σ^2	κ	ρ
H_0	0.7993	0.2698	–	3.7967	0.0417	5.2930	0.9412
H_1	0.7993	0.2739	-0.0039	3.7966	0.0414	5.2938	0.9305

Adapted from Table 1 in Kim et al 2012 [28].

3.5 Bibliographic notes

This is the first project that the author worked on back in the year 2000, and this introduced the author to the field of cancer screening. The major methodology papers are Shen et al 2001 [48] and Kim et al 2012 [28]. There is not much research in this area. One reason may be that not many screening programs use two diagnostic procedures, and data were limited as well.

4

Lead Time Distribution in Cancer Screening

CONTENTS

Lead time, the length of time that the diagnosis is advanced by screening, is an important indicator of a screening program. In this chapter, we derive the probability distribution of the lead time in periodic cancer screenings under a few different model assumptions. In general, the lead time is distributed as a mixture of a point mass at zero and a positive piecewise continuous random variable. The components of this mixture represent two aspects of screening benefits, namely, a reduction in the number of interval cases and the extent by which screening advanced the time of diagnosis. Simulations and applications provide estimates of the lead time in different situations.

DOI: 10.1201/9781003404125-4

4.1 Introduction

When evaluating the effectiveness of a screening program, one should account for the fact that the age at diagnosis is earlier if the disease is detected by screening rather than by the onset of clinical symptoms. The difference between the age of diagnosis with screening and the future onset of clinical disease without screening is called the *lead time*. Even in the absence of effective therapy, the screening will appear to lengthen the time from diagnosis until death. If one does not account for the lead time when analyzing the benefit of screening, then one's inference is subject to lead time bias (Kafadar and Prorok 1994, 1996, 2003 [22, 23, 24]).

We assume the commonly followed disease progression model as before[87], where the disease develops by progressing through three states, $S_0 \rightarrow S_p \rightarrow S_c$. These are the disease-free state S_0; the preclinical disease state S_p, in which an asymptomatic individual unknowingly has the disease that a screening exam can detect; and the clinical state S_c in which the disease manifests itself in clinical symptoms.

If a person enters the preclinical state (S_p) at age t_1 and becomes clinically incident (S_c) later at age t_2, then $(t_2 - t_1)$ is the sojourn time in the preclinical state. If this person undergoes a screening exam at a time t within the time interval (t_1, t_2) and cancer is diagnosed, then the length of time $(t_2 - t)$ is the person's lead time. This is illustrated in Figures 4.1 and 2.2.

As mentioned earlier, the rationale behind screening is that early detection and effective treatment hopefully lead to better survival. For a particular case detected by the screening exam, the lead time is, of course, unobservable. The distribution of the lead time depends on the distributions of the sojourn time, the sensitivity, and the transition probability into the preclinical state. Our model may be an aid in characterizing the effectiveness of screening programs and determining the optimal interval of future screening time.

Many researchers have proposed methods to make inferences on the lead time among participants in a screening program, whether within a randomized study or not. Prorok 1982 [42] made a major contribution by deriving the conditional probability distribution of the lead time, given someone was detected at the i-th screening exam, and this is called the *local lead time*. He

FIGURE 4.1
Illustration of disease development and the lead time.

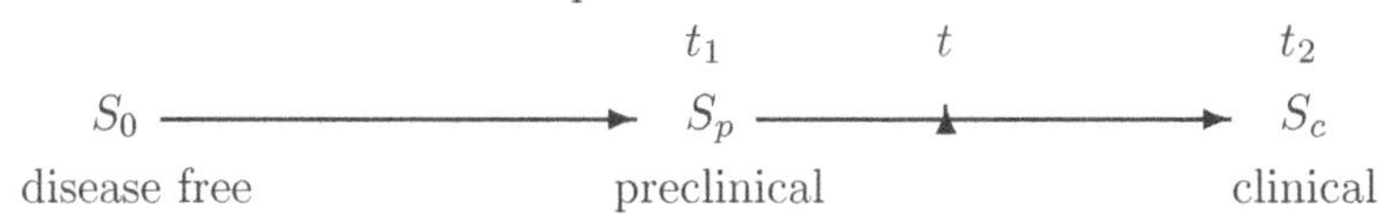

$x =$ onset of S_p, $y =$ onset of S_c.

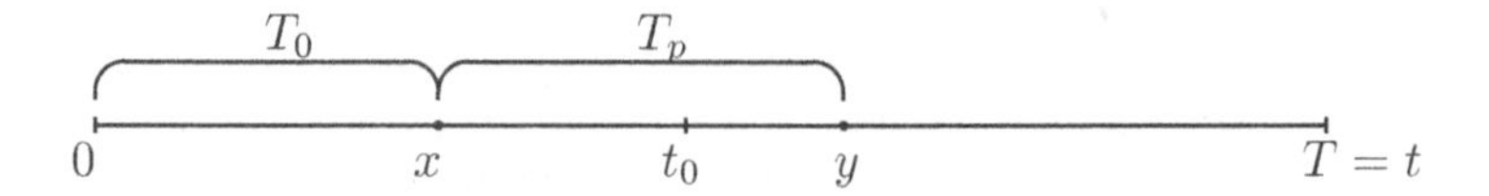

FIGURE 4.2
Illustration of the incidence time.

applied his model in simulations to study the properties of the lead time, assuming different sojourn time distributions. He noted that when one increases the number of exams, keeping the time interval between any two consecutive exams fixed, the local lead time properties appeared to stop changing after four or five screening exams in his simulation. The stabilization of the local lead time properties suggested a stopping rule for comparative studies, in that further screenings will not yield more information about the benefit of screening versus no screening. His work, however, has limited applicability. He considered only the screen-detected cases, ignoring the interval cases for whom the lead time is zero. His results apply to cases who are screen-detected at the i-th screening exam. He did not estimate the whole proportion of cases that were not detected by the periodic screening.

Straatman et al 1997 [51] estimated the mean lead time among participants in a screening program, applying ideas similar to Prorok (1982). They assumed an exponential distribution for the sojourn time in the preclinical state. Because of the memoryless nature of the exponential distribution, the lead time had the same exponential distribution as the sojourn time in their models. Walter and Day (1983) considered other distributions, such as a log-normal distribution and a step-function for the sojourn time, in addition to an exponential distribution [54]. They derived a formula to estimate the mean lead time. Other publications have estimated the mean lead time and the variance of the lead time [22, 23, 24, 86, 85] The main focus of these papers was on the screen-detected cases and on the survival benefits, rather than on the inference of the lead time.

In this chapter, we derive the probability distribution of the lead time in a few steps, beginning from the simplest and moving on to the more complicated (but close to reality) models. In section 4.2, we derive the lead time for the whole cohort, including both screen-detected cases and interval-incident cases, when one's lifetime is fixed; and we greatly simplified the deriving procedure of Prorok (1982) when one was diagnosed at the i-th exam. In section 4.3, we extend this model to the situation when one's lifetime is a random variable, where the distribution of the human lifetime is derived from the US Social

Security Administration's actuarial life table. The above two models are for participants without any screening history at their current age. In section 4.4, we extend the lead time model to the case when participants have a screening history already and plan for their future screening exams. The above models are derived when the sensitivity depends on one's age, but is independent of the sojourn time. Finally, we provide updated formulas when the sensitivity depends on the ratio of time one has stayed in the preclinical state and the sojourn time.

4.2 Lead time distribution when lifetime is fixed

Consider a cohort of initially asymptomatic individuals who enroll in a screening program. We let $\beta(t)$ be the screening sensitivity, where t is an individual's age at the exam. We let $w(t)$ be the probability density function of the time duration in the disease-free state S_0; that is, $w(t)dt$ is the probability of making a transition from S_0 to S_p in $(t, t+dt)$. We let $q(x)$ be the probability density function of the sojourn time in the preclinical state S_p, and let $Q(z) = \int_z^\infty q(x)dx$ be the survival function of the sojourn time in the S_p. Throughout this chapter, the time variable t represents a participating individual's age.

When we consider the concept of lead time, we assume that the person will develop symptomatic cancer. Therefore, the lead time distribution is, in fact, a conditional distribution, given that someone will ultimately develop the clinical disease during one's lifetime. Using breast cancer as an example, we will study the case of an initially asymptomatic woman with no history of cancer and has not taken any screening so far, who will go through a series of periodic screening exams and develops breast cancer later in her life.

We assume that a woman is asymptomatic at her age t_0 and without any screening so far. We define D as a binary random variable, with $D = 1$ indicating the development of clinical disease and $D = 0$ indicating the absence of the clinical disease before death. We let L be the lead time. The lead time is 0 for individuals whose disease is not detected by the screening, but who develops clinical symptoms between two scheduled exams. The distribution of the lead time for a woman will be a mixture of a point mass at zero (i.e., the clinical incident case between screenings) and the density of a positive piecewise continuous random variable (i.e., the screen-detected case):

$$\begin{aligned} P(L = 0|D = 1, T = t) &= \frac{P(L = 0, D = 1|T = t)}{P(D = 1|T = t)}, \\ f_L(z|D = 1, T = t) &= \frac{f_L(z, D = 1|T = t)}{P(D = 1|T = t)}, \quad z > 0. \end{aligned} \tag{4.1}$$

Where the lifetime $T = t(> t_0)$ is a fixed value in this section, and we will expand to the situation when T is a random variable in the next. We need to derive $P(D = 1|T = t)$, the probability of developing breast cancer during one's lifetime after age t_0, the joint probability $P(L = 0, D = 1|T = t)$, and the joint probability density function $f_L(z, D = 1|T = t)$ for $z > 0$.

To derive the probability of developing breast cancer $P(D = 1|T = t)$, that is, a woman will have clinical symptoms at some age $y \in (t_0, T)$, we let x be her age at the onset of the preclinical state S_p, let T_0, T_p represent the time spent in the disease-free state S_0 and the preclinical state S_p, respectively, then the PDF of the incidence at $T_c = T_0 + T_p = y$ is

$$I(y) = \int_0^y w(x)q(y - x)dx$$

See Figure 4.2.

The lifetime risk of breast cancer after age t_0 is simply an integration over all possible values of y, i.e., a clinical incidence case in (t_0, T), Hence,

$$\begin{aligned} P(D = 1|T = t) &= \int_{t_0}^t I(y)dy = \int_{t_0}^t \int_0^y w(x)q(y - x)dxdy \\ &= \int_0^{t_0} w(x)[Q(t_0 - x) - Q(t - x)]dx + \int_{t_0}^t w(x)[1 - Q(t - x)]dx, \end{aligned} \tag{4.2}$$

where $T = t$ is the fixed lifetime.

4.2.1 Lead time distribution with two exams

We use a screening program with two exams as an example to illustrate the key ideas underlying the formulation of $P(L = 0, D = 1|T = t)$ and $f_L(z, D = 1|T = t)$. We will expand to the case of any number of exams afterward.

Consider a woman who goes through two screening exams at her ages $t_0 < t_1$. Her lead time is zero, if and only if she has symptomatic cancer (i.e. in the clinical state S_c) in the intervals (t_0, t_1) or $(t_1, T = t)$. Hence,

$$P(L = 0, D = 1|T = t) = I_{2,1} + I_{2,2},$$

where $I_{2,1}$ is the probability of being an interval case in (t_0, t_1), and $I_{2,2}$ is the probability of being an interval case in $(t_1, T = t)$. The first subscription index reminds us that she has taken two exams. We define $t_{-1} = 0$.

For a woman to be a clinical incident case in (t_0, t_1), let x represent the onset age of the preclinical state S_p and t represent the onset age of the clinical state S_c and $(t - x)$ is the sojourn time. See Figure 4.3.

If she is an incident case in (t_0, t_1), then there are only two possibilities: either she enters the preclinical state at $x \in (0, t_0)$, her cancer was not detected

x = onset of S_p, y = onset of S_c

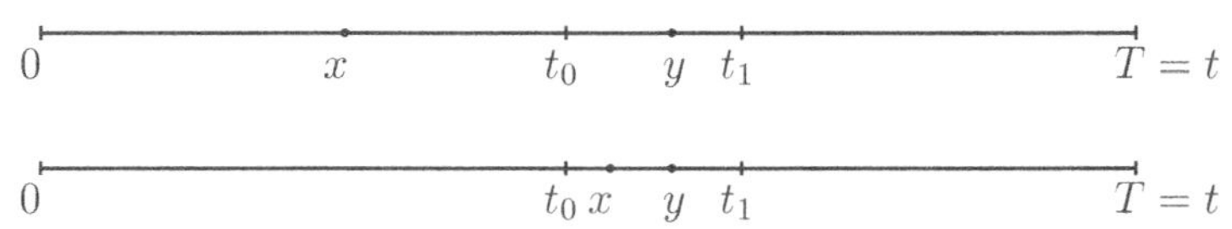

FIGURE 4.3
Calculation of probability of incidence in (t_0, t_1).

at t_0, and her sojourn time is between $(t_0 - x, t_1 - x)$; or she enters the preclinical state at $x \in (t_0, t_1)$, and her sojourn time is less than $t_1 - x$. These two events are mutually exclusive, hence the probability is

$$
\begin{aligned}
I_{2,1} &= (1-\beta_0)\int_{t_0}^{t_1}\int_0^{t_0} w(x)q(y-x)dxdy + \int_{t_0}^{t_1}\int_{t_0}^{y} w(x)q(y-x)dxdy \\
&= (1-\beta_0)\int_0^{t_0} w(x)\{Q(t_0-x) - Q(t_1-x)\}dx \\
&\quad + \int_{t_0}^{t_1} w(x)\{1 - Q(t_1-x)\}dx,
\end{aligned}
$$

where $\beta_i = \beta(t_i)$ is the sensitivity at age t_i.

Similarly, to calculate $I_{2,2}$, the probability of incidence in $(t_1, T = t)$, there are three mutually exclusive events: (i) she enters the preclinical state in $(0, t_0)$, her cancer was missed at t_0, t_1; or (ii) she enters the preclinical state in (t_0, t_1), her cancer was missed at t_1; or (iii) she enters the preclinical state in $(t_1, T = t)$. See Figure 4.4. Therefore,

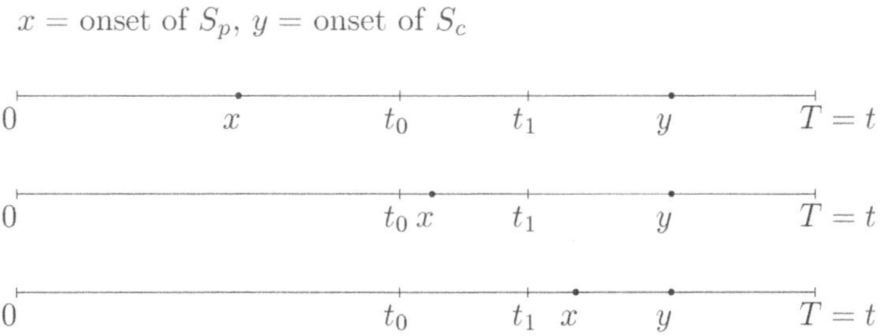

x = onset of S_p, y = onset of S_c

0 x t_0 t_1 y $T = t$

0 t_0 x t_1 y $T = t$

0 t_0 t_1 x y $T = t$

FIGURE 4.4
Calculation of probability of incidence in $(t_1, T = t)$.

$$
\begin{aligned}
I_{2,2} &= (1-\beta_0)(1-\beta_1)\int_{t_1}^{t}\int_{0}^{t_0} w(x)q(y-x)dxdy \\
&\quad +(1-\beta_1)\int_{t_1}^{t}\int_{t_0}^{t_1} w(x)q(y-x)dxdy + \int_{t_1}^{t}\int_{t_1}^{y} w(x)q(y-x)dxdy \\
&= (1-\beta_0)(1-\beta_1)\int_{0}^{t_0} w(x)\{Q(t_1-x)-Q(t-x)\}dx \\
&\quad +(1-\beta_1)\int_{t_0}^{t_1} w(x)\{Q(t_1-x)-Q(t-x)\}dx \\
&\quad +\int_{t_1}^{t} w(x)\{1-Q(t-x)\}dx.
\end{aligned}
$$

The lead time will be greater than zero for the screen-detected cases. These are the people who might benefit from the periodic screening exams, since their diseases are diagnosed at an early stage, and if effective treatments exist, they could have a better choice of treatment and live longer. To derive the probability density function $f_L(z, D=1|T=t)$, we need to decide the domain of the lead time z. Since the lifetime is assumed to be a fixed value, the lead time cannot be longer than $(T-t_0)$. That is, the domain of lead time should be $(0, T-t_0]$. We partition the domain into two parts: $(0, T-t_1]$ and $(T-t_1, T-t_0]$.

When the lead time $z \in (0, T-t_1]$, there are two possibilities: this person was diagnosed either at t_0 or at t_1. In both cases, she would have entered the clinical state S_c at age $t_c = t_i + z, i = 0, 1$ if she were not screened at t_i. See Figure 4.5, where x is the onset of the S_p, and t_c indicates the onset of S_c if no screening. Therefore, the density is

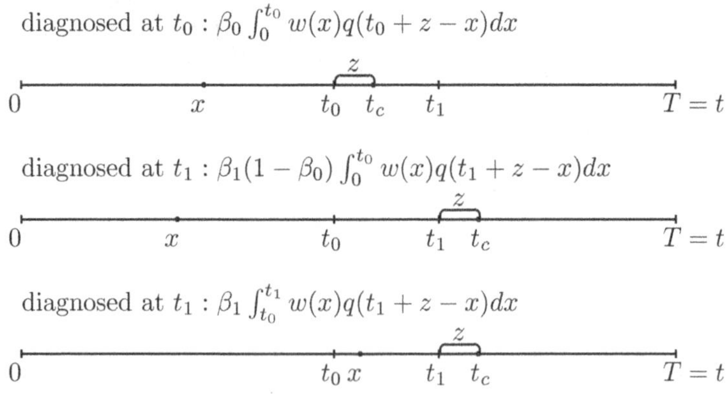

diagnosed at t_0 : $\beta_0 \int_0^{t_0} w(x)q(t_0+z-x)dx$

0 x t_0 t_c t_1 $T=t$ (z between t_0 and t_c)

diagnosed at t_1 : $\beta_1(1-\beta_0)\int_0^{t_0} w(x)q(t_1+z-x)dx$

0 x t_0 t_1 t_c $T=t$ (z between t_1 and t_c)

diagnosed at t_1 : $\beta_1 \int_{t_0}^{t_1} w(x)q(t_1+z-x)dx$

0 t_0 x t_1 t_c $T=t$ (z between t_1 and t_c)

FIGURE 4.5
The joint PDF $f_L(z, D=1|T=t)$ when $K=2$.

$$
\begin{aligned}
& f_L(z, D=1|T=t) \\
= \;& P(\text{detected at } t_0 \text{ and would incident at } t_0+z \text{ if not screened}) \\
& +P(\text{detected at } t_1 \text{ and would incident at } t_1+z \text{ if not screened}) \\
= \;& \beta_0 \int_0^{t_0} w(x)q(t_0+z-x)dx + \beta_1(1-\beta_0)\int_0^{t_0} w(x)q(t_1+z-x)dx \\
& +\beta_1 \int_{t_0}^{t_1} w(x)q(t_1+z-x)dx, \qquad \text{for } z \in (0, t-t_1].
\end{aligned}
$$

When the lead time $z \in (T-t_1, T-t_0]$, that is, her lead time is longer than $(T-t_1)$, there is only one possibility: she must have been detected at t_0 since her lifetime is bounded by T. Therefore,

$$
f_L(z, D=1|T=t) = \beta_0 \int_0^{t_0} w(x)q(t_0+z-x)dx, \qquad \text{for } z \in (t-t_1, t-t_0]
$$

Combining the above results and plugging into equation (4.1), the distribution for the lead time has been derived.

Exercise 4.1. Prove that

$$
P(L=0|D=1, T=t) + \int_0^{T-t_0} f_L(z|D=1, T=t)dz = 1.
$$

Hence, the mixture distribution is a valid PDF.

4.2.2 Lead time distribution with any number of exams

We generalize the result to any number of screening exams when lifetime T is fixed. Assume a woman will take K ordered screening exams that occur at her age $t_0 < t_1 < \cdots < t_{K-1}$. We call her i-th generation if she enters S_p between t_{i-1} and t_i, $i = 1, 2, \ldots, K-1$. We call her 0-th generation if she enters S_p before her first exam at t_0. We define $t_{-1} \equiv 0$, and let $t_K = T$.

The distribution of the lead time is a mixture of a point mass at zero and a positive continuous random variable, which is defined in equations (4.1). The denominator $P(D=1|T=t)$ is the same as in equation (4.2), we only need to calculate the joint probability $P(L=0, D=1|T=t)$ and the joint probability density function $f_L(z, D=1|T=t)$.

The lead time is zero if and only if an individual is an interval case. Let $I_{K,i}$ denote the probability of being an interval case in the i-th screening interval (t_{i-1}, t_i) in a sequence of K screening exams. Then

$$
P(L=0, D=1|T=t) = I_{K,1} + I_{K,2} + \cdots + I_{K,K}, \tag{4.3}
$$

where

$$\begin{aligned} I_{K,j} &= \sum_{i=0}^{j-1}(1-\beta_i)\cdots(1-\beta_{j-1})\int_{t_{i-1}}^{t_i} w(x)[Q(t_{j-1}-x)-Q(t_j-x)]dx \\ &+ \int_{t_{j-1}}^{t_j} w(x)[1-Q(t_j-x)]dx, \qquad \text{for } j=1,\cdots,K. \end{aligned} \tag{4.4}$$

It can be proved by mathematical induction that, if the sensitivity is less than 1, then for any fixed sequence $t_0 < t_1 < \cdots < t_{K-1} < T$,

$$I_{1,1} \geq (I_{2,1} + I_{2,2}) \geq \cdots \geq (I_{K,1} + \cdots + I_{K,K}). \tag{4.5}$$

In other words, more screening reduces the probability of interval cases (i.e., the case whose lead time equals zero) among women who would develop cancer in their lifetime.

When the lead time is greater than zero, we derive the joint probability density function $f_L(z, D = 1|T = t)$, where $z \in (0, t - t_0]$. We denote $T = t = t_K$. When $t - t_1 < z \leq t - t_0$, detection can only occur at t_0. In general, when $t - t_j < z \leq t - t_{j-1}, j = 2, 3, \cdots, K$, one could be screen-detected at $t_i, i = 0, \cdots, j - 1$. Thus, when $t - t_j < z \leq t - t_{j-1}, j = 2, 3, \cdots, K$ (i.e., $t_c = t_i + z < T = t, i = 0, \cdots, j - 1$),

$$\begin{aligned} &f_L(z, D=1|T=t) \\ &= \sum_{i=1}^{j-1}\beta_i\left\{\sum_{r=0}^{i-1}(1-\beta_r)\cdots(1-\beta_{i-1})\int_{t_{r-1}}^{t_r} w(x)q(t_i+z-x)dx\right. \\ &\left.+\int_{t_{i-1}}^{t_i} w(x)q(t_i+z-x)dx\right\} + \beta_0\int_0^{t_0} w(x)q(t_0+z-x)dx. \end{aligned} \tag{4.6}$$

When $j = 1$ and $t - t_1 < z \leq t - t_0$ (i.e., one must have been detected at t_0), the above formula becomes

$$f_L(z, D=1|T=t) = \beta_0\int_0^{t_0} w(x)q(t_0+z-x)dx. \tag{4.7}$$

Exercise 4.2. Prove that for any screening sequence $t_0 < t_1 < \cdots < t_{K-1}$, if the lifetime $T = t > t_{K-1}$, then

$$P(L=0, D=1|T=t) + \int_0^{t-t_0} f_L(z, D=1|T=t)dz = P(D=1|T=t).$$

Hence,

$$Pr(L=0|D=1, T=t) + \int_0^{T-t_0} f_L(z|D=1, T=t)dz = 1.$$

Therefore, the mixture distribution of the lead time is a valid PDF.

The probability density function of the lead time is not continuous at the points $(T - t_j), j = 1, \cdots, K - 1$, which can be easily verified from equations (4.6) and (4.7).

4.2.3 Lead time distribution at the j-th exam

Prorok (1982) derived the lead time distribution if one was diagnosed at the j-th screening exam. The derivation used properties of the forward and backward recurrence times from the renewal process theory, and the procedure was lengthy. We obtain the same result as in Prorok (1982) by conditioning on detection at the j-th screening exam, with a simplified procedure.

Assume there are K screening exams and define events

$$A_j = \{\text{one is diagnosed at the } (j{+}1)\text{-th exam at her age } t_j\},\ j = 0, \cdots, K{-}1.$$

The (conditional) probability density function for the lead time given A_j is

$$f_L(z|A_j) = \frac{f_L(z, A_j)}{P(A_j)}, \quad z > 0. \tag{4.8}$$

The denominator is the probability of being detected at t_j, and we have derived the general formula in equation (2.13) of Chapter 2, we only need to change the index by letting $k = j + 1$, i.e., $P(A_j)$ is the D_{j+1,t_0} in equation (2.13):

$$\begin{aligned} P(A_j) = \beta_j \Bigg\{ &\sum_{i=0}^{j-1} (1-\beta_i)\cdots(1-\beta_{j-1}) \int_{t_{i-1}}^{t_i} w(x)Q(t_j - x)dx \\ &+ \int_{t_{j-1}}^{t_j} w(x)Q(t_j - x)dx \Bigg\}. \end{aligned} \tag{4.9}$$

For the numerator, there are $(j + 1)$ mutually exclusive events: (i) she enters the preclinical state at age $x \in (t_{i-1}, t_i), i = 0, 1, \ldots, j-1$, her sojourn time is $(t_j{+}z{-}x)$ and her cancer was not diagnosed in the previous exams except at t_j, these are j cases; and (ii) she enters the preclinical state at age $x \in (t_{j-1}, t_j)$, and her cancer was diagnosed at t_j. We just add up all these probabilities:

$$\begin{aligned} f_L(z, A_j) &= \sum_{i=0}^{j} f_L(z, A_j, \text{she enters } S_p \text{ in } (t_{i-1}, t_i)\ ) \\ &= \beta_j \Bigg\{ \sum_{i=0}^{j-1} (1-\beta_i)\cdots(1-\beta_{j-1}) \int_{t_{i-1}}^{t_i} w(x)q(t_j + z - x)dx \\ &\quad + \int_{t_{j-1}}^{t_j} w(x)q(t_j + z - x)dx \Bigg\}. \end{aligned} \tag{4.10}$$

This is exactly the same result as in formula (2) in Prorok 1982 (which he called the *local lead time* PDF). Our procedure is much simple without using the forward and backward recurrence times.

Exercise 4.3. Prove that

$$\int_0^{\infty} f_L(z, A_j)dz = P(A_j).$$

Therefore,

$$\int_0^\infty f_L(z|A_j)dz = 1.$$

which means that $f_L(z|A_j)$ is a valid PDF.

4.2.4 Application: The HIP for breast cancer

The lead time distribution depends on the sensitivity $\beta(t)$, the transition probability $w(t)$, and the sojourn time distribution $q(x)$. Hence, an accurate estimation of these parameters is essential in the estimation of the lead time.

We applied our method to the Health Insurance Plan of Greater New York (HIP) data (Shapiro et al 1988 [47]). Wu, Rosner, and Broemeling 2005 estimated the age-dependent sensitivity $\beta(t)$, the transition density $w(t)$, and the sojourn time distribution $q(x)$ using the HIP data [79]. The unknown parameters were $\theta = (b_0, b_1, \mu, \sigma^2, \kappa, \rho)$. We used Markov Chain Monte Carlo (MCMC) to draw posterior samples from the posterior $f(\theta|HIP)$. The posterior sample size was 2000 from two parallel chains with over-dispersed initial values [79], see section 2.4.3 for details.

Given the HIP data, the posterior predictive distribution of the lead time can be estimated as

$$\begin{aligned} f(L|HIP) &= \int f(L, \theta|HIP)d\theta = \int f(L|\theta, HIP)f(\theta|HIP)d\theta \\ &= \int f(L|\theta)f(\theta|HIP)d\theta \approx \frac{1}{n}\sum_i f(L|\theta_i^*), \end{aligned} \tag{4.11}$$

where θ_i^* is a posterior sample drawn from the posterior distribution $f(\theta|HIP)$, and the last step is Monte Carlo integration.

Table 4.1 summarizes the Bayesian posterior inference of the lead time when human life is fixed at 80 years old [80]. The screening time interval Δ was 6, 9, 12, 18, and 24 months from age $t_0 = 50$ to $T = 80$. The density curves of the lead time for different screening intervals are shown in Figure 4.6. The mode, the mean, and the standard deviation (SD) in the table are for the mixture distribution.

From these results, we see that if a woman begins annual screening (i.e., $\Delta = 12$ months) when she is 50 years old and continues until she reaches 80, then there is a 23.37% chance that she will be an interval incident case, and not benefit from early detection by the screening program if she develops breast cancer during those 30 years. Her chance of no benefit from the screening program decreases to 8.95% if the exams are 6 months apart.

Table 4.1 shows that the mean lead time increases as the screening time interval decreases. In other words, more screening exams will contribute to a longer lead time, which would translate to treatment of the disease at an earlier stage and, potentially improved prognosis. The increase in the mean

TABLE 4.1
Application for the HIP data using Bayesian posterior samples.

Δ	^aK	$^bP_0$	$1-P_0$	Mode	^{c}Mean	SD
6 mo.	60	8.95	91.05	0.50	1.418	2.111
9 mo.	40	16.04	83.96	0.38	1.282	2.075
12 mo.	30	23.37	76.63	0.30	1.168	2.040
18 mo.	20	36.52	63.48	0.16	0.988	1.969
24 mo.	15	46.68	53.32	0.08	0.856	1.901

[a]Total number of screening from 50 to 80.
[b]$P_0 = P(L = 0|D = 1)$ is the probability that the lead time is zero, Both columns 3 and 4 are in percentages.
[c]The mode, the mean, and the standard deviation (SD) in the table are for the mixture distribution, in years.
Adapted from Table 1 in Wu et al 2007 [80].

lead time is partly due to the smaller point mass for zero lead time when screening exams are closer together.

The standard error of the lead time decreases as the time between screening exams increases. Table 4.1 also reveals that the standard deviation for the program's lead time is larger than the mean lead time. In the table, the largest mode is 0.5 years (6 months), corresponding to screening exams every 6 months. With annual exams, the mode value for the lead time is 0.3 years (3.6 months). The change of the mode is shown clearly in Figure 4.6.

4.2.5 Application: The Minnesota Colorectal Cancer study

We applied the method to the Minnesota colorectal data. Wu, Erwin, and Rosner 2009a estimated the age-dependent sensitivity $\beta(t)$, the age-dependent transition probability $w(t)$ and the sojourn time distribution $q(x)$ from the MCCCS study group from a Bayesian approach [65]. The parametric models for $\beta(t), w(t)$ and $q(x)$ has six unknown parameters, that is, $\theta = (b_0, b_1, \mu, \sigma^2, \kappa, \rho)$. We used the Markov Chain Monte Carlo simulations to obtain 1000 posterior samples for θ. See section 2.4.4 for details.

Given the Minnesota study group data, the posterior predictive distribution of the lead time z can be estimated by

$$f_L(z|MCCCS) \approx \frac{1}{n} \sum_i f_L(z|\theta_i^*)$$

where $\theta_i^*, i = 1, \ldots, 1000$ are the Bayesian posterior samples.

We applied the method to make predictive inferences in the case of a program consisting of periodic fecal occult blood tests for males and females aged 50 to 80 years. We estimated what the results would be if people were

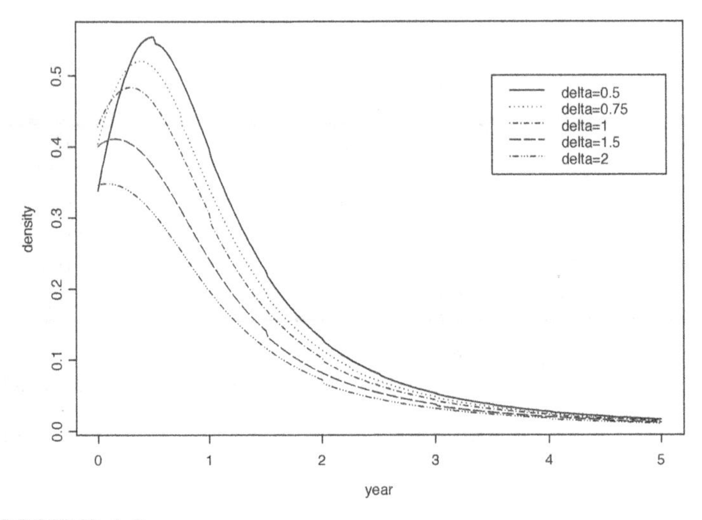

FIGURE 4.6
The lead time density using the HIP posterior samples. Adapted from Figure 3 in Wu et al 2007 [80].

screened at different screening intervals. The results are summarized in Table 4.2. The time interval between screens was 6, 9, 12, 18, and 24 months, between ages 50 (t_0) and 80 years (T). The density curves for the lead time are shown in Figure 4.7 for different screening intervals for both males and females. From these results, we see that if a man begins annual screening when he is 50 years old and continues until he reaches 80, then there is an 18.87% chance that he will not benefit from early detection by the screening program if he develops colorectal cancer during those 30 years. His chance of no benefit from the screening program decreases to 6.45% if the exams are 6 months apart. While for the females, the chance of no early detection is 9.48% for annual test and 2.39% for 6-month test.

Table 4.2 shows that the mean lead time increases as the screening time interval decreases for both genders. In other words, more screening exams will contribute to a longer lead time, which would translate to treatment of the disease at an earlier stage and potentially improved prognosis. The increase in the mean lead time is partly due to the smaller point mass for zero lead time when screening exams are closer together. The standard error of the lead time decreases as the time between screening exams increases. Table 4.2 also reveals that the standard deviation for the program's lead time is larger than the mean lead time. The mode of the lead time, which is the value that is most likely taken by the lead time when it is positive, is 0.68 years (or 8 months), corresponding to screening exams every 6 months for males, and 0.96 years (or 11.5 months) for females. With annual exams, the mode value for the lead

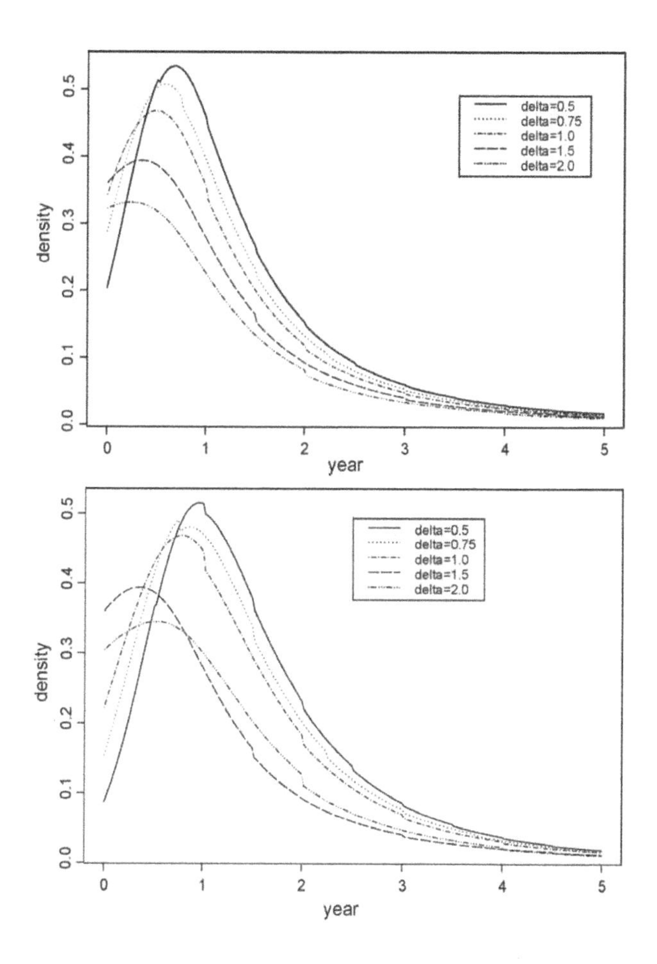

FIGURE 4.7
The lead time density using the Minnesota posterior samples, the top panel is the males. Adapted from Figures 2 and 3 in Wu et al 2009b [66].

time is 0.6 years (6 months) for males and 0.78 years (9.4 months) for females. The density curve of the lead time when it is positive is plotted in Figure 4.7.

4.3 Lead time distribution when lifetime is random

We extend the model to the case when human lifetime T is a random variable. For an asymptomatic individual currently at age t_0, we don't know the lifetime in the future, so it is more realistic to assume that the lifetime is random.

TABLE 4.2
Lead time estimation for males and females using the Minnesota study data.

Δ	Males			Females		
	$^aP_0$	Mode	^{b}Mean(s.d.)	P_0	Mode	^{c}Mean(s.d.)
6 mo.	6.45	0.68	1.640 (2.408)	2.39	0.96	1.699 (1.690)
9 mo.	12.22	0.58	1.474 (2.331)	5.31	0.86	1.552 (1.665)
12 mo.	18.87	0.50	1.333 (2.265)	9.48	0.78	1.419 (1.643)
18 mo.	32.15	0.34	1.111 (2.151)	20.33	0.64	1.192 (1.599)
24 mo.	43.11	0.24	0.949 (2.051)	31.51	0.52	1.015 (1.550)

[a] $P_0 = P(L = 0|D = 1)$ is the probability that the lead time is zero, in percentages.
[b] The mode, the mean, and the standard deviation (s.d.) in the table are in years.
Adapted from Table 2 in Wu et al 2009b [66].

4.3.1 Probability formulae

For an initially asymptomatic individual currently at age t_0, assume there will be K screening exams in her lifetime, occurring at her ages $t_0 < t_1 < \cdots < t_{K-1}$, and her lifetime T is random, with a probability density function $f_T(t)$. The conditional distribution of the lead time, given that one's lifetime $T = t (> t_{K-1})$, would be

$$\begin{aligned} P(L = 0|D = 1, T = t) &= \frac{P(L = 0, D = 1|T = t)}{P(D = 1|T = t)}, \\ f_L(z|D = 1, T = t) &= \frac{f_L(z, D = 1|T = t)}{P(D = 1|T = t)}, \quad z > 0, \end{aligned}$$

where $P(D = 1|T = t)$ was given in equation (4.2), $P(L = 0, D = 1|T = t)$ was given in (4.3) and (4.4), and $f_L(z, D = 1|T = t)$ was given in (4.6) and (4.7).

For an individual at her current age t_0, since the duration of her life is a random variable, her number of screenings in the future would be random. However, if she has a pre-planned screening schedule (e.g., if she plans to take the screening exam every 12 months, 18 months, etc.), then the distribution of the lead time when lifetime T is larger than t_0 can be obtained by

$$\begin{aligned} P(L = 0|D = 1, T > t_0) &= \int_{t_0}^{\infty} P(L = 0|D = 1, T = t) f_T(t|T > t_0) dt, \\ f_L(z|D = 1, T > t_0) &= \int_{t_0+z}^{\infty} f_L(z|D = 1, T = t) f_T(t|T > t_0) dt, z > 0. \end{aligned} \tag{4.12}$$

Where the conditional PDF of the lifetime $f_T(t|T \geq t_0)$ is

$$f_T(t|T > t_0) = \begin{cases} \frac{f_T(t)}{P(T>t_0)} = \frac{f_T(t)}{1-F_T(t_0)}, & \text{if } t > t_0; \\ 0, & \text{otherwise.} \end{cases} \tag{4.13}$$

The lower bound for the integration in (4.12) should be $t_0 + z$ instead of t_0 because z is always less than $(t - t_0)$ for any fixed lifetime t; hence, t should be larger than $t_0 + z$. We can prove that this is a valid mixed probability distribution, because

$$\begin{aligned} & P(L = 0|D = 1, T \geq t_0) + \int_0^\infty f_L(z|D = 1, T \geq t_0)dz \\ = & \int_{t_0}^\infty P(L = 0|D = 1, T = t) f_T(t|T \geq t_0)dt \\ & + \int_0^\infty \int_{t_0+z}^\infty f_L(z|D = 1, T = t) f_T(t|T \geq t_0)dtdz \\ = & \int_{t_0}^\infty P(L = 0|D = 1, T = t) f_T(t|T \geq t_0)dt \\ & + \int_{t_0}^\infty \int_0^{t-t_0} f_L(z|D = 1, T = t) f_T(t|T \geq t_0)dzdt \\ = & \int_{t_0}^\infty f_T(t|T \geq t_0)dt = 1. \end{aligned}$$

The number of screening $K = K(T) = \lceil (T - t_0)/\Delta \rceil$, is the largest integer that is smaller than or equal to $(T - t_0)/\Delta$, where Δ is the pre-planned screening interval in the future. In fact, for any future screening schedule, such as $t_0 < t_1 < \ldots$, the screening number $K = n$ if $t_{n-1} < T \leq t_n$. Hence, K is a random variable as well, taking integer values and is changing with one's lifetime T in the equations (4.12).

4.3.2 The conditional lifetime distribution

We used the actuarial life table from the US Social Security Administration (SSA) to obtain information on the lifetime distribution $f_T(t|T \geq t_0)$. This life table is published at `http://ssa.gov/OACT/STATS/table4c6.html` and it is updated every 6 months, in April and November every year, although the changes are negligible. It is based on information from all Social Security area populations, including all 50 states, DC, and surrounding islands of the United States. Due to the SSA's calculation method, there is a time lag of 4 years in the life table, The period life table is based on population mortality, it provides the conditional probability of death within 1 year from age 0 to age 119, that is, $P(T < n+1|T \geq n), n = 0, 1, 2, \ldots, 119$. We used the version that was published by the SSA in April 2010 when we first derived the method in this section.

We let $b_n = P(T < n+1|T \geq n)$, which is given in the life table. We let $a_n = P(T \geq n+1|T \geq n) = 1 - b_n$. Using the conditional probability formula,

$$\begin{aligned} P(T \geq n+2|T \geq n) &= P(T \geq n+2, T \geq n+1|T \geq n) \\ &= P(T \geq n+1|T \geq n)P(T \geq n+2|T \geq n+1, T \geq n) \\ &= a_n a_{n+1} \end{aligned} \tag{4.14}$$

By mathematical induction, for any integer age t_0,

$$\begin{aligned} P(T \geq t_0+n|T \geq t_0) &= \prod_{i=1}^{n} P(T \geq t_0+i|T \geq t_0+i-1) \\ &= \prod_{i=1}^{n} a_{t_0+i-1}, \quad \forall n = 1, 2, \ldots, (120-t_0). \end{aligned} \tag{4.15}$$

Using approximation, we have

$$\begin{aligned} f_T(t_0+n|T \geq t_0) &= \lim_{\epsilon \to 0} \frac{P(t_0+n \leq T < t_0+n+\epsilon|T \geq t_0)}{\epsilon} \\ &\approx P(t_0+n \leq T < t_0+n+1|T \geq t_0) \\ &= P(T \geq t_0+n|T \geq t_0) - P(T \geq t_0+n+1|T \geq t_0) \\ &= (1-a_{t_0+n}) \prod_{i=1}^{n} a_{t_0+i-1}, \quad \forall n = 1, 2, \ldots, (120-t_0). \end{aligned} \tag{4.16}$$

A special case is when $n = 0$: since $P(T \geq t_0|T \geq t_0) = 1$, we obtain

$$\begin{aligned} f_T(t_0|T \geq t_0) &= \lim_{\epsilon \to 0} \frac{P(t_0 \leq T < t_0+\epsilon|T \geq t_0)}{\epsilon} \\ &\approx P(t_0 \leq T < t_0+1|T \geq t_0) \\ &= P(T \geq t_0|T \geq t_0) - P(T \geq t_0+1|T \geq t_0) = 1 - a_{t_0}. \end{aligned} \tag{4.17}$$

Finally, for any real value $t \in (n, n+1)$, where $n = t_0, t_0+1, \ldots, 119$, we use a step function to approximate: $f_T(t|T \geq t_0) \approx f_T(n|T \geq t_0)$. We note that this approximation is a valid PDF, as

$$\begin{aligned} \int_{t_0}^{\infty} f_T(t|T \geq t_0)dt &= \sum_{n=0}^{120-t_0} f_T(t_0+n|T \geq t_0) \\ &= \sum_{n=0}^{120-t_0} [P(T \geq t_0+n|T \geq t_0) - P(T \geq t_0+n+1|T \geq t_0)] \\ &= P(T \geq t_0|T \geq t_0) = 1. \end{aligned}$$

The conditional PDF of the lifetime T for females is plotted in Figure 4.8 at three different initial ages $t_0 = 40, 50, 60$.

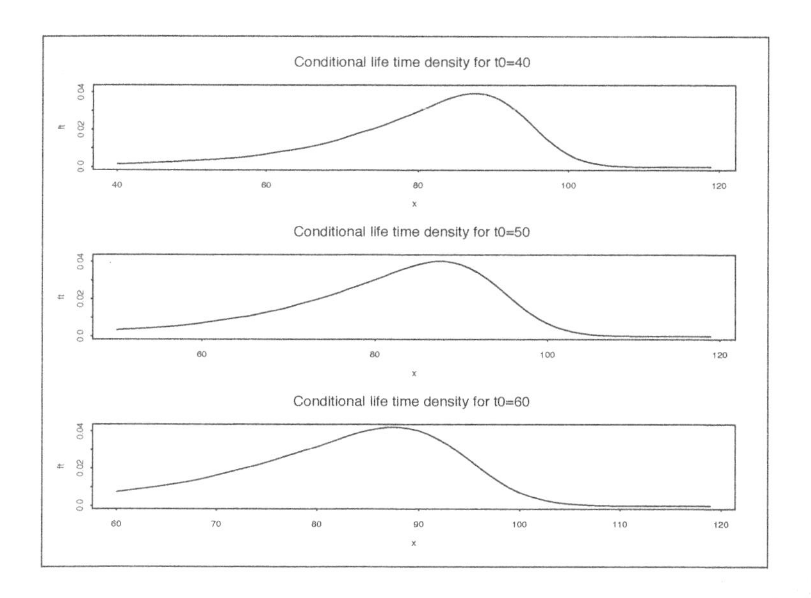

FIGURE 4.8
The PDF of female lifetime derived from the life table when $t_0 = 40$, 50, and 60. Adapted from Figure 1 in Wu et al 2012 [72].

4.3.3 Application: The HIP for breast cancer

The lead time distribution is a function of the sensitivity $\beta(t)$, the transition probability density $w(t)$, the sojourn time distribution $q(x)$, a person's current age t_0, and future screening frequency or schedule. Thus inference on the lead time distribution requires estimates of $\beta(t), w(t)$ and $q(x)$, which are available from the HIP study using likelihoods and Bayesian inference (Wu et al 2005).

We use the 2000 Bayesian posterior samples θ_i^* in the inference for the lead time [72]. The posterior predictive distribution of the lead time is

$$\begin{aligned} f_L(l|HIP) &= \int f_L(l, \theta|HIP)d\theta \\ &= \int f_L(l|\theta)f(\theta|HIP)d\theta \approx \frac{1}{n}\sum_{i=1}^{n} f_L(l|\theta_i^*), \end{aligned} \tag{4.18}$$

where θ_i^* is the posterior sample ($i = 1, \cdots, 2000$) and $f_L(l|\theta_i^*)$ is the mixture distribution defined by Equations (4.12).

Three hypothetical cohorts of initially asymptomatic women, with initial screening age $t_0 = 40$, 50, and 60 are assumed in the simulation. For each cohort, we examined four screening intervals Δ =12, 18, 24, and 30 months. The number of screenings $K = \lceil (T - t_0)/\Delta \rceil$ is a function of the lifetime T; therefore, it is a random variable in the simulation. From Equation (4.18),

TABLE 4.3
Projected lead time distribution using posterior samples from the HIP data.

Δ	$^aP_0(C.I.)$	1-P_0 (s.e.)	^bEL (s.e.)	$^cMed/IQR$
		Age at initial screen $t_0 = 40$		
12 mo.	26.29 (16.48, 39.68)	73.71 (5.99)	1.04(1.69)	0.71
18 mo.	39.25 (27.10, 50.72)	60.75 (5.96)	0.87(1.63)	0.61
24 mo.	49.04 (36.19, 59.00)	50.96 (5.95)	0.75(1.58)	0.61
30 mo.	56.34 (42.66, 65.99)	43.66 (5.87)	0.66(1.52)	0.57
		Age at initial screen $t_0 = 50$		
12 mo.	23.76 (12.39, 41.42)	76.24 (7.07)	1.07(1.70)	0.71
18 mo.	36.51 (22.19, 52.25)	63.49 (7.35)	0.91(1.65)	0.61
24 mo.	46.32 (29.37, 59.98)	53.68 (7.35)	0.79(1.60)	0.61
30 mo.	53.71 (35.75, 65.76)	46.29 (7.18)	0.70(1.55)	0.57
		Age at initial screen $t_0 = 60$		
12 mo.	21.98 (8.22, 45.49)	78.02 (8.47)	1.08(1.68)	0.65
18 mo.	34.28 (16.78, 55.15)	65.72 (9.06)	0.92(1.63)	0.65
24 mo.	43.91 (22.88, 61.45)	56.09 (9.08)	0.81(1.59)	0.61
30 mo.	51.21 (29.42, 66.50)	48.79 (8.84)	0.72(1.55)	0.61

$^aP_0 = P(L = 0|D = 1)$. Columns 2 and 3 are in percentages.
^{b}the mean and the standard deviation(S.E.) of the mixture distribution in column 4 are in years.
^{c}the median over the inter-quartile range (IQR) when the lead time is greater than zero.
Adapted from Table 1 in Wu et al 2012 [72].

the distribution of the lead time is simply a weighted average of the different lengths of lifetimes.

Table 4.3 summarizes the inference for the lead time. The probability that the lead time is zero (with the corresponding 95% C.I.), the probability that the lead time is positive, and the corresponding standard errors are reported as percentages The mean lead time and its standard error were reported in years. Since the lead time distribution is very skewed, we also report the ratio of the median and the IQR as more sensible summaries of location and spread. The median of the lead time (when it is positive) is about 0.85 years for all 12 situations; the first quartile of the lead time ranges from 0.35 to 0.45 years, and the third quartile ranges from 1.65 to 1.85 years. The density curves for the lead time are shown in Figure 4.9 for different screening intervals when $t_0 = 50$, as the density curves when the t_0 is 40 or 60 are similar.

The results suggest that a woman who begins annual screening (i.e., $\Delta = 12$ months) when she is 50 years old and develops breast cancer in her life would have a 23.76% chance that her cancer would not be detected by the scheduled exams. The probability of no early detection from the screening

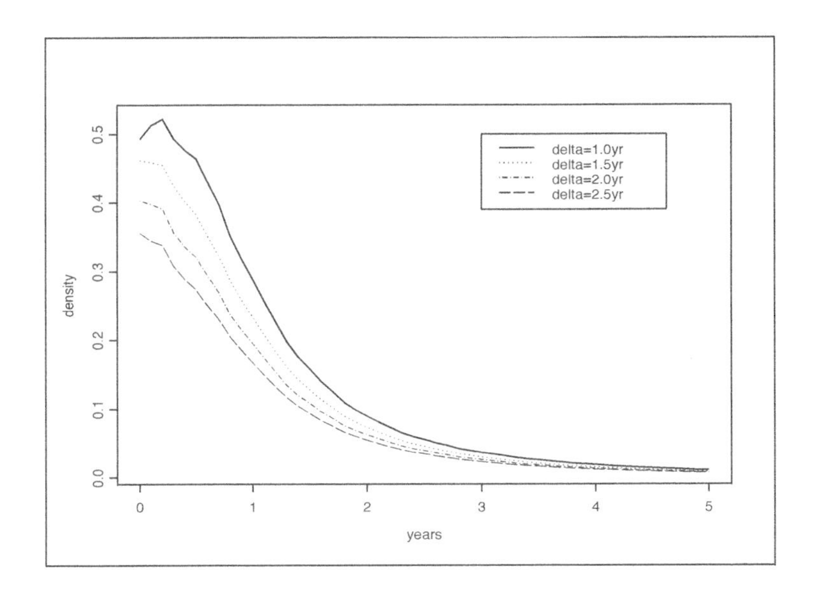

FIGURE 4.9
The lead time density using the HIP when the lifetime is random. Adapted from Figure 2 in Wu et al 2012 [72].

program increases to 46.32% if the exams are biennial. For a woman with initial screening age of 40 (respectively, 60), the probability of no early detection with annual screens will be 26.29% (respectively 21.98% for age 60). The probability of no early detection is monotonically increasing when the screening interval increases within the same age group. This probability is monotonically decreasing as the initial age increases for the same screening interval. We also reported the 95% credible intervals for the probability of "no early detection" in this table. The difference between the initial age of 50 and 60 is smaller than the corresponding difference between the initial age of 40 and 50 groups.

The mean lead time decreases as the screening time interval increases in Table 4.3; i.e., more frequent screening exams result in longer lead times. The increase in the mean lead time is due partly to the smaller point mass at zero lead time when screening exams are closer together. The standard deviation of the lead time decreases as the time between screening exams increases. Table 4.3 also reveals that the standard deviation for the lead time is larger than the mean lead time due to the skewed distribution. Hence, we evaluated the ratio of median/IQR. This ratio decreases as the screening interval increases, and lies between 0.57 and 0.71 for different cases in Table 4.3.

The mode of the lead time is less than 0.1 year (or 1 month) when the screening interval is 2 or 2.5 years for all three groups; when the screening interval is 1.5 years, the mode is slightly above 0.1 years (or 1.2 months) for all three age groups; when the screening interval is 1 year, the mode is around 0.24 years (or 2.8 months) for all three age groups.

We ran another simulation according to the recommendation of the US Preventive Services Task Force, that is, biennial screening for women aged 50 to 74. The result does not bode well for screening. The probability of no-early-detection (the interval case) is 56.36% (standard error $\approx$ 5.24%), or effectively about 50-50 odds. In another simulation with annual screening from ages 50 to 60, followed by biennial screening from 60 to 80 (and no further screens), the probability of zero lead time is 42.93%; it is very similar to the case of starting age at 50 or 60 in Table 4.3, with biennial screenings. This may be due to the fact that the screening sensitivity was lower in the 1960s compared with today's technology.

4.4 Lead time distribution for people with a screening history

All of the above methods are developed based on the assumption that an asymptomatic individual has not taken any screening exams at his/her current age; that is, there is no screening history. While in reality, participants aged 55 and older may already have taken at least one (previous) screening exam with negative results in the past and look healthy at their current age, they are called participants with a screening history. In this section, we will develop a lead time model which can incorporate one's screening history and derive the lead time distribution when the lifetime is fixed, and then when it is random. And we will present some simulation results.

We use the disease progressive model: $S_0 \to S_p \to S_c$ [87], where S_0 is the disease-free state, S_p refers to the preclinical disease state, and S_c represents the clinical disease state, that clinical symptoms have presented.

If an individual at current age a_0, has taken K_1 exams before, at ages $t_0 < t_1 < \cdots < t_{K_1-1}$, all exam results were negative, and she plans to take K more screens at her age $t_{K_1} < t_{K_1+1} < t_{K_1+2} < \cdots < t_{K_1+K-1}$ in the future, assume $t_{K_1-1} \leq a_0 < t_{K_1}$. To derive the lead time distribution, we proceed as follows:

- We derive the lead time distribution for the simplest case when $K_1 = K = 1$ (one previous screen and one future screen) with the lifetime T fixed. Then we allow the lifetime T to be random.

- We derive the lead time distribution to any fixed positive integers K_1 and K, when the lifetime T is fixed. Finally, we allow the lifetime T to be random; and hence the number of future screening exams K is random as well.

Let $\beta(t)$ be the sensitivity of the exam at age t, i.e., the probability that the screening is positive given that the individual is in the preclinical state S_p at age t, and let $\beta_i = \beta(t_i)$. We let X be the time duration in the disease-free state S_0, with a sub-PDF (or transition density) $w(x)$; and let Y be the sojourn time, with a PDF $q(y)$; and $Q(y) = \int_y^\infty q(x)dx$ be the survival function of the sojourn time Y. We assume that the sojourn time Y and the duration of the disease-free state X are independent.

Let D be a binary random variable, with $D = 1$ indicating the true clinical disease status, and $D = 0$ indicating no clinical disease status for the whole lifetime. Let L represent the lead time for an individual who develops the symptomatic disease. The distribution of the lead time is a mixture of a point mass at zero and a positive probability density, depending on whether the cancer is a clinical incident case, or is detected by screening.

4.4.1 Lead time distribution when $K_1 = K = 1$

We will use female lung cancer as an example in the problem solving, while the result is equally valid for other kinds of cancer screening. Suppose an asymptomatic woman at current age a_0, previously had only one screening exam at age $t_0 (< a_0)$, and it was negative. We define the event:

$$H_1 = \left\{ \begin{array}{l} \text{A woman had one exam at age } t_0, \text{ no lung cancer was found,} \\ \text{and she is asymptomatic at her current age } a_0. \end{array} \right\}.$$

Suppose that she plans to take an exam at $t_1 (\geq a_0)$, and her lifetime $T = t (> t_1)$ is a fixed value, then

$$\begin{aligned} P(L = 0|D = 1, H_1, T = t) &= \frac{P(L = 0, D = 1, H_1|T = t)}{P(D = 1, H_1|T = t)}, \\ f_L(z|D = 1, H_1, T = t) &= \frac{f_L(z, D = 1, H_1|T = t)}{P(D = 1, H_1|T = t)}. \end{aligned} \tag{4.19}$$

To calculate $P(D = 1, H_1|T = t)$, the probability of no lung cancer appearing before/at age a_0 but would develop lung cancer later in one's lifetime, i.e., cancer appears in (a_0, T), it could happen in one of three disjoint cases: she enters the preclinical state in $(0, t_0)$, (t_0, a_0), or (a_0, T); and the onset of the clinical state is in (a_0, T). See Figure 4.10.

Hence,

$$\begin{aligned} & P(D = 1, H_1|T = t) \\ &= (1 - \beta_0) \int_0^{t_0} w(x)[Q(a_0 - x) - Q(t - x)]dx \\ &\quad + \int_{t_0}^{a_0} w(x)[Q(a_0 - x) - Q(t - x)]dx + \int_{a_0}^{t} w(x)[1 - Q(t - x)]dx. \end{aligned} \tag{4.20}$$

To calculate $P(L=0, D=1, H_1|T=t)$, the probability of clinical incidence in (a_0, T) with a screening at t_1, it equals the probability of incidence in (a_0, t_1) and (t_1, T). It could happen in six possible ways: (i) she is an incident case in (a_0, t_1), and she enters the preclinical state in one of the three intervals $(0, t_0), (t_0, a_0), (a_0, t_1)$; (ii) she is an incident case in (t_1, T), and she enters the preclinical state in one of the three intervals $(0, t_0), (t_0, t_1), (t_1, T)$. Hence,

$$\begin{aligned} & P(L=0, D=1, H_1|T=t) \\ = \; & (1-\beta_0)\int_0^{t_0} w(x)[Q(a_0-x)-Q(t_1-x)]dx \\ & + \int_{t_0}^{a_0} w(x)[Q(a_0-x)-Q(t_1-x)]dx + \int_{a_0}^{t_1} w(x)[1-Q(t_1-x)]dx \\ & +(1-\beta_0)(1-\beta_1)\int_0^{t_0} w(x)[Q(t_1-x)-Q(t-x)]dx \qquad (4.21) \\ & +(1-\beta_1)\int_{t_0}^{t_1} w(x)[Q(t_1-x)-Q(t-x)]dx \\ & + \int_{t_1}^{t} w(x)[1-Q(t-x)]dx. \end{aligned}$$

Finally, to obtain $f_L(z, D=1, H_1|T=t)$, the probability density function of lead time when it is positive, it means that her lung cancer was caught at t_1, and if she were not screened, her cancer symptoms would have appeared at (t_1+z). Depending on when she enters the preclinical state, it could happen in two possible ways: she enters the preclinical state either in $(0, t_0)$ or in (t_0, t_1), either way, her sojourn time in the preclinical state would be (t_1+z-x), where x is the onset time/age of her preclinical state. Hence, for $0 < z \leq (t-t_1)$,

$$\begin{aligned} & f_L(z, D=1, H_1|T=t) \qquad (4.22) \\ = \; & \beta_1\left\{(1-\beta_0)\int_0^{t_0} w(x)q(t_1+z-x)dx + \int_{t_0}^{t_1} w(x)q(t_1+z-x)dx\right\}. \end{aligned}$$

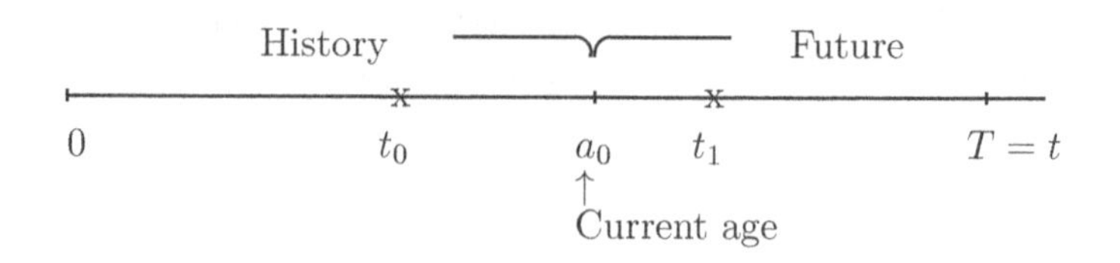

FIGURE 4.10
Screening history and future schedule when $K_1 = K = 1$.

A special case is when $a_0 = t_1$, the equation (4.21) will be simplified to

$$\begin{aligned}
&P(L = 0, D = 1, H_1|T = t) \\
&= (1 - \beta_0)(1 - \beta_1) \int_0^{t_0} w(x)[Q(t_1 - x) - Q(t - x)]dx \\
&\quad + (1 - \beta_1) \int_{t_0}^{t_1} w(x)[Q(t_1 - x) - Q(t - x)]dx \\
&\quad + \int_{t_1}^{t} w(x)[1 - Q(t - x)]dx.
\end{aligned} \tag{4.23}$$

And the other two equations (4.20) and (4.22) will be the same.

Exercise 4.4. Prove that

$$\begin{aligned}
&P(L = 0, D = 1, H_1|T = t) + \int_0^{t-t_1} f_L(z, D = 1, H_1|T = t)dz \\
&= P(D = 1, H_1|T = t).
\end{aligned}$$

Hence

$$P(L = 0|D = 1, H_1, T = t) + \int_0^{t-t_1} f_L(z|D = 1, H_1, T = t)dz = 1.$$

And the mixture distribution is a valid PDF.

When $K = 0$, that is, there is no screening exam after a_0, or we can consider it the same as $a_0 < T < t_1$. In this case, since $P(L = 0, D = 1, H_1|T = t) = P(D = 1, H_1|T = t)$, the distribution of the lead time is a point mass at 0 with probability 1, that is,

$$P(L = 0|D = 1, H_1, T = t) = 1$$

And the density $f_L(z|D = 1, H_1, T = t) = 0$ for any $z > 0$.

When lifetime T is random and is greater than the current age a_0, the lead time distribution would be

$$\begin{aligned}
&P(L = 0|D = 1, H_1, T > a_0) \\
&= \int_{a_0}^{\infty} P(L = 0|D = 1, H_1, T = t) f_T(t|T > a_0)\, dt,
\end{aligned} \tag{4.24}$$

$$\begin{aligned}
&f_L(z|D = 1, H_1, T > a_0) \\
&= \int_{a_0+z}^{\infty} f_L(z|D = 1, H_1, T = t) f_T(t|T > a_0)\, dt, \ \ z > 0,
\end{aligned} \tag{4.25}$$

where $f_T(t|T > a_0) = f_T(t)/P(T > a_0)$ if $t > a_0$ is the conditional PDF of the lifetime.

Exercise 4.5. Prove that

$$P(L=0|D=1,H_1,T>a_0)+\int_0^\infty f_L(z|D=1,H_1,T>a_0)dz=1.$$

Therefore, the mixture distribution of the lead time is valid.

4.4.2 Lead time distribution for any K_1 and K

Now we generalize the method to any positive integer K_1 and K, with K_1 and K representing previous (historic) and future screening numbers respectively. We let D be the binary random variable indicating the true disease status. The time variable t represents a fixed value of age, and T represents a person's lifetime. For a person who already had K_1 screening exams and looks healthy right now, we define the event

$$H_{K_1}=\left\{\begin{array}{l}\text{A woman has taken } K_1 \text{ exams at her age}\\ t_0<t_1<\cdots<t_{K_1-1}, \text{ no cancer was diagnosed,}\\ \text{and she is asymptomatic at her current age } a_0\end{array}\right\}.$$

Suppose that she plans to continue with K screenings in the future at her age $t_{K_1}<t_{K_1+1}<t_{K_1+2}<\cdots<t_{K_1+K-1}$, with $t_{K_1}\geq a_0$. See Figure 4.11. First, we solve the problem assuming that the lifetime T is fixed, then we allow T to be random. When her lifetime $T=t>t_{K_1+K-1}$, the lead time distribution is

$$\begin{aligned}P(L=0|D=1,H_{K_1},T=t)&=\frac{P(L=0,D=1,H_{K_1}|T=t)}{P(D=1,H_{K_1}|T=t)},\\ f_L(z|D=1,H_{K_1},T=t)&=\frac{f_L(z,D=1,H_{K_1}|T=t)}{P(D=1,H_{K_1}|T=t)}.\end{aligned}\tag{4.26}$$

The denominator, $P(D=1,H_{K_1}|T=t)$, is the probability that an asymptomatic person develops clinical cancer from her current age to the end of life T, whether she takes screening or not in the future, with a sequence of exams in the past at the age $t_0<t_1<\cdots<t_{K_1-1}$. This could happen in (K_1+2) mutually exclusive ways: (i) she enters the preclinical state S_p in

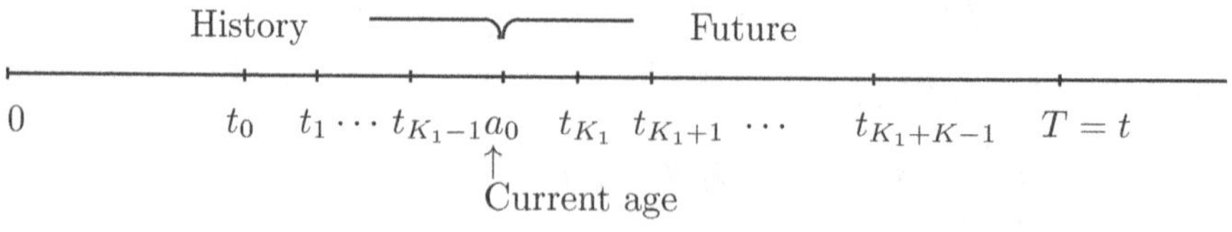

History — Future

0 t_0 $t_1\cdots t_{K_1-1}a_0$ t_{K_1} t_{K_1+1} $\cdots$ t_{K_1+K-1} $T=t$

↑ Current age

FIGURE 4.11
A course of screening exams in the past and the future.

$(t_{i-1}, t_i), i = 0, 1, \ldots, K_1 - 1$, her cancer was not detected by the exams at $t_i, \ldots, t_{K_1-1}$; (ii) she enters the S_p in (t_{K_1-1}, a_0); and (iii) she enters the S_p in (a_0, t). And in cases (i) and (ii), her sojourn time is longer than $(a_0 - x)$, but shorter than $(t - x)$, where x is the onset of the preclinical state S_p; and in case (iii), her sojourn time is simply shorter than $(t - x)$. Since these are mutually exclusive events, we add these probabilities:

$$\begin{aligned} &P(D = 1, H_{K_1} | T = t) \\ &= \sum_{i=0}^{K_1-1} (1 - \beta_i) \cdots (1 - \beta_{K_1-1}) \int_{t_{i-1}}^{t_i} w(x)[Q(a_0 - x) - Q(t - x)]\, dx \\ &\quad + \int_{t_{K_1-1}}^{a_0} w(x)[Q(a_0 - x) - Q(t - x)]\, dx \\ &\quad + \int_{a_0}^{t} w(x)[1 - Q(t - x)]\, dx. \end{aligned} \tag{4.27}$$

The numerator $P(L = 0, D = 1, H_{K_1} | T = t)$ is the probability of all possible interval cases in the (future) intervals (a_0, t_{K_1}) and $(t_{K_1+j-1}, t_{K_1+j}), j = 1, 2, \ldots, K$, where the last interval is (t_{K_1+K-1}, t). And it is

$$P(L = 0, D = 1, H_{K_1} | T = t) = I_{(a_0, t_{K_1})} + \sum_{j=K_1+1}^{K_1+K} I_{K_1+K,j} \tag{4.28}$$

where $I_{(a_0, t_{K_1})}$ is the probability of incidence in (a_0, t_{K_1}), and it is

$$\begin{aligned} &I_{(a_0, t_{K_1})} \\ &= \sum_{i=0}^{K_1-1} (1 - \beta_i) \cdots (1 - \beta_{K_1-1}) \int_{t_{i-1}}^{t_i} w(x)[Q(a_0 - x) - Q(t_{K_1} - x)]dx \\ &\quad + \int_{t_{K_1-1}}^{a_0} w(x)[Q(a_0 - x) - Q(t_{K_1} - x)]dx \\ &\quad + \int_{a_0}^{t_{K_1}} [1 - Q(t_{K_1} - x)]dx. \end{aligned} \tag{4.29}$$

And $I_{K_1+K,j}$ is the probability of incidence in $(t_{j-1}, t_j), j = K_1 + 1, \ldots, (K_1 + K)$, and it is

$$\begin{aligned} &I_{K_1+K,j} \\ &= \sum_{i=0}^{j-1} (1 - \beta_i) \cdots (1 - \beta_{j-1}) \int_{t_{i-1}}^{t_i} w(x)[Q(t_{j-1} - x) - Q(t_j - x)]\, dx \\ &\quad + \int_{t_{j-1}}^{t_j} w(x)[1 - Q(t_j - x)]\, dx, \text{ for } j = K_1 + 1, \ldots, K_1 + K. \end{aligned} \tag{4.30}$$

And for $0 < z \leq t - t_{K_1}$, the joint lead time density is

$$\begin{aligned} & f_L(z, D=1, H_{K_1}|T=t) \\ & = \sum_{i=K_1}^{j-1} \beta_i \left\{ \sum_{r=0}^{i-1} (1-\beta_r)\cdots(1-\beta_{i-1}) \int_{t_{r-1}}^{t_r} w(x)q(t_i+z-x)dx \right. \\ & \left. + \int_{t_{i-1}}^{t_i} w(x)q(t_i+z-x)\,dx \right\}, \quad \text{if } t-t_j < z \leq t-t_{j-1}, \\ & \qquad \text{for } j = K_1+1, \ldots, K_1+K. \end{aligned} \tag{4.31}$$

Note that when $a_0 = t_{K_1}$, the probability $I_{(a_0, t_{K_1})} = 0$; therefore, the probability $P(L=0, D=1, H_{K_1}|T=t)$ is greatly simplified. However, the denominator $P(D=1, H_{K_1}|T=t)$ and the joint density $f_L(z, D=1, H_{K_1}|T=t)$ will not change at all.

Exercise 4.6. Prove that

$$\begin{aligned} & P(L=0, D=1, H_{K_1}|T=t) + \int_0^{t-t_{K_1}} f_L(z, D=1, H_{K_1}|T=t)dz \\ & = P(D=1, H_{K_1}|T=t). \end{aligned}$$

Therefore, this mixture probability distribution is valid, that is,

$$\begin{aligned} & P(L=0|D=1, H_{K_1}, T=t) \\ & \qquad + \int_0^{t-t_{K_1}} f_L(z|D=1, H_{K_1}, T=t)\,dz \equiv 1. \end{aligned}$$

When there is no screening exam after a_0, the distribution of the lead time is a point mass at zero with probability 1.

When lifetime $T > a_0$ is a random variable, the lead time distribution can be obtained by

$$\begin{aligned} & P(L=0|D=1, H_{K_1}, T > a_0) \\ & = \int_{a_0}^{\infty} P(L=0|D=1, H_{K_1}, T=t) f_T(t|T>a_0)\,dt, \end{aligned} \tag{4.32}$$

$$\begin{aligned} & f_L(z|D=1, H_{K_1}, T > a_0) \\ & = \int_{a_0+z}^{\infty} f_L(z|D=1, H_{K_1}, T=t) f_T(t|T>a_0)\,dt, \; z > 0. \end{aligned} \tag{4.33}$$

And the conditional lifetime distribution density $f_T(t|T > a_0)$ is estimated using the actuarial life table [72]. For a person at her current age a_0, if she plans to follow a future screening schedule, such as $t_{K_1} < t_{K_1+1} < \ldots$, then the number of screenings in the future $K = n$ if $t_{K_1+n-1} < T \leq t_{K_1+n}$; therefore the future screening number $K = K(T)$ is random if the lifetime T is random. If the future screening exam is equally spaced with a time interval Δ, then $K = K(T) = \lceil (T - t_{K_1})/\Delta \rceil$.

4.4.3 Lead time distribution at the t_j

We derive the PDF of the lead time if one was diagnosed with cancer for the first time at t_j, for $j = K_1, K_1+1, \ldots$. We define events:

$$A_j = \{\text{One is diagnosed at } t_j \text{ for the first time}\} \cap H_{K_1}.$$

The PDF of the lead time at t_j, given that A_j happened is

$$f_L(z|A_j) = \frac{f_L(z, A_j)}{P(A_j)}, \quad z > 0, j = K_1, K_1+1, \ldots.$$

In fact, this is the same distribution as that in section 4.2.3, and the only difference is the index of j, and we simply repeat here:

$$\begin{aligned} P(A_j) =& \beta_j \left\{ \sum_{i=0}^{j-1} (1-\beta_i)\cdots(1-\beta_{j-1}) \int_{t_{i-1}}^{t_i} w(x)Q(t_j - x)dx \right. \\ &+ \left. \int_{t_{j-1}}^{t_j} w(x)Q(t_j - x)dx \right\}, \quad j = K_1, K_1+1, \ldots. \end{aligned} \tag{4.34}$$

And the numerator is

$$\begin{aligned} f_L(z, A_j) =& \sum_{i=0}^{j} f_L(z, A_j, \text{she enters } S_p \text{ in } (t_{i-1}, t_i)\,) \\ =& \beta_j \left\{ \sum_{i=0}^{j-1} (1-\beta_i)\cdots(1-\beta_{j-1}) \int_{t_{i-1}}^{t_i} w(x)q(t_j + z - x)dx \right. \\ &+ \left. \int_{t_{j-1}}^{t_j} w(x)q(t_j + z - x)dx \right\}, z > 0, j = K_1, K_1+1, K_1+K-1. \end{aligned} \tag{4.35}$$

Exercise 4.7. Prove that for any $j = K_1, K_1+1, \ldots,$

$$\int_0^\infty f_L(z|A_j)dz = 1.$$

4.4.4 Simulation study

The simulation study was carried out when the current age $a_0 = t_{k_1}$, for more details, see Liu et al 2021[34]. We used the following setup:

1. Three initial screening ages: $t_0 = 56, 60, 64$.
2. For each t_0, four current ages: $t_{K_1} = t_0+4, t_0+8, t_0+12, t_0+16$.
3. Two fixed screening sensitivities independent of age: $\beta = 0.7$, and 0.9.
4. Three mean sojourn time: MST = 2, 5, and 10 years.

5. Four screening intervals in the past (Δ_1) and in the future (Δ_2):

$$(\Delta_1, \Delta_2) = (1,1), (2,1), (1,2), \text{ and } (2,2).$$

The $(\Delta_1, \Delta_2) = (1,2)$ means that an individual received annual screening exams in the past and will take biennial exams in the future. We used the male's lifetime PDF derived from the actuarial lifetime table in this simulation as females show a similar pattern. We use the following parametric functions [33, 34]

$$\begin{aligned} w(t|\mu,\sigma^2) &= \frac{0.3}{\sqrt{2\pi}\sigma t}\exp\{-(\log t-\mu)^2/(2\sigma^2)\}, \\ q(x|\lambda,\alpha) &= \alpha\lambda x^{\alpha-1}\exp\left(-\lambda x^{\alpha}\right), \quad \lambda>0, \alpha>0, \\ Q(x|\lambda,\alpha) &= \exp\left(-\lambda x^{\alpha}\right), \quad \lambda>0, \alpha>0. \end{aligned} \tag{4.36}$$

The input parameters of μ and σ^2 were chosen, such that the mode is around 70, as most lung cancer cases were diagnosed around that age. Different values of λ, α were chosen such that the mean sojourn time would be 2, 5, and 10 years, these are listed in Table 4.4.

Simulation results for MST = 2, 5, and 10 are shown in Tables 4.5-4.7. In each table, P_0, the probability that the lead time is zero, is in percentage. When the lead time is positive, the mean lead time EL, its standard deviation, the median, and the mode of lead time are reported in years.

The mean lead time is positively related to the sojourn time: a larger mean sojourn time will lead to a larger mean lead time. The mean lead time is around 1 year if the mean sojourn time (MST) is 2 years; and it is around 2 to 3 years (or 3 to 6 years) if the MST is 5 years (or 10 years) correspondingly.

The probability of no-early-detection P_0 is negatively correlated with the MST: longer MST means smaller P_0, showing that people with slow-growing tumors will benefit more from screening. For example, if an individual started a biennial screening exam at the age of 56, and will continue screening annually

TABLE 4.4
Values of input parameters in the simulation study.

	Parameter	Settings	Value
Sensitivity	N/A	fixed value	0.7 or 0.9
Transition PDF	μ	Mode of log-normal	4.4
	σ^2	distribution is 70	0.16
Sojourn time	λ	MST=2	0.1963
		MST=5	0.0314
		MST=10	0.0079
	α	fixed value	2

Adapted from Table 1 in Liu et al 2021[34].

from her current age $t_{K_1} = 64$, with screening sensitivity $\beta = 0.7$, the P_0 will be 20.23%, 6.87%, and 3.82% correspondingly under the different MSTs of 2, 5, and 10 years. The P_0 is negatively correlated to the screening sensitivity: higher sensitivity will lead to lower P_0. Comparing the results for $\beta = 0.7$ and 0.9 under the same conditions, the probability P_0 is almost doubled in the case of the lower sensitivity. Therefore, higher sensitivity will contribute to early detection.

The lead time distribution tends to be the same for different t_0 if the current age t_{K_1} is fixed. To illustrate, simply look at the results of $t_{K_1} = 68$ and $t_{K_1} = 72$. In Tables 4.5-4.7, the results of (t_0, t_{K_1}) =(56, 68), (60, 68) and (64, 68) are almost the same. This indicates that the t_0 does not seem to affect the lead time distribution so much as long as the person still looks healthy at the current age. Figure 4.12 shows the density plots of the lead time for $t_{K_1} = 68$ and $t_{K_1} = 72$. In the figure, each curve actually represents the density of three different initial screening ages (i.e., $t_0 = 56$, 60, and 64), because the curves completely overlap each other, so we can only observe four curves in each panel. However, the length of the past and future screening intervals do affect the lead time density, with the future intervals causing more differences.

The P_0 is slightly increasing with a participant's current age given that all other factors are the same. This means that the younger participants may benefit slightly more from the screening program. This increase is more obvious when the MST is larger. For example, in Table 4.6, the probability P_0 is 17.21% and the mean lead time is 2.80 years for an individual who started the annual screening exam at age 56 and will begin screening biennially from current age $t_{K_1} = 60$, if the sensitivity $\beta = 0.7$. The probability P_0 goes up to 20.19% and the mean lead time becomes 2.36 years when the individual's current age is 72. Figure 4.13 gives percentages of P_0 and $P_1 = 1 - P_0$. We can see that P_0 increases as the current age t_{K_1} increases for all screening schedules. Since the results are the same for different t_0, we put results of all t_{K_1} together in the bar plots regardless of t_0.

For a given combination of sensitivity, the initial age, and the current age, we compare the results of different screening schedules. For the cases with the same Δ_2 (future screening interval) but different Δ_1 (historic screening interval), the lead time distribution tends to be very similar. For example, we compare the results of $(\Delta_1, \Delta_2) = (1, 1)$, $(1, 2)$ and $(2, 1)$. It is easy to see that the results of $(\Delta_1, \Delta_2) = (1, 1)$ are significantly different from the results of $(\Delta_1, \Delta_2) = (1, 2)$, but the results for $(\Delta_1, \Delta_2) = (1, 1)$ and $(\Delta_1, \Delta_2) = (2, 1)$ are very close. We can also see this from the PDF curves of lead time shown in Figure 4.14. As the results are similar, we only present curves of $t_0 = 56$, $\beta = 0.7$ and MST is 5 years for different t_{K_1}. The PDF curves for lead time with the same future screening interval Δ_2 almost overlap each other for the given initial screening age, the current age, the sensitivity, and the mean sojourn time.

However, we can still find a trend that larger Δ_1 will result in smaller P_0 and longer mean lead time if Δ_2 remains the same, and it is more obvious

TABLE 4.5

The lead time distribution when MST = 2 years.

(Δ_1, Δ_2)	$\beta = 0.7$				$\beta = 0.9$			
(years)	P_0	EL (s.d.)	Median	Mode	P_0	EL (s.d.)	Median	Mode
	initial screening age $t_0 = 56$, current age $t_{K_1} = 60$							
(1,1)	20.10	1.14 (1.05)	1.25	0.85	10.32	1.33 (1.04)	1.35	0.95
(2,1)	20.02	1.13 (1.04)	1.25	0.75	10.05	1.32 (1.04)	1.35	0.95
(1,2)	41.26	0.76 (0.97)	1.15	0.35	28.00	0.95 (1.01)	1.15	0.45
(2,2)	40.69	0.76 (0.96)	1.15	0.35	27.08	0.96 (1.00)	1.15	0.45
	initial screening age $t_0 = 56$, current age $t_{K_1} = 64$							
(1,1)	20.34	1.12 (1.04)	1.25	0.75	10.45	1.31 (1.03)	1.35	0.95
(2,1)	20.23	1.11 (1.03)	1.25	0.65	10.10	1.30 (1.03)	1.35	0.95
(1,2)	41.34	0.75 (0.96)	1.15	0.15	28.09	0.94 (1.00)	1.15	0.45
(2,2)	40.63	0.75 (0.96)	1.05	0.15	26.96	0.94 (0.99)	1.15	0.45
	initial screening age $t_0 = 56$, current age $t_{K_1} = 68$							
(1,1)	20.69	1.09 (1.03)	1.25	0.65	10.63	1.29 (1.03)	1.25	0.85
(2,1)	20.53	1.08 (1.02)	1.25	0.65	10.19	1.27 (1.02)	1.25	0.85
(1,2)	41.46	0.74 (0.95)	1.05	0.15	28.21	0.92 (0.99)	1.15	0.45
(2,2)	40.58	0.74 (0.94)	1.05	0.15	26.81	0.93 (0.98)	1.05	0.15
	initial screening age $t_0 = 56$, current age $t_{K_1} = 72$							
(1,1)	21.15	1.06 (1.01)	1.15	0.65	10.88	1.25 (1.01)	1.25	0.85
(2,1)	20.93	1.05 (1.01)	1.15	0.65	10.32	1.24 (1.01)	1.25	0.65
(1,2)	41.58	0.72 (0.93)	1.05	0.15	28.36	0.90 (0.97)	1.05	0.15
(2,2)	40.50	0.72 (0.93)	1.05	0.15	26.61	0.91 (0.97)	1.05	0.15
	initial screening age $t_0 = 60$, current age $t_{K_1} = 64$							
(1,1)	20.34	1.12 (1.04)	1.25	0.75	10.45	1.31 (1.03)	1.35	0.95
(2,1)	20.23	1.11 (1.03)	1.25	0.65	10.10	1.30 (1.03)	1.35	0.95
(1,2)	41.34	0.75 (0.96)	1.15	0.15	28.09	0.94 (1.00)	1.15	0.45
(2,2)	40.63	0.75 (0.96)	1.05	0.15	26.96	0.94 (0.99)	1.15	0.45
	initial screening age $t_0 = 60$, current age $t_{K_1} = 68$							
(1,1)	20.69	1.09 (1.03)	1.25	0.65	10.63	1.29 (1.02)	1.25	0.85
(2,1)	20.53	1.08 (1.02)	1.25	0.65	10.19	1.27 (1.02)	1.25	0.85
(1,2)	41.46	0.74 (0.95)	1.05	0.15	28.21	0.92 (0.99)	1.15	0.45
(2,2)	40.58	0.74 (0.94)	1.05	0.15	26.81	0.93 (0.98)	1.05	0.15
	initial screening age $t_0 = 60$, current age $t_{K_1} = 72$							
(1,1)	21.15	1.06 (1.01)	1.15	0.65	10.88	1.25 (1.01)	1.25	0.85
(2,1)	20.93	1.05 (1.01)	1.15	0.65	10.32	1.24 (1.01)	1.25	0.65
(1,2)	41.58	0.72 (0.93)	1.05	0.15	28.36	0.90 (0.97)	1.05	0.15
(2,2)	40.50	0.72 (0.93)	1.05	0.15	26.61	0.91 (0.97)	1.05	0.15
	initial screening age $t_0 = 60$, current age $t_{K_1} = 76$							
(1,1)	21.77	1.01 (0.99)	1.15	0.45	11.22	1.20 (1.00)	1.25	0.65
(2,1)	21.46	1.00 (0.98)	1.15	0.15	10.49	1.18 (0.99)	1.15	0.65
(1,2)	41.77	0.69 (0.91)	1.05	0.15	28.55	0.87 (0.95)	1.05	0.15
(2,2)	40.43	0.70 (0.91)	0.95	0.05	26.38	0.88 (0.94)	1.05	0.15
	initial screening age $t_0 = 64$, current age $t_{K_1} = 68$							
(1,1)	20.69	1.09 (1.03)	1.25	0.65	10.63	1.29 (1.02)	1.25	0.85
(2,1)	20.53	1.08 (1.02)	1.25	0.65	10.19	1.27 (1.02)	1.25	0.85
(1,2)	41.46	0.74 (0.95)	1.05	0.15	28.21	0.92 (0.99)	1.15	0.45
(2,2)	40.58	0.74 (0.94)	1.05	0.15	26.81	0.93 (0.98)	1.05	0.15
	initial screening age $t_0 = 64$, current age $t_{K_1} = 72$							
(1,1)	21.15	1.06 (1.01)	1.15	0.65	10.88	1.25 (1.01)	1.25	0.85
(2,1)	20.93	1.05 (1.01)	1.15	0.65	10.32	1.24 (1.01)	1.25	0.65
(1,2)	41.58	0.72 (0.93)	1.05	0.15	28.36	0.90 (0.97)	1.05	0.15
(2,2)	40.50	0.72 (0.93)	1.05	0.15	26.61	0.91 (0.97)	1.05	0.15
	initial screening age $t_0 = 64$, current age $t_{K_1} = 76$							
(1,1)	21.77	1.01 (0.99)	1.15	0.45	11.22	1.20 (1.00)	1.25	0.65
(2,1)	21.46	1.00 (0.98)	1.15	0.15	10.49	1.18 (0.99)	1.15	0.65
(1,2)	41.77	0.69 (0.91)	1.05	0.15	28.55	0.87 (0.95)	1.05	0.15
(2,2)	40.43	0.70 (0.91)	0.95	0.05	26.38	0.88 (0.94)	1.05	0.15
	initial screening age $t_0 = 64$, current age $t_{K_1} = 80$							
(1,1)	22.60	0.95 (0.96)	1.05	0.15	11.68	1.13 (0.97)	1.15	0.45
(2,1)	22.15	0.94 (0.95)	1.05	0.15	10.71	1.12 (0.96)	1.15	0.15
(1,2)	41.88	0.66 (0.88)	0.95	0.05	28.68	0.82 (0.92)	1.05	0.15
(2,2)	40.21	0.66 (0.88)	0.95	0.05	25.97	0.84 (0.92)	0.95	0.05

Adapted from Table 2 in Liu et al 2021 [34].

TABLE 4.6
The lead time distribution when MST = 5 years.

(Δ_1, Δ_2)	$\beta = 0.7$				$\beta = 0.9$			
(years)	P_0	EL (s.d.)	Median	Mode	P_0	EL (s.d.)	Median	Mode
	initial screening age $t_0 = 56$, current age $t_{K_1} = 60$							
(1,1)	6.47	3.44 (2.50)	3.35	2.45	2.77	3.72 (2.48)	3.45	2.75
(2,1)	6.44	3.42 (2.50)	3.35	2.45	2.55	3.71 (2.47)	3.45	2.75
(1,2)	17.21	2.80 (2.49)	2.95	1.85	8.81	3.21 (2.48)	3.15	2.25
(2,2)	16.73	2.80 (2.49)	2.95	1.85	8.09	3.23 (2.47)	3.15	2.25
	initial screening age $t_0 = 56$, current age $t_{K_1} = 64$							
(1,1)	6.95	3.31 (2.46)	3.25	2.15	3.00	3.59 (2.44)	3.35	2.45
(2,1)	6.87	3.29 (2.46)	3.15	2.15	2.72	3.58 (2.44)	3.35	2.45
(1,2)	17.93	2.69 (2.44)	2.85	1.45	9.31	3.09 (2.44)	3.05	1.95
(2,2)	17.28	2.70 (2.44)	2.85	1.45	8.38	3.12 (2.43)	3.05	1.95
	initial screening age $t_0 = 56$, current age $t_{K_1} = 68$							
(1,1)	7.64	3.14 (2.41)	3.05	1.95	3.34	3.41 (2.39)	3.15	1.95
(2,1)	7.51	3.12 (2.41)	3.05	1.95	2.95	3.41 (2.39)	3.15	1.95
(1,2)	18.91	2.54 (2.38)	2.75	1.45	10.01	2.93 (2.38)	2.85	1.95
(2,2)	18.05	2.56 (2.38)	2.75	1.15	8.79	2.97 (2.38)	2.85	1.95
	initial screening age $t_0 = 56$, current age $t_{K_1} = 72$							
(1,1)	8.58	2.93 (2.33)	2.85	1.65	3.80	3.18 (2.32)	2.95	1.95
(2,1)	8.37	2.91 (2.33)	2.85	1.65	3.28	3.19 (2.32)	2.95	1.95
(1,2)	20.19	2.36 (2.29)	2.55	0.15	10.93	2.73 (2.30)	2.65	1.45
(2,2)	19.06	2.39 (2.29)	2.55	0.15	9.32	2.78 (2.30)	2.75	0.15
	initial screening age $t_0 = 60$, current age $t_{K_1} = 64$							
(1,1)	6.96	3.31 (2.46)	3.25	2.15	3.00	3.59 (2.44)	3.35	2.45
(2,1)	6.90	3.28 (2.46)	3.15	2.15	2.72	3.58 (2.44)	3.35	2.45
(1,2)	17.93	2.69 (2.44)	2.85	1.45	9.31	3.09 (2.44)	3.05	1.95
(2,2)	17.29	2.69 (2.44)	2.85	1.45	8.38	3.12 (2.43)	3.05	1.95
	initial screening age $t_0 = 60$, current age $t_{K_1} = 68$							
(1,1)	7.64	3.14 (2.41)	3.05	1.95	3.34	3.41 (2.39)	3.15	1.95
(2,1)	7.51	3.12 (2.41)	3.05	1.95	2.95	3.41 (2.39)	3.15	1.95
(1,2)	18.91	2.54 (2.38)	2.75	1.45	10.01	2.93 (2.38)	2.85	1.95
(2,2)	18.05	2.56 (2.38)	2.75	1.15	8.79	2.97 (2.38)	2.85	1.95
	initial screening age $t_0 = 60$, current age $t_{K_1} = 72$							
(1,1)	8.58	2.93 (2.33)	2.85	1.65	3.80	3.18 (2.32)	2.95	1.95
(2,1)	8.37	2.91 (2.33)	2.85	1.65	3.28	3.19 (2.32)	2.95	1.95
(1,2)	20.19	2.36 (2.29)	2.55	0.15	10.93	2.73 (2.30)	2.65	1.45
(2,2)	19.06	2.39 (2.29)	2.55	0.15	9.32	2.78 (2.30)	2.75	0.15
	initial screening age $t_0 = 60$, current age $t_{K_1} = 76$							
(1,1)	9.84	2.65 (2.23)	2.55	0.15	4.42	2.90 (2.22)	2.65	1.45
(2,1)	9.50	2.64 (2.23)	2.55	0.15	3.71	2.92 (2.23)	2.65	0.15
(1,2)	21.85	2.14 (2.17)	2.35	0.15	12.13	2.47 (2.19)	2.45	0.15
(2,2)	20.35	2.17 (2.18)	2.35	0.05	10.01	2.55 (2.20)	2.45	0.15
	initial screening age $t_0 = 64$, current age $t_{K_1} = 68$							
(1,1)	7.65	3.14 (2.41)	3.05	1.95	3.34	3.41 (2.39)	3.15	1.95
(2,1)	7.54	3.11 (2.41)	3.05	1.95	2.95	3.41 (2.39)	3.15	1.95
(1,2)	18.91	2.54 (2.38)	2.75	1.45	10.01	2.93 (2.38)	2.85	1.95
(2,2)	18.06	2.55 (2.38)	2.75	1.15	8.78	2.97 (2.38)	2.85	1.95
	initial screening age $t_0 = 64$, current age $t_{K_1} = 72$							
(1,1)	8.58	2.93 (2.33)	2.85	1.65	3.80	3.18 (2.32)	2.95	1.95
(2,1)	8.37	2.91 (2.33)	2.85	1.65	3.28	3.19 (2.32)	2.95	1.95
(1,2)	20.19	2.36 (2.29)	2.55	0.15	10.93	2.73 (2.30)	2.65	1.45
(2,2)	19.06	2.39 (2.29)	2.55	0.15	9.32	2.78 (2.30)	2.75	0.15
	initial screening age $t_0 = 64$, current age $t_{K_1} = 76$							
(1,1)	9.84	2.65 (2.23)	2.55	0.15	4.42	2.90 (2.22)	2.65	1.45
(2,1)	9.50	2.64 (2.23)	2.55	0.15	3.71	2.92 (2.23)	2.65	0.15
(1,2)	21.85	2.14 (2.17)	2.35	0.15	12.13	2.47 (2.19)	2.45	0.15
(2,2)	20.35	2.17 (2.18)	2.35	0.05	10.01	2.55 (2.20)	2.45	0.15
	initial screening age $t_0 = 64$, current age $t_{K_1} = 80$							
(1,1)	11.58	2.32 (2.08)	2.25	0.15	5.29	2.55 (2.08)	2.35	0.15
(2,1)	11.06	2.32 (2.09)	2.25	0.05	4.31	2.58 (2.09)	2.35	0.05
(1,2)	23.94	1.86 (2.01)	2.05	0.05	13.67	2.17 (2.04)	2.15	0.15
(2,2)	21.98	1.91 (2.02)	2.05	0.05	10.87	2.26 (2.05)	2.15	0.05

Adapted from Table 3 in Liu et al 2021 [34].

TABLE 4.7
The lead time distribution when MST = 10 years.

(Δ_1, Δ_2)	$\beta = 0.7$				$\beta = 0.9$			
(years)	P_0	EL (s.d.)	Median	Mode	P_0	EL (s.d.)	Median	Mode
			initial screening age $t_0 = 56$, current age $t_{K_1} = 60$					
(1,1)	3.43	6.32 (4.41)	5.95	3.95	1.47	6.60 (4.39)	6.05	4.25
(2,1)	3.38	6.32 (4.44)	5.95	3.95	1.24	6.66 (4.41)	6.15	4.25
(1,2)	9.19	5.58 (4.42)	5.45	2.85	4.48	6.07 (4.39)	5.75	3.85
(2,2)	8.64	5.63 (4.44)	5.45	2.85	3.78	6.17 (4.41)	5.75	3.85
			initial screening age $t_0 = 56$, current age $t_{K_1} = 64$					
(1,1)	4.00	5.87 (4.23)	5.45	3.65	1.73	6.13 (4.21)	5.65	3.75
(2,1)	3.82	5.92 (4.26)	5.55	3.65	1.44	6.22 (4.24)	5.65	3.75
(1,2)	10.31	5.15 (4.23)	5.05	2.65	5.14	5.61 (4.21)	5.25	2.65
(2,2)	9.52	5.25 (4.26)	5.15	2.65	4.24	5.75 (4.23)	5.35	3.25
			initial screening age $t_0 = 56$, current age $t_{K_1} = 68$					
(1,1)	4.82	5.31 (4.01)	4.95	2.95	2.11	5.57 (3.99)	5.05	2.95
(2,1)	4.55	5.38 (4.04)	5.05	2.95	1.72	5.67 (4.02)	5.15	3.15
(1,2)	11.79	4.64 (3.98)	4.55	0.15	6.04	5.07 (3.97)	4.75	1.95
(2,2)	10.74	4.76 (4.03)	4.65	0.15	4.84	5.23 (4.01)	4.85	2.65
			initial screening age $t_0 = 56$, current age $t_{K_1} = 72$					
(1,1)	5.92	4.68 (3.72)	4.35	0.15	2.63	4.92 (3.70)	4.45	2.15
(2,1)	5.54	4.76 (3.77)	4.45	0.15	2.09	5.04 (3.75)	4.55	0.15
(1,2)	13.70	4.05 (3.68)	4.05	0.15	7.23	4.45 (3.68)	4.15	0.15
(2,2)	12.31	4.20 (3.73)	4.15	0.15	5.63	4.63 (3.73)	4.25	0.15
			initial screening age $t_0 = 60$, current age $t_{K_1} = 64$					
(1,1)	4.00	5.86 (4.23)	5.45	3.65	1.73	6.13 (4.21)	5.65	3.75
(2,1)	3.93	5.87 (4.27)	5.45	3.65	1.44	6.21 (4.24)	5.65	3.75
(1,2)	10.27	5.15 (4.23)	5.05	2.65	5.14	5.61 (4.21)	5.25	2.65
(2,2)	9.55	5.21 (4.26)	5.05	2.65	4.21	5.74 (4.23)	5.35	3.25
			initial screening age $t_0 = 60$, current age $t_{K_1} = 68$					
(1,1)	4.82	5.31 (4.01)	4.95	2.95	2.11	5.57 (3.99)	5.05	2.95
(2,1)	4.56	5.38 (4.05)	4.95	2.95	1.72	5.67 (4.02)	5.15	3.15
(1,2)	11.79	4.64 (3.98)	4.55	0.15	6.04	5.07 (3.97)	4.75	1.95
(2,2)	10.74	4.76 (4.03)	4.65	0.15	4.84	5.23 (4.01)	4.85	2.65
			initial screening age $t_0 = 60$, current age $t_{K_1} = 72$					
(1,1)	5.92	4.68 (3.72)	4.35	0.15	2.63	4.92 (3.70)	4.45	2.15
(2,1)	5.54	4.76 (3.77)	4.45	0.15	2.09	5.04 (3.75)	4.55	0.15
(1,2)	13.70	4.05 (3.68)	4.05	0.15	7.23	4.45 (3.68)	4.15	0.15
(2,2)	12.31	4.20 (3.73)	4.15	0.15	5.63	4.63 (3.73)	4.25	0.15
			initial screening age $t_0 = 60$, current age $t_{K_1} = 76$					
(1,1)	7.38	3.99 (3.37)	3.65	0.15	3.33	4.21 (3.35)	3.75	0.15
(2,1)	6.86	4.08 (3.43)	3.75	0.05	2.59	4.34 (3.41)	3.85	0.15
(1,2)	16.11	3.42 (3.31)	3.45	0.15	8.76	3.78 (3.32)	3.55	0.15
(2,2)	14.29	3.57 (3.38)	3.55	0.05	6.62	3.98 (3.38)	3.65	0.15
			initial screening age $t_0 = 64$, current age $t_{K_1} = 68$					
(1,1)	4.82	5.31 (4.01)	4.95	2.95	2.11	5.57 (3.99)	5.05	2.95
(2,1)	4.70	5.32 (4.05)	4.95	0.15	1.71	5.66 (4.03)	5.15	3.15
(1,2)	11.73	4.64 (3.98)	4.55	0.15	6.04	5.07 (3.97)	4.75	1.95
(2,2)	10.76	4.72 (4.02)	4.55	0.15	4.80	5.22 (4.01)	4.85	0.15
			initial screening age $t_0 = 64$, current age $t_{K_1} = 72$					
(1,1)	5.92	4.68 (3.72)	4.35	0.15	2.63	4.92 (3.70)	4.45	2.15
(2,1)	5.55	4.76 (3.77)	4.45	0.15	2.09	5.04 (3.75)	4.55	0.15
(1,2)	13.70	4.05 (3.68)	4.05	0.15	7.23	4.45 (3.68)	4.15	0.15
(2,2)	12.31	4.19 (3.73)	4.15	0.15	5.63	4.63 (3.73)	4.25	0.15
			initial screening age $t_0 = 64$, current age $t_{K_1} = 76$					
(1,1)	7.38	3.99 (3.37)	3.65	0.15	3.33	4.21 (3.35)	3.75	0.15
(2,1)	6.86	4.08 (3.43)	3.75	0.05	2.59	4.34 (3.41)	3.85	0.15
(1,2)	16.11	3.42 (3.31)	3.45	0.15	8.76	3.78 (3.32)	3.55	0.15
(2,2)	14.30	3.57 (3.38)	3.55	0.05	6.62	3.98 (3.38)	3.65	0.15
			initial screening age $t_0 = 64$, current age $t_{K_1} = 80$					
(1,1)	9.38	3.26 (2.97)	3.05	0.05	4.29	3.47 (2.96)	3.05	0.15
(2,1)	8.67	3.35 (3.03)	3.05	0.05	3.28	3.60 (3.02)	3.15	0.05
(1,2)	19.09	2.76 (2.89)	2.85	0.05	10.72	3.08 (2.91)	2.85	0.15
(2,2)	16.76	2.92 (2.97)	2.85	0.05	7.86	3.28 (2.99)	2.95	0.05

Adapted from Table 4 in Liu et al 2021 [34].

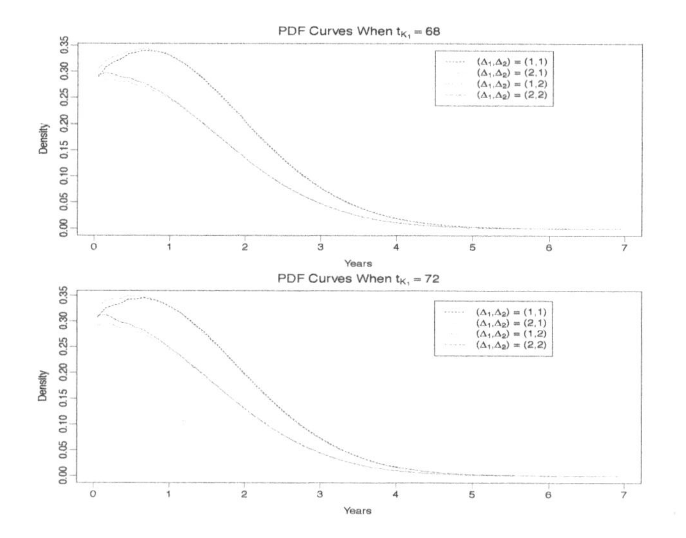

FIGURE 4.12
The PDF curves of the lead time for $t_{K_1} = 68$ and $t_{K_1} = 72$ with different t_0: 12 curves representing different (Δ_1, Δ_2) and different initial age t_0 are plotted for $t_{K_1} = 68$ (upper) and $t_{K_1} = 72$ (bottom), respectively. Curves with the same t_0 overlap, so only one curve for each t_0 shows. $\beta = 0.7$, MST = 2 yrs. Adapted from Figure 1 in Liu et al 2021 [34].

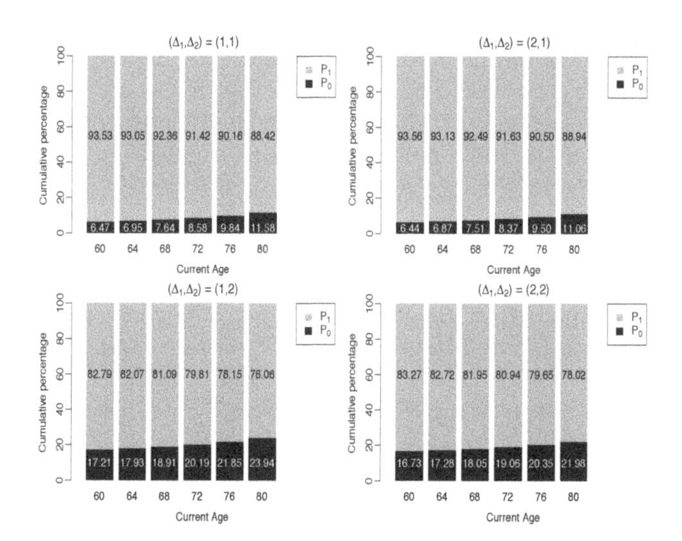

FIGURE 4.13
The bar plots of percentage changes for P_0 and P_1 with different t_{K_1}: Six bars representing different current ages are plotted for each of the four screening schedules, $(\Delta_1, \Delta_2) = (1, 1)$ (upper left), $(\Delta_1, \Delta_2) = (2, 1)$ (upper right), $(\Delta_1, \Delta_2) = (1, 2)$ (bottom left) and $(\Delta_1, \Delta_2) = (2, 2)$ (bottom right). $\beta = 0.7$, MST = 5, any $t_0 (< t_{K_1})$. Adapted from Figure 2 in Liu et al 2021 [34].

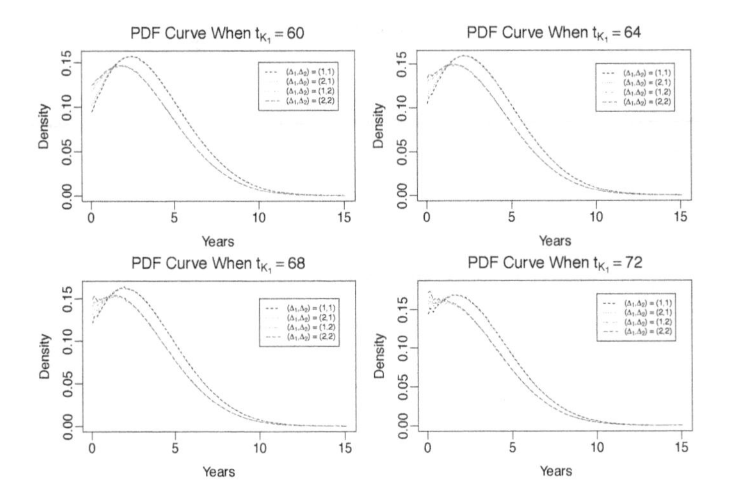

FIGURE 4.14
The sub-PDF curves of the lead time for $t_0 = 56$, $\beta = 0.7$, MST $= 5$. Adapted from Figure 4 in Liu et al 2021 [34].

when MST is longer. In Table 4.7, the probability P_0 is 9.19% and the mean lead time is 5.58 for an individual whose initial screening age $t_0 = 56$ and current age $t_{K_1} = 60$ with screening schedules $(\Delta_1, \Delta_2) = (1, 2)$ given the screening sensitivity $\beta = 0.7$. The probability P_0 decreases to 8.64% and the mean lead time increases to 5.63 if the individual's past screening interval $\Delta_1 = 2$. We can see the trend more clearly in Figure 4.15.

4.4.5 Application: NLST CT data

The National Lung Screening Trial (NLST) study was designed to compare two screening modalities for the early detection of lung cancer among heavy smokers: low-dose computed tomography (CT) versus standard chest X-rays [53].

We apply the method to the NLST low-dose CT data, it was assumed that the current age a_0 equals t_{K_1}. We used the parametric model for the sensitivity, $\beta(t) = \{1 + \exp[-b_0 - b_1(t - \bar{t})]\}^{-1}$ and the same equations in (4.36) for the $w(t), q(x)$, and $Q(x)$. The six unknown parameters $\theta = (b_0, b_1, \mu, \sigma^2, \lambda, \alpha)$ were estimated using Markov Chain Monte Carlo (MCMC) and a likelihood function based on NLST-LDCT data [32]. Two MCMC chains were simulated with overdispersed initial values. Each chain was 130,000 iterations, with 30,000 burn-in, and after the burn-in, the posteriors were sampled every 200 steps, providing 500 posteriors θ for each chain. We then used the pooled

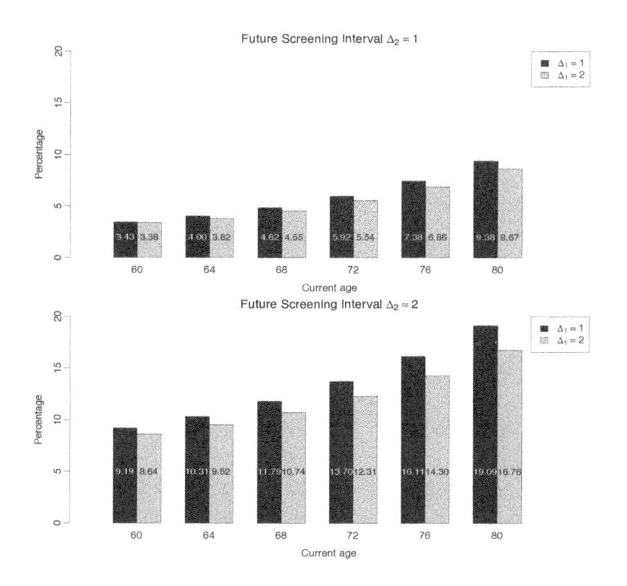

FIGURE 4.15
The bar plots of percentage changes for P_0 with different Δ_1 and the same Δ_2: Bars grouped by six different current ages are plotted for two future schedules, $\Delta_2 = 1$ (upper) and $\Delta_2 = 2$ (bottom). $\beta = 0.7$, MST $= 10$, any t_0. Adapted from Figure 6 in Liu et al 2021 [34].

1,000 posterior samples, to estimate the lead time for hypothetic cohorts. The posterior predictive distribution of the lead time is a weighted average at each θ_j^*:

$$f_L(l|NLST) \approx \frac{1}{n} \sum_{j=1}^{n} f_L(l|\theta_j^*), \ n = 1000.$$

For each gender, there are four cohorts of initially asymptomatic individuals, with current age $t_{K_1} = 60$, 64, 68, and 72, respectively. And within each cohort, we examined six different screening schedules $(\Delta_1, \Delta_2) = (1, 1)$, $(2, 1)$, $(-, 1)$, $(1, 2)$, $(2, 2)$, and $(-, 2)$, The symbol $\Delta_1 = -$ means that the individuals have no screening history; this is added for comparison purposes. The initial screening age is $t_0 = 56$ for all cases (except those without any screening history, in which case, their current age t_{K_1} is their initial screening age). As the simulation study in Section 4.4.4 showed that the t_0 has little impact on the future lead time distribution, we only tried one t_0 here. Simulation results of the 24 scenarios for each gender are presented in Tables 4.8 and 4.9.

The results of $(\Delta_1, \Delta_2) = (1, 1)$, $(2, 1)$, and $(-, 1)$ are similar for both genders, and the results of $(\Delta_1, \Delta_2) = (1, 2)$, $(2, 2)$, and $(-, 2)$ are also similar. This means the future screening schedule plays a more important role than

TABLE 4.8
Application: Lead time distribution for male heavy smokers with initial screening age $t_0 = 56$.

(Δ_1, Δ_2)	P_0 (95% C.I.)	$1 - P_0$ (s.d.)	EL (s.d.)	Med/IQR
		current age $t_{K_1} = 60$		
(1,1)	11.83 (7.37, 17.93)	88.17 (2.66)	0.87 (0.69)	1.06
(2,1)	11.67 (7.28, 17.79)	88.33 (2.62)	0.86 (0.68)	0.94
(-,1)	11.65 (7.28, 17.76)	88.35 (2.61)	0.86 (0.68)	0.94
(1,2)	36.91 (28.21, 45.48)	63.09 (4.49)	0.54 (0.66)	0.83
(2,2)	36.30 (27.59, 44.99)	63.70 (4.53)	0.54 (0.66)	0.83
(-,2)	36.35 (27.67, 45.06)	63.65 (4.54)	0.55 (0.66)	0.83
		current age $t_{K_1} = 64$		
(1,1)	11.86 (6.93, 19.12)	88.14 (3.04)	0.86 (0.68)	0.94
(2,1)	11.62 (6.82, 18.83)	88.38 (3.00)	0.85 (0.68)	0.94
(-,1)	11.58 (6.82, 18.77)	88.42 (2.99)	0.85 (0.68)	0.94
(1,2)	36.60 (27.69, 45.84)	63.40 (4.72)	0.55 (0.66)	0.83
(2,2)	35.68 (26.67, 45.19)	64.32 (4.78)	0.54 (0.65)	0.83
(-,2)	35.68 (26.42, 45.11)	64.32 (4.83)	0.55 (0.66)	0.83
		current age $t_{K_1} = 68$		
(1,1)	12.00 (6.47, 20.89)	88.00 (3.62)	0.85 (0.68)	0.94
(2,1)	11.66 (6.42, 20.48)	88.34 (3.59)	0.84 (0.68)	0.94
(-,1)	11.61 (6.39, 20.48)	88.39 (3.58)	0.83 (0.67)	0.94
(1,2)	36.31 (27.09, 46.40)	63.69 (5.08)	0.54 (0.65)	0.83
(2,2)	35.01 (25.60, 45.55)	64.99 (5.18)	0.54 (0.65)	0.83
(-,2)	34.96 (25.23, 45.45)	65.04 (5.26)	0.54 (0.65)	0.94
		current age $t_{K_1} = 72$		
(1,1)	12.29 (6.07, 23.67)	87.71 (4.43)	0.83 (0.68)	0.94
(2,1)	11.84 (5.96, 23.35)	88.16 (4.43)	0.81 (0.67)	0.94
(-,1)	11.77 (5.96, 23.33)	88.23 (4.43)	0.81 (0.67)	1.06
(1,2)	36.04 (26.18, 47.83)	63.96 (5.60)	0.54 (0.65)	0.83
(2,2)	34.34 (24.37, 46.75)	65.66 (5.78)	0.54 (0.64)	0.94
(-,2)	34.22 (23.88, 46.78)	65.78 (5.89)	0.54 (0.64)	0.81

Adapted from Table 5 in Liu et al 2021 [34].

the past screening schedule regarding the lead time distribution. For example, in Table 4.8, the probability P_0 is 11.83% and the mean lead time is 0.87 years for screening schedules $(\Delta_1, \Delta_2) = (1, 1)$, and P_0 is 11.67% and the mean lead time is 0.86 for $(\Delta_1, \Delta_2) = (2, 1)$ given the person's current age $t_{K_1} = 60$. The probability P_0 is 11.65% and the mean lead time is 0.86 years if the person's future screening interval is 1 year and the person had no screening history. We also present the density curves of lead time for males and females in Figures 4.16 and 4.17, respectively. In each figure, four panels represent four

TABLE 4.9
Application: Lead time distribution for female heavy smokers with initial screening age $t_0 = 56$.

(Δ_1, Δ_2)	P_0 (95% C.I.)	$1 - P_0$ (s.d.)	EL (s.d.)	Med/IQR
		current age $t_{K_1} = 60$		
(1,1)	6.87 (3.94, 10.93)	93.13 (1.81)	1.06 (0.72)	1.17
(2,1)	6.78 (3.91, 10.73)	93.22 (1.77)	1.05 (0.72)	1.17
(-,1)	6.76 (3.91, 10.68)	93.24 (1.76)	1.05 (0.72)	1.17
(1,2)	28.69 (19.83, 38.26)	71.31 (4.64)	0.69 (0.73)	0.94
(2,2)	28.15 (19.39, 37.77)	71.85 (4.63)	0.69 (0.73)	0.94
(-,2)	28.26 (19.41, 37.85)	71.74 (4.65)	0.69 (0.73)	0.94
		current age $t_{K_1} = 64$		
(1,1)	6.84 (3.82, 10.98)	93.16 (1.90)	1.05 (0.72)	1.17
(2,1)	6.69 (3.74, 10.68)	93.31 (1.85)	1.04 (0.72)	1.17
(-,1)	6.67 (3.74, 10.60)	93.33 (1.84)	1.04 (0.72)	1.05
(1,2)	28.44 (19.38, 37.99)	71.56 (4.65)	0.69 (0.73)	0.94
(2,2)	27.63 (18.76, 37.18)	72.37 (4.65)	0.69 (0.72)	0.94
(-,2)	27.69 (18.71, 37.29)	72.31 (4.69)	0.69 (0.72)	0.94
		current age $t_{K_1} = 68$		
(1,1)	6.85 (3.70, 11.24)	93.15 (2.06)	1.04 (0.72)	1.17
(2,1)	6.64 (3.59, 10.99)	93.36 (2.00)	1.03 (0.72)	1.05
(-,1)	6.60 (3.59, 10.96)	93.40 (1.99)	1.02 (0.72)	1.17
(1,2)	28.20 (19.36, 37.59)	71.80 (4.68)	0.69 (0.72)	0.94
(2,2)	27.06 (18.24, 36.58)	72.94 (4.69)	0.69 (0.72)	0.94
(-,2)	27.06 (18.00, 36.61)	72.94 (4.77)	0.68 (0.72)	0.94
		current age $t_{K_1} = 72$		
(1,1)	6.92 (3.57, 12.24)	93.08 (2.31)	1.03 (0.72)	1.17
(2,1)	6.63 (3.39, 11.78)	93.37 (2.26)	1.00 (0.72)	1.06
(-,1)	6.59 (3.39, 11.63)	93.41 (2.25)	1.00 (0.71)	1.06
(1,2)	27.97 (19.11, 37.41)	72.03 (4.76)	0.69 (0.72)	0.94
(2,2)	26.45 (17.74, 35.99)	73.55 (4.78)	0.68 (0.71)	0.94
(-,2)	26.39 (17.20, 36.03)	73.61 (4.90)	0.68 (0.71)	0.75

Adapted from Table 6 in Liu et al 2021 [34].

different current ages ($t_{K_1} = 60$, 64, 68, and 72). In each panel, the six curves are the corresponding lead time densities for six different screening intervals: $(\Delta_1, \Delta_2) =$ (1,1), (1,2), (-,1), (2,1), (2,2), and (-,2). The density curves of lead time for the same future screening interval Δ_2 almost overlap each other given the same current age.

There is a similar trend as in the simulation study that larger Δ_1 will result in smaller P_0 if Δ_2 is the same. In Table 4.8, the probability P_0 is 11.83% for current age $t_{K_1} = 60$ with screening schedules $(\Delta_1, \Delta_2) = (1, 1)$, and it decreases to 11.67% if the individual's past screening interval $\Delta_1 = 2$.

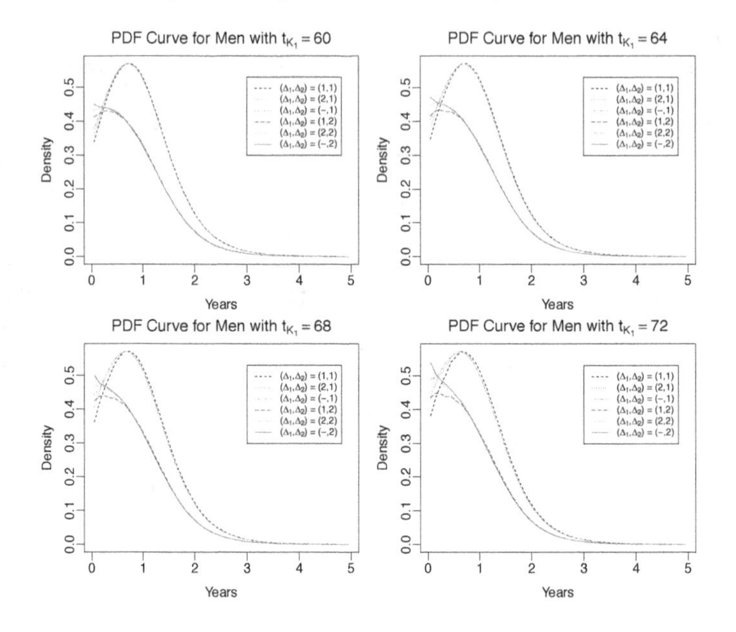

FIGURE 4.16
The lead time curve for male heavy smokers with screening history when $t_0 = 56$: 6 curves of different (Δ_1, Δ_2) are provided at four current ages, $t_{K_1} = 60$, 64, 68, and 72. Adapted from Figure 7 in Liu et al 2021 [34].

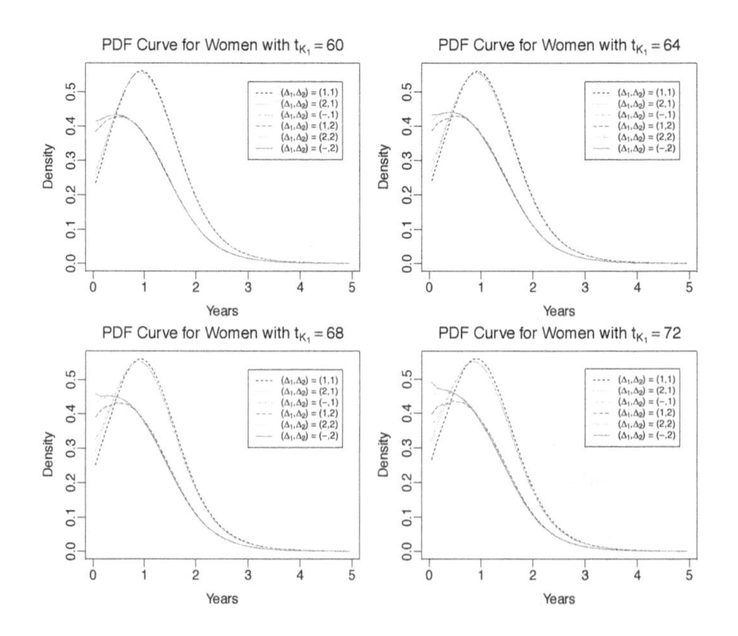

FIGURE 4.17
The lead time curve for female heavy smokers with screening history when $t_0 = 56$: 6 curves of different (Δ_1, Δ_2) are provided at four current ages, $t_{K_1} = 60$, 64, 68, and 72. Adapted from Figure 8 in Liu et al 2021 [34].

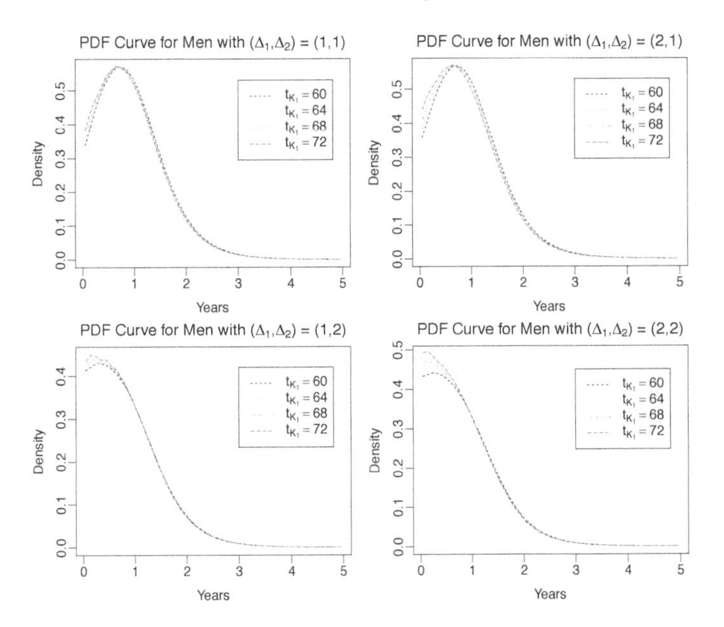

FIGURE 4.18
The lead time curve for male heavy smokers with screening history when $t_0 = 56$: 4 curves of different current ages are provided for four screening schedules, $(\Delta_1, \Delta_2) =$ (1,1), (2,1), (1,2), and (2,2). Adapted from Figure 9 in Liu et al 2021 [34].

For both genders, it is obvious that the probability P_0 increases and the mean lead time decreases as the future screening interval Δ_2 increases within the same age group. Across the (current) age groups, the probability P_0 and the mean lead time does not change much. To illustrate, the lead time density curves of males and females are plotted in Figures 4.18 and 4.19, respectively. Four panels represent four different screening schedules, and four curves represent four current ages in each panel. In each panel, the curves do not differ too much except in the very beginning.

The projected lead time is significantly affected by gender. Compared to females, males usually have a larger P_0 and a shorter mean lead time, given the same age and the same screening schedule. It seems that male heavy smokers have a smaller chance to be detected early by LDCT screening than their female counterparts do.

4.5 Model extension: When sensitivity is a function of sojourn time

As we have pointed out, sensitivity may not only depend on one's age. In practice, it may depend more on how long an individual has stayed in the

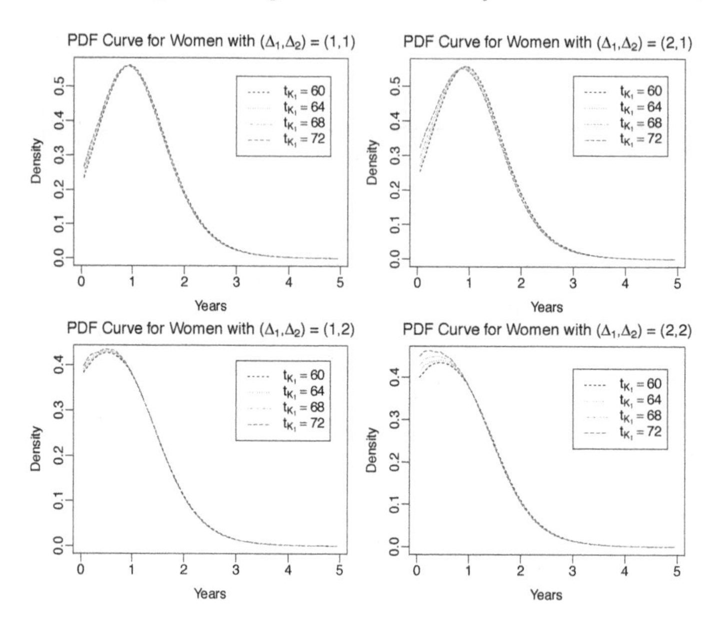

FIGURE 4.19
The lead time curve for female heavy smokers with screening history when $t_0 = 56$: 4 curves of different current ages are provided for four screening schedules, $(\Delta_1, \Delta_2) =$ (1,1), (2,1), (1,2), and (2,2). Adapted from Figure 10 in Liu et al 2021 [34].

preclinical state, relative to the whole duration of the sojourn time in the S_p. In other words, it depends on how far the tumor cells have developed. It is very hard to diagnose the tumors until they have reached a macroscopic dimension that usually have a cell population of about 10^9 and are at least 31 generations from the first post-malignant division [6]. Therefore, we modeled sensitivity as a function of the time spent in the preclinical state and the sojourn time [12]. The method allows us to provide an accurate estimation of the onset age of the preclinical state, the sojourn time in the preclinical state, and screening sensitivity at the onset and late stage of the preclinical state. This lays a foundation for all other parameter estimation and modeling. See section 2.5.2 for details.

We will expand the lead time methods by allowing the sensitivity to be a function of the ratio of time spent in the preclinical state and the sojourn time. We let $\beta(s|S), 0 \leq s \leq S$ be the sensitivity, where s is the length of time that one has stayed in the state S_p, and the sojourn time in the preclinical state S is a random variable. Intuitively, β will increase as s increases and will decrease as S increases. We define $w(t), q(x)$, and $Q(x)$ as before, representing the transition density, the sojourn time density, and its survival function, respectively. All probability calculations will change from one-dimensional integral to two-dimensional integral appropriately.

4.5.1 Lead time distribution without any screening history

Consider an asymptomatic woman at her current age t_0 without a history of lung cancer, and plans to undergo K ordered screenings at her age $t_0 < t_1 < \cdots < t_{K-1}$. We first derive the lead time distribution when her lifetime $T = t > t_{K-1}$ is fixed, then we allow her lifetime T to be random.

Let L denote the lead time, and let D represent disease status, with $D = 1$ indicating the development of clinical disease, and $D = 0$ indicating the absence of the disease. When $T = t > t_{K-1}$ is fixed, the lead time distribution is a mixture of a point mass at zero and a piece-wise continuous density [72]:

$$\begin{aligned} P(L=0|D=1,T=t) &= \frac{P(L=0,D=1|T=t)}{P(D=1|T=t)}, \\ f_L(z|D=1,T=t) &= \frac{f_L(z,D=1|T=t)}{P(D=1|T=t)}. \end{aligned} \tag{4.37}$$

Where the denominator is the same as in equation (4.2):

$$\begin{aligned} &P(D=1|T=t) \\ &= \int_0^{t_0} w(x)[Q(t_0-x)-Q(t-x)]dx + \int_{t_0}^{t} w(x)[1-Q(t-x)]dx. \end{aligned}$$

The probability that the lead time is zero in equation (4.37) is

$$\begin{aligned} P(L=0,D=1|T=t) &= I_{K,1}+I_{K,2}+\cdots+I_{K,K}, \\ I_{K,j} &= \sum_{i=0}^{j-1}\int_{t_{i-1}}^{t_i} w(x)\int_{t_{j-1}-x}^{t_j-x} q(t)\left\{\prod_{r=i}^{j-1}[1-\beta(t_r-x|t)]\right\}dtdx \\ &\quad + \int_{t_{j-1}}^{t_j} w(x)[1-Q(t_j-x)]dx, \text{ for all } j=1,\cdots,K. \end{aligned} \tag{4.38}$$

The joint probability density when the lead time is positive:

$$\begin{aligned} &f_L(z,D=1|T=t) \\ &= \int_0^{t_0} w(x)q(t_0+z-x)\beta(t_0-x|t_0+z-x)dx, \text{ if } t-t_1 < z \leq t-t_0. \\ &f_L(z,D=1|T=t) \\ &= \sum_{i=1}^{j-1}\left\{\sum_{r=0}^{i-1}\int_{t_{r-1}}^{t_r} w(x)q(t_i+z-x)\beta(t_i-x|t_i+z-x)\right. \\ &\quad \times\left(\prod_{m=r}^{i-1}[1-\beta(t_r-x|t_i+z-x)]\right)dx \\ &\quad \left.+\int_{t_{i-1}}^{t_i} w(x)q(t_i+z-x)\beta(t_i-x|t_i+z-x)dx\right\} \\ &\quad + \int_0^{t_0} w(x)q(t_0+z-x)\beta(t_0-x|t_0+z-x)dx. \\ &\quad \text{if } t-t_j < z \leq t-t_{j-1}, j=2,3,\cdots,K. \end{aligned} \tag{4.39}$$

Exercise 4.8. Prove that

$$P(L=0|D=1,T=t)+\int_0^{t-t_0} f_L(z|D=1,T=t)dz=1.$$

Hence the mixed distribution is valid.

When the lifetime T is a random variable, the lead time distribution can be obtained by

$$\begin{aligned}
&P(L=0|D=1,T>t_0)\\
&=\int_{t_0}^{\infty} P(L=0|D=1,T=t)f_T(t|T>t_0)dt,\\
&f_L(z|D=1,T>t_0)\\
&=\int_{t_0+z}^{\infty} f_L(z|D=1,T=t)f_T(t|T>t_0)dt, \quad z\in(0,\infty),
\end{aligned} \tag{4.40}$$

where the conditional PDF of human life was derived from the actuarial life table on the US Social Security Administration (SSA) website [72]:

$$f_T(t|T>t_0)=\begin{cases} \frac{f_T(t)}{P(T>t_0)}=\frac{f_T(t)}{1-F_T(t_0)}, & \text{if } t>t_0\\ 0, & \text{otherwise}\end{cases} \tag{4.41}$$

And we can prove that

$$P(L=0|D=1,T>t_0)+\int_0^{\infty} f_L(z|D=1,T>t_0)dz=1,$$

showing that it is a valid mixture distribution.

4.5.2 Lead time distribution with a screening history

Assume a woman at current age t_{K_1} has gone through K_1 exams before, at her age $t_0<t_1<\cdots<t_{K_1-1}$, all test results were negative, and she plans to take K more exams at the future age $t_{K_1}<t_{K_1+1}<t_{K_1+2}<\cdots<t_{K_1+K-1}$. We consider the general case for any positive integer $K_1\geq 1$ and $K\geq 1$, and define the event:

$$H_{K_1}=\left\{\begin{array}{l}\text{A woman had screening exams at her age}\\ t_0<t_1<\cdots<t_{K_1-1}, \text{no cancer was detected,}\\ \text{and she is asymptomatic at her current age } t_{K_1}\end{array}\right\}.$$

We first derive the distribution of lead time when human lifetime T is fixed, then we allow T to be random. When the lifetime $T=t(>t_{K_1-1})$ is fixed, the distribution of lead time is

$$\begin{aligned}
P(L=0|D=1,H_{K_1},T=t)&=\frac{P(L=0,D=1,H_{K_1}|T=t)}{P(D=1,H_{K_1}|T=t)},\\
f_L(z|D=1,H_{K_1},T=t)&=\frac{f_L(z,D=1,H_{K_1}|T=t)}{P(D=1,H_{K_1}|T=t)}.
\end{aligned} \tag{4.42}$$

To obtain $P(D=1, H_{K_1}|T=t)$, the probability of having clinical cancer in (t_{K_1}, t) and with a sequence of exams at age $t_0 < t_1 < \cdots < t_{K_1-1}$), this could happen in (K_1+2) disjoint ways: (i) She enters the preclinical state S_p in $(t_{i-1}, t_i), i = 0, 1, \ldots, K_1 - 1$, and her cancer was not detected by the exams at $t_i, \ldots, t_{K_1-1}$; (ii) she enters S_p in (t_{K_1-1}, t_{K_1}); and (iii) she enters S_p in (t_{K_1}, t). And in cases (i) and (ii), her sojourn time is longer than $t_{K_1} - x$, but shorter than $(t-x)$, where x is the onset of the S_p; in case (iii) her sojourn time is shorter than $(t-x)$. Since the sensitivity depends on the sojourn time, we have to put it inside the integral. And we add these probabilities:

$$
\begin{aligned}
&P(D=1, H_{K_1}|T=t) \\
&= \sum_{i=0}^{K_1-1} \int_{t_{i-1}}^{t_i} w(x) \int_{t_{K_1}-x}^{t-x} q(t) \prod_{r=i}^{K_1-1} [1-\beta(t_r - x|t)] dt\, dx \\
&+ \int_{t_{K_1-1}}^{t_{K_1}} w(x)[Q(t_{K_1}-x) - Q(t-x)]\, dx \\
&+ \int_{t_{K_1}}^{t} w(x)[1-Q(t-x)]\, dx.
\end{aligned} \tag{4.43}
$$

To calculate $P(L=0, D=1, H_{K_1}|T=t)$, we denote $T = t = t_{K_1+K}$ to simplify notation, but keep in mind that $t = t_{K_1+K}$ is not a screening time, but the lifetime. We $I_{K_1+K,j}$ represent the probability of incidence in (t_{j-1}, t_j), $j = K_1+1, K_1+2, \ldots, K_1+K$, then

$$
\begin{aligned}
&P(L=0, D=1, H_{K_1}|T=t) \\
=&I_{K_1+K,K_1+1} + I_{K_1+K,K_1+2} + \cdots + I_{K_1+K,K_1+K},
\end{aligned} \tag{4.44}
$$

where

$$
\begin{aligned}
I_{K_1+K,\, j} =& \sum_{i=0}^{j-1} \int_{t_{i-1}}^{t_i} w(x) \int_{t_{j-1}-x}^{t_j - x} q(t) \prod_{r=i}^{j-1} [1-\beta(t_r - x|t) dt\, dx \\
&+ \int_{t_{j-1}}^{t_j} w(x)[1-Q(t_j - x)]\, dx, \\
&\text{for } j = K_1+1, \cdots, K_1+K.
\end{aligned} \tag{4.45}
$$

Finally, if $t - t_j < z \le t - t_{j-1}$, for $j = K_1+1, \ldots, K_1+K$, the PDF of lead time at z is

$$
\begin{aligned}
&f_L(z, D=1, H_{K_1}|T=t) \\
&= \sum_{i=K_1}^{j-1} \left\{ \sum_{n=0}^{i-1} \int_{t_{n-1}}^{t_n} w(x) q(t_i + z - x) \beta(t_i - x|t_i + z - x) \right. \\
&\times \prod_{r=n}^{i-1} [1-\beta(t_r - x|t_i + z - x)]\, dx \\
&\left. + \int_{t_{i-1}}^{t_i} w(x) q(t_i + z - x) \beta(t_i - x|t_i + z - x)\, dx \right\}.
\end{aligned} \tag{4.46}
$$

Exercise 4.9. Prove that

$$P(L=0|D=1,H_{K_1},T=t)+\int_0^{T-t_{K_1}} f_L(z|D=1,H_{K_1},T=t)\,dz \equiv 1.$$

Therefore, this mixed probability distribution is valid. When the lifetime T is random, the lead time distribution when T is greater than the current age t_{K_1} can be obtained by

$$\begin{aligned}
&P(L=0|D=1,H_{K_1},T>t_{K_1})\\
&=\int_{t_{K_1}}^{\infty} P(L=0|D=1,H_{K_1},T=t)f_T(t|T>t_{K_1})\,dt,\\
&f_L(z|D=1,H_{K_1},T>t_{K_1})\\
&=\int_{t_{K_1}+z}^{\infty} f_L(z|D=1,H_{K_1},T=t)f_T(t|T>t_{K_1})\,dt,\\
&z\in(0,\infty),
\end{aligned} \tag{4.47}$$

where

$$f_T(t|T>t_{K_1})=\begin{cases} \frac{f_T(t)}{P(T>t_{K_1})}=\frac{f_T(t)}{1-F_T(t_{K_1})}, & \text{if } t>t_{K_1},\\ 0, & \text{otherwise.}\end{cases}$$

And the lifetime distribution density $f_T(t|T>t_{K_1})$ can be obtained by using the US Social Security Administration's actuarial life table [72].

Exercise 4.10. Prove that

$$P(L=0|D=1,H_{K_1},T>t_{K_1})+\int_0^{\infty} f_L(z|D=1,H_{K_1},T>t_{K_1})dz=1.$$

For a person at her current age t_{K_1}, if she plans to follow a future screening schedule, such as $t_{K_1}<t_{K_1+1}<\ldots$, then the number of screenings in the future $K=n$ if $t_{K_1+n-1}<T\le t_{K_1+n}$; therefore the future screening number $K=K(T)$ is random if the lifetime T is random. If the future screening exam is equally spaced with a time interval Δ, then $K=K(T)=\lceil (T-t_{K_1})/\Delta\rceil$.

4.6 Bibliographic notes

The methods in the chapter were published in three papers: Wu et al 2007 [80], Wu et al 2012 [72], and Liu et al 2021 [34].

The idea of developing a lead time model including both screen-detected and interval cases was started in 2021 after I read the paper of Prorok 1982

[42]. The first result was published in the 2006 JSM proceedings [81]. The method of the lead time distribution when the lifetime is fixed (section 4.2) was published in Wu et al 2007 [80]. Wu et al 2012 extended the method to the case when the lifetime is random [72] (section 4.3). The lead time distribution for people with a screening history (section 4.4) was derived by Liu et al 2021 [34], and it was part of Dr. Liu's PhD dissertation. I laid out the probability calculation in section 4.5, it is ongoing research, I have not done much simulation for the methods in section 4.5, and readers may explore that further.

There were some research articles that applied the methods in this chapter to different cancer screening data. Wu et al 2009 estimated the lead time distribution for colorectal cancer using the Minnesota colorectal data [66]. Wu et al 2011 applied the lead time method to lung cancer screening using the Mayo Lung Project data [67]. The lifetime was assumed to be a fixed value in both papers. Jang et al 2013 estimated the lead time distribution using the Johns Hopkins Lung Project (JHLP) data when the lifetime is random [21]. Liu et al 2018 estimated the projected lead time for male and female heavy smokers using the NLST low-dose CT data with the lifetime as a random variable [33].

There are some publications that focus on simulations of the lead time. Shows and Wu 2011 carried out the lead time simulation under the stable disease model, where the sensitivity and the transition density are both constants across all age groups [50]. Kendrick et al 2015 implemented simulation studies on the lead time when the human lifetime is random [25]. Liu et al 2017 is a good review article on the estimation of three key parameters and the lead time modeling [31].

4.7 Solution for some exercises

Exercise 4.2

Proof: We want to prove

$$P(L=0, D=1|T=t) + \int_0^{t-t_0} f_L(z, D=1|T=t)dz = P(D=1|T=t)$$

$$= \int_0^{t_0} w(x)[Q(t_0-x) - Q(t-x)]dx + \int_{t_0}^{t} w(x)[1 - Q(t-x)dx.$$

We let $T = t = t_K$ and organize the probability of interval cases into four parts of $\mathbf{A}, \mathbf{B}, \mathbf{C}, \mathbf{D}$:

$$P(L=0, D=1|T=t) = I_{K,1} + I_{K,2} + \cdots + I_{K,K}$$

$$
\begin{aligned}
&= \sum_{j=1}^{K}\left\{\sum_{i=0}^{j-1}(1-\beta_i)\cdots(1-\beta_{j-1})\int_{t_{i-1}}^{t_i} w(x)\{Q(t_{j-1}-x)-Q(t_j-x)\}dx \right.\\
&\quad \left. + \int_{t_{j-1}}^{t_j} w(x)\{1-Q(t_j-x)\}dx\right\}\\
&= \sum_{j=1}^{K}\sum_{i=0}^{j-1}(1-\beta_i)\cdots(1-\beta_{j-1})\int_{t_{i-1}}^{t_i} w(x)Q(t_{j-1}-x)dx\\
&\quad -\sum_{j=1}^{K}\sum_{i=0}^{j-1}(1-\beta_i)\cdots(1-\beta_{j-1})\int_{t_{i-1}}^{t_i} w(x)Q(t_j-x)dx\\
&\quad + \int_{t_0}^{t} w(x)dx - \sum_{j=1}^{K}\int_{t_{j-1}}^{t_j} w(x)Q(t_j-x)dx\\
&\equiv \mathbf{A}-\mathbf{B}+\mathbf{C}-\mathbf{D}.
\end{aligned}
$$

For the integration part, we break it down at $(t-t_j, t-t_{j-1})$, and swap dx and dz:

$$
\begin{aligned}
&\int_0^{t-t_0} f_L(z, D=1|T=t_K)dz\\
&= \sum_{j=2}^{K}\int_{t-t_j}^{t-t_{j-1}} f_L(z, D=1|T=t_K)dz + \int_{t-t_1}^{t-t_0} f_L(z, D=1|T=t_K)dz\\
&= \sum_{j=2}^{K}\int_{t-t_j}^{t-t_{j-1}}\sum_{i=1}^{j-1}\beta_i\left\{\sum_{r=0}^{i-1}(1-\beta_r)\cdots(1-\beta_{i-1})\int_{t_{r-1}}^{t_r} w(x)q(t_i+z-x)dx\right.\\
&\quad \left. + \int_{t_{i-1}}^{t_i} w(x)q(t_i+z-x)dx\right\} + \beta_0\int_0^{t_0} w(x)q(t_0+z-x)dxdz\\
&\quad + \int_{t-t_1}^{t-t_0}\beta_0\int_0^{t_0} w(x)q(t_0+z-x)dxdz
\end{aligned}
$$

$$
\begin{aligned}
&= \sum_{j=2}^{K}\int_{t-t_j}^{t-t_{j-1}}\sum_{i=1}^{j-1}\beta_i\left\{\sum_{r=0}^{i-1}(1-\beta_r)\cdots(1-\beta_{i-1})\int_{t_{r-1}}^{t_r} w(x)q(t_i+z-x)dx\right.\\
&\quad \left. + \int_{t_{i-1}}^{t_i} w(x)q(t_i+z-x)dx\right\}dz \qquad \text{(swap dx and dz)}\\
&\quad + \int_0^{t-t_0}\beta_0\int_0^{t_0} w(x)q(t_0+z-x)dxdz
\end{aligned}
$$

$$
\begin{aligned}
= & \sum_{j=2}^{K}\sum_{i=1}^{j-1}\beta_i\left\{\sum_{r=0}^{i-1}(1-\beta_r)\cdots(1-\beta_{i-1})\int_{t_{r-1}}^{t_r} w(x)\right. \\
& \left.\times\int_{t-t_j}^{t-t_{j-1}} q(t_i+z-x)dzdx + \int_{t_{i-1}}^{t_i} w(x)\int_{t-t_j}^{t-t_{j-1}} q(t_i+z-x)dzdx\right\} \\
& +\beta_0\int_0^{t_0} w(x)[Q(t_0-x)-Q(t-x)]dx \\
= & \sum_{j=2}^{K}\sum_{i=1}^{j-1}\beta_i\left\{\sum_{r=0}^{i-1}(1-\beta_r)\cdots(1-\beta_{i-1}) \text{ next: swap sum of j and i}\right. \\
& \times\int_{t_{r-1}}^{t_r} w(x)[Q(t_i-x+t-t_j)-Q(t_i-x+t-t_{j-1})]dx \\
& \left.+\int_{t_{i-1}}^{t_i} w(x)[Q(t_i-x+t-t_j)-Q(t_i-x+t-t_{j-1})]dx\right\} \\
& +\beta_0\int_0^{t_0} w(x)[Q(t_0-x)-Q(t-x)]dx
\end{aligned}
$$

$$
\begin{aligned}
= & \sum_{i=1}^{K-1}\sum_{j=i+1}^{K}\beta_i\left\{\sum_{r=0}^{i-1}(1-\beta_r)\cdots(1-\beta_{i-1}) \text{ next: swap sum of j and r}\right. \\
& \times\int_{t_{r-1}}^{t_r} w(x)[Q(t_i-x+t-t_j)-Q(t_i-x+t-t_{j-1})]dx \\
& \left.+\int_{t_{i-1}}^{t_i} w(x)[Q(t_i-x+t-t_j)-Q(t_i-x+t-t_{j-1})]dx\right\} \\
& +\beta_0\int_0^{t_0} w(x)[Q(t_0-x)-Q(t-x)]dx \\
= & \sum_{i=1}^{K-1}\beta_i\sum_{r=0}^{i-1}(1-\beta_r)\cdots(1-\beta_{i-1}) \\
& \times\sum_{j=i+1}^{K}\int_{t_{r-1}}^{t_r} w(x)[Q(t_i-x+t-t_j)-Q(t_i-x+t-t_{j-1})]dx \\
& +\sum_{i=1}^{K-1}\beta_i\sum_{j=i+1}^{K}\int_{t_{i-1}}^{t_i} w(x)[Q(t_i-x+t-t_j)-Q(t_i-x+t-t_{j-1})]dx \\
& +\beta_0\int_0^{t_0} w(x)[Q(t_0-x)-Q(t-x)]dx
\end{aligned}
$$

$$= \sum_{i=1}^{K-1}\beta_i\sum_{r=0}^{i-1}(1-\beta_r)\cdots(1-\beta_{i-1})\sum_{j=i+1}^{K}\int_{t_{r-1}}^{t_r} w(x)Q(t_i-x+t-t_j)dx$$
$$-\sum_{i=1}^{K-1}\beta_i\sum_{r=0}^{i-1}(1-\beta_r)\cdots(1-\beta_{i-1})\sum_{j=i+1}^{K}\int_{t_{r-1}}^{t_r} w(x)Q(t_i-x+t-t_{j-1})dx$$
$$+\sum_{i=1}^{K-1}\beta_i\sum_{j=i+1}^{K}\int_{t_{i-1}}^{t_i} w(x)Q(t_i-x+t-t_j)dx$$
$$-\sum_{i=1}^{K-1}\beta_i\sum_{j=i+1}^{K}\int_{t_{i-1}}^{t_i} w(x)Q(t_i-x+t-t_{j-1})dx$$
$$+\beta_0\int_0^{t_0} w(x)[Q(t_0-x)-Q(t-x)]dx.$$

Now we change index by letting $l = j-1$ in the second and fourth items above:

$$\int_0^{t-t_0} f_L(z, D=1|T=t=t_K)dz$$
$$= \sum_{i=1}^{K-1}\beta_i\sum_{r=0}^{i-1}(1-\beta_r)\cdots(1-\beta_{i-1})\sum_{j=i+1}^{K}\int_{t_{r-1}}^{t_r} w(x)Q(t_i-x+t-t_j)dx$$
$$-\sum_{i=1}^{K-1}\beta_i\sum_{r=0}^{i-1}(1-\beta_r)\cdots(1-\beta_{i-1})\sum_{l=i}^{K-1}\int_{t_{r-1}}^{t_r} w(x)Q(t_i-x+t-t_l)dx$$
$$+\sum_{i=1}^{K-1}\beta_i\sum_{j=i+1}^{K}\int_{t_{i-1}}^{t_i} w(x)Q(t_i-x+t-t_j)dx$$
$$-\sum_{i=1}^{K-1}\beta_i\sum_{l=i}^{K-1}\int_{t_{i-1}}^{t_i} w(x)Q(t_i-x+t-t_l)dx$$
$$+\beta_0\int_0^{t_0} w(x)[Q(t_0-x)-Q(t-x)]dx$$
$$= \sum_{i=1}^{K-1}\beta_i\sum_{r=0}^{i-1}(1-\beta_r)\cdots(1-\beta_{i-1})\int_{t_{r-1}}^{t_r} w(x)Q(t_i-x)dx \ (i\to j, r\to i)$$
$$-\sum_{i=1}^{K-1}\beta_i\sum_{r=0}^{i-1}(1-\beta_r)\cdots(1-\beta_{i-1})\int_{t_{r-1}}^{t_r} w(x)Q(t-x)dx$$
$$+\sum_{i=1}^{K-1}\beta_i\int_{t_{i-1}}^{t_i} w(x)Q(t_i-x)dx-\sum_{i=1}^{K-1}\beta_i\int_{t_{i-1}}^{t_i} w(x)Q(t-x)dx$$

$$
\begin{aligned}
&+\beta_0 \int_0^{t_0} w(x)[Q(t_0 - x) - Q(t - x)]dx \\
= &\sum_{j=1}^{K-1} \beta_j \sum_{i=0}^{j-1} (1-\beta_i)\cdots(1-\beta_{j-1}) \int_{t_{i-1}}^{t_i} w(x)Q(t_j - x)dx \\
&- \sum_{j=1}^{K-1} \beta_j \sum_{i=0}^{j-1} (1-\beta_i)\cdots(1-\beta_{j-1}) \int_{t_{i-1}}^{t_i} w(x)Q(t - x)dx \\
&+ \sum_{i=1}^{K-1} \beta_i \int_{t_{i-1}}^{t_i} w(x)Q(t_i - x)dx - \sum_{i=1}^{K-1} \beta_i \int_{t_{i-1}}^{t_i} w(x)Q(t - x)dx \\
&+\beta_0 \int_0^{t_0} w(x)[Q(t_0 - x) - Q(t - x)]dx \\
= &\mathbf{E} - \mathbf{F} + \mathbf{G} - \mathbf{H} + \mathbf{I}
\end{aligned}
$$

Compare with the $P(L = 0, D = 1) = \mathbf{A} - \mathbf{B} + \mathbf{C} - \mathbf{D}$, we have

$$
\begin{aligned}
\mathbf{E} - \mathbf{B} = &\sum_{j=1}^{K-1} (\beta_j - 1) \sum_{i=0}^{j-1} (1-\beta_i)\cdots(1-\beta_{j-1}) \int_{t_{i-1}}^{t_i} w(x)Q(t_j - x)dx \\
&- \sum_{i=0}^{K-1} (1-\beta_i)\cdots(1-\beta_{K-1}) \int_{t_{i-1}}^{t_i} w(x)Q(t_K - x)dx \\
= &- \sum_{j=1}^{K-1} \sum_{i=0}^{j-1} (1-\beta_i)\cdots(1-\beta_j) \int_{t_{i-1}}^{t_i} w(x)Q(t_j - x)dx \\
&- \sum_{i=0}^{K-1} (1-\beta_i)\cdots(1-\beta_{K-1}) \int_{t_{i-1}}^{t_i} w(x)Q(t - x)dx.
\end{aligned}
$$

Now combine with $\mathbf{A}$, and let $l = j - 1$:

$$
\begin{aligned}
\mathbf{A} + \mathbf{E} - \mathbf{B} = &\sum_{j=1}^{K} \sum_{i=0}^{j-1} (1-\beta_i)\cdots(1-\beta_{j-1}) \int_{t_{i-1}}^{t_i} w(x)Q(t_{j-1} - x)dx \\
&- \sum_{j=1}^{K-1} \sum_{i=0}^{j-1} (1-\beta_i)\cdots(1-\beta_j) \int_{t_{i-1}}^{t_i} w(x)Q(t_j - x)dx \\
&- \sum_{i=0}^{K-1} (1-\beta_i)\cdots(1-\beta_{K-1}) \int_{t_{i-1}}^{t_i} w(x)Q(t - x)dx
\end{aligned}
$$

$$
\begin{aligned}
&= \sum_{l=0}^{K-1}\sum_{i=0}^{l}(1-\beta_i)\cdots(1-\beta_l)\int_{t_{i-1}}^{t_i} w(x)Q(t_l-x)dx \\
&\quad -\sum_{j=1}^{K-1}\sum_{i=0}^{j-1}(1-\beta_i)\cdots(1-\beta_j)\int_{t_{i-1}}^{t_i} w(x)Q(t_j-x)dx \\
&\quad -\sum_{i=0}^{K-1}(1-\beta_i)\cdots(1-\beta_{K-1})\int_{t_{i-1}}^{t_i} w(x)Q(t-x)dx \\
&= \sum_{j=1}^{K-1}\sum_{i=0}^{j}(1-\beta_i)\cdots(1-\beta_j)\int_{t_{i-1}}^{t_i} w(x)Q(t_j-x)dx \\
&\quad +(1-\beta_0)\int_{0}^{t_0} w(x)Q(t_0-x)dx \\
&\quad -\sum_{j=1}^{K-1}\sum_{i=0}^{j-1}(1-\beta_i)\cdots(1-\beta_j)\int_{t_{i-1}}^{t_i} w(x)Q(t_j-x)dx \\
&\quad -\sum_{i=0}^{K-1}(1-\beta_i)\cdots(1-\beta_{K-1})\int_{t_{i-1}}^{t_i} w(x)Q(t-x)dx
\end{aligned}
$$

$$
\begin{aligned}
&= \sum_{j=1}^{K-1}(1-\beta_j)\int_{t_{j-1}}^{t_j} w(x)Q(t_j-x)dx + (1-\beta_0)\int_{0}^{t_0} w(x)Q(t_0-x)dx \\
&\quad -\sum_{i=0}^{K-1}(1-\beta_i)\cdots(1-\beta_{K-1})\int_{t_{i-1}}^{t_i} w(x)Q(t-x)dx
\end{aligned}
$$

Now combine more terms:

$$
\begin{aligned}
\mathbf{A}-\mathbf{B}+\mathbf{E}+\mathbf{G} &= \sum_{j=1}^{K-1}(1-\beta_j)\int_{t_{j-1}}^{t_j} w(x)Q(t_j-x)dx \\
&\quad +(1-\beta_0)\int_{0}^{t_0} w(x)Q(t_0-x)dx \\
&\quad -\sum_{i=0}^{K-1}(1-\beta_i)\cdots(1-\beta_{K-1})\int_{t_{i-1}}^{t_i} w(x)Q(t-x)dx \\
&\quad +\sum_{i=1}^{K-1}\beta_i\int_{t_{i-1}}^{t_i} w(x)Q(t_i-x)dx
\end{aligned}
$$

$$
\begin{aligned}
&= \sum_{j=1}^{K-1} \int_{t_{j-1}}^{t_j} w(x)Q(t_j - x)dx + (1-\beta_0)\int_0^{t_0} w(x)Q(t_0 - x)dx \\
&\quad - \sum_{i=0}^{K-1} (1-\beta_i)\cdots(1-\beta_{K-1}) \int_{t_{i-1}}^{t_i} w(x)Q(t-x)dx.
\end{aligned}
$$

Hence,

$$
\begin{aligned}
&\mathbf{A} - \mathbf{B} + \mathbf{E} + \mathbf{G} + \mathbf{I} \\
&= \sum_{j=1}^{K-1} \int_{t_{j-1}}^{t_j} w(x)Q(t_j - x)dx + (1-\beta_0)\int_0^{t_0} w(x)Q(t_0 - x)dx \\
&\quad - \sum_{i=0}^{K-1} (1-\beta_i)\cdots(1-\beta_{K-1}) \int_{t_{i-1}}^{t_i} w(x)Q(t-x)dx \\
&\quad +\beta_0 \int_0^{t_0} w(x)[Q(t_0 - x) - Q(t-x)]dx \\
&= \sum_{j=1}^{K-1} \int_{t_{j-1}}^{t_j} w(x)Q(t_j - x)dx + \int_0^{t_0} w(x)Q(t_0 - x)dx \\
&\quad - \sum_{i=0}^{K-1} (1-\beta_i)\cdots(1-\beta_{K-1}) \int_{t_{i-1}}^{t_i} w(x)Q(t-x)dx \\
&\quad -\beta_0 \int_0^{t_0} w(x)Q(t-x)dx.
\end{aligned}
$$

$$
\begin{aligned}
&\mathbf{A} - \mathbf{B} + \mathbf{E} + \mathbf{G} + \mathbf{I} - \mathbf{D} \\
&= \sum_{j=1}^{K-1} \int_{t_{j-1}}^{t_j} w(x)Q(t_j - x)dx + \int_0^{t_0} w(x)Q(t_0 - x)dx \\
&\quad - \sum_{i=0}^{K-1} (1-\beta_i)\cdots(1-\beta_{K-1}) \int_{t_{i-1}}^{t_i} w(x)Q(t-x)dx \\
&\quad -\beta_0 \int_0^{t_0} w(x)Q(t-x)dx - \sum_{j=1}^{K} \int_{t_{j-1}}^{t_j} w(x)Q(t_j - x)dx \\
&= \int_0^{t_0} w(x)Q(t_0 - x)dx - \int_{t_{K-1}}^{t_K} w(x)Q(t-x)dx \\
&\quad - \sum_{i=0}^{K-1} (1-\beta_i)\cdots(1-\beta_{K-1}) \int_{t_{i-1}}^{t_i} w(x)Q(t-x)dx \\
&\quad -\beta_0 \int_0^{t_0} w(x)Q(t-x)dx.
\end{aligned}
$$

Now rewrite $-\mathbf{F}$:

$$
\begin{aligned}
-\mathbf{F} &= \sum_{j=1}^{K-1}(-\beta_j)\sum_{i=0}^{j-1}(1-\beta_i)\cdots(1-\beta_{j-1})\int_{t_{i-1}}^{t_i} w(x)Q(t-x)dx \\
&= \sum_{j=1}^{K-1}(1-\beta_j-1)\sum_{i=0}^{j-1}(1-\beta_i)\cdots(1-\beta_{j-1})\int_{t_{i-1}}^{t_i} w(x)Q(t-x)dx \\
&= \sum_{j=1}^{K-1}(1-\beta_j)\sum_{i=0}^{j-1}(1-\beta_i)\cdots(1-\beta_{j-1})\int_{t_{i-1}}^{t_i} w(x)Q(t-x)dx \\
&\quad - \sum_{j=1}^{K-1}\sum_{i=0}^{j-1}(1-\beta_i)\cdots(1-\beta_{j-1})\int_{t_{i-1}}^{t_i} w(x)Q(t-x)dx \\
&= \sum_{j=1}^{K-1}\sum_{i=0}^{j-1}(1-\beta_i)\cdots(1-\beta_{j-1})(1-\beta_j)\int_{t_{i-1}}^{t_i} w(x)Q(t-x)dx \\
&\quad - \sum_{j=1}^{K-1}\sum_{i=0}^{j-1}(1-\beta_i)\cdots(1-\beta_{j-1})\int_{t_{i-1}}^{t_i} w(x)Q(t-x)dx \\
&= \sum_{j=1}^{K-1}\left\{\sum_{i=0}^{j}(1-\beta_i)\cdots(1-\beta_{j-1})(1-\beta_j)\int_{t_{i-1}}^{t_i} w(x)Q(t-x)dx\right. \\
&\quad \left. - (1-\beta_j)\int_{t_{j-1}}^{t_j} w(x)Q(t-x)dx\right\} \\
&\quad - \sum_{j=1}^{K-1}\sum_{i=0}^{j-1}(1-\beta_i)\cdots(1-\beta_{j-1})\int_{t_{i-1}}^{t_i} w(x)Q(t-x)dx \\
&= \sum_{j=1}^{K-1}\sum_{i=0}^{j}(1-\beta_i)\cdots(1-\beta_j)\int_{t_{i-1}}^{t_i} w(x)Q(t-x)dx \\
&\quad - \sum_{j=1}^{K-1}\sum_{i=0}^{j-1}(1-\beta_i)\cdots(1-\beta_{j-1})\int_{t_{i-1}}^{t_i} w(x)Q(t-x)dx \\
&\quad - \sum_{j=1}^{K-1}(1-\beta_j)\int_{t_{j-1}}^{t_j} w(x)Q(t-x)dx \\
&= \sum_{j=1}^{K-1}\sum_{i=0}^{j}(1-\beta_i)\cdots(1-\beta_j)\int_{t_{i-1}}^{t_i} w(x)Q(t-x)dx \\
&\quad - \sum_{l=0}^{K-2}\sum_{i=0}^{l}(1-\beta_i)\cdots(1-\beta_l)\int_{t_{i-1}}^{t_i} w(x)Q(t-x)dx
\end{aligned}
$$

$$
\begin{aligned}
& -\sum_{j=1}^{K-1}(1-\beta_j)\int_{t_{j-1}}^{t_j} w(x)Q(t-x)dx \\
= & \sum_{i=0}^{K-1}(1-\beta_i)\cdots(1-\beta_{K-1})\int_{t_{i-1}}^{t_i} w(x)Q(t-x)dx \\
& -(1-\beta_0)\int_0^{t_0} w(x)Q(t-x)dx - \sum_{j=1}^{K-1}(1-\beta_j)\int_{t_{j-1}}^{t_j} w(x)Q(t-x)dx.
\end{aligned}
$$

Now look at $-\mathbf{F}-\mathbf{H}$:

$$
\begin{aligned}
-\mathbf{F}-\mathbf{H} = & \sum_{i=0}^{K-1}(1-\beta_i)\cdots(1-\beta_{K-1})\int_{t_{i-1}}^{t_i} w(x)Q(t-x)dx \\
& -(1-\beta_0)\int_0^{t_0} w(x)Q(t-x)dx - \sum_{j=1}^{K-1}\int_{t_{j-1}}^{t_j} w(x)Q(t-x)dx. \\
= & \sum_{i=0}^{K-1}(1-\beta_i)\cdots(1-\beta_{K-1})\int_{t_{i-1}}^{t_i} w(x)Q(t-x)dx \\
& -(1-\beta_0)\int_0^{t_0} w(x)Q(t-x)dx - \int_{t_0}^{t_{K-1}} w(x)Q(t-x)dx.
\end{aligned}
$$

Finally, we put all the pieces together, and recall that $T = t = t_K$:

$$
\begin{aligned}
& P(L=0, D=1|T=t) + \int_0^{t-t_0} f_L(z, D=1|T=t)dz \\
= & \mathbf{C} + (\mathbf{A}-\mathbf{B}+\mathbf{E}+\mathbf{G}+\mathbf{I}-\mathbf{D}) - \mathbf{F} - \mathbf{H} \\
= & \int_{t_0}^{t} w(x)dx + \int_0^{t_0} w(x)Q(t_0-x)dx - \int_{t_{K-1}}^{t_K} w(x)Q(t-x)dx \\
& -\sum_{i=0}^{K-1}(1-\beta_i)\cdots(1-\beta_{K-1})\int_{t_{i-1}}^{t_i} w(x)Q(t-x)dx \\
& -\beta_0\int_0^{t_0} w(x)Q(t-x)dx \\
& +\sum_{i=0}^{K-1}(1-\beta_i)\cdots(1-\beta_{K-1})\int_{t_{i-1}}^{t_i} w(x)Q(t-x)dx \\
& -(1-\beta_0)\int_0^{t_0} w(x)Q(t-x)dx - \int_{t_0}^{t_{K-1}} w(x)Q(t-x)dx.
\end{aligned}
$$

$$
\begin{aligned}
&= \int_{t_0}^{t} w(x)dx + \int_0^{t_0} w(x)Q(t_0-x)dx - \int_{t_{K-1}}^{t_K} w(x)Q(t-x)dx \\
&\quad - \int_0^{t_0} w(x)Q(t-x)dx - \int_{t_0}^{t_{K-1}} w(x)Q(Tt-x)dx. \\
&= \int_{t_0}^{t} w(x)dx + \int_0^{t_0} w(x)Q(t_0-x)dx - \int_{t_0}^{t} w(x)Q(t-x)dx \\
&\quad - \int_0^{t_0} w(x)Q(t-x)dx \\
&= \int_0^{t_0} w(x)[Q(t_0-x) - Q(t-x)]dx + \int_{t_0}^{t} w(x)[1-Q(t-x)dx \\
&= P(D=1|T=t=t_K).
\end{aligned}
$$

This finishes the proof.

Exercise 4.4

Proof:

$$
\begin{aligned}
&\int_0^{t-t_1} f_L(z, D=1, H_1|T=t)dz \\
&\quad = \int_0^{t-t_1} \left[\beta_1(1-\beta_0)\int_0^{t_0} w(x)q(t_1+z-x)dx \right. \\
&\quad\quad \left. + \beta_1 \int_{t_0}^{t_1} w(x)q(t_1+z-x)dx\right] dz \\
&\quad = \beta_1(1-\beta_0)\int_0^{t_0} w(x)\int_0^{t-t_1} q(t_1+z-x)dzdx \\
&\quad\quad + \beta_1 \int_{t_0}^{t_1} w(x)\int_0^{t-t_1} q(t_1+z-x)dzdx \\
&\quad = \beta_1(1-\beta_0)\int_0^{t_0} w(x)[Q(t_1-x) - Q(t-x)]dx \\
&\quad\quad + \beta_1 \int_{t_0}^{t_1} w(x)[Q(t_1-x) - Q(t-x)]dx
\end{aligned}
$$

Now start from the left size:

$$
\begin{aligned}
&P(L=0, D=1, H_1|T=t) + \int_0^{t-t_1} f_L(z, D=1, H_1|T=t)dz \\
&\quad = (1-\beta_0)\int_0^{t_0} w(x)[Q(a_0-x) - Q(t_1-x)]dx \\
&\quad\quad + \int_{t_0}^{a_0} w(x)[Q(a_0-x) - Q(t_1-x)]dx
\end{aligned}
$$

$$
\begin{aligned}
& + \int_{a_0}^{t_1} w(x)[1 - Q(t_1 - x)]dx \\
& +(1-\beta_0)(1-\beta_1) \int_0^{t_0} w(x)[Q(t_1 - x) - Q(t - x)]dx \\
& +(1-\beta_1) \int_{t_0}^{t_1} w(x)[Q(t_1 - x) - Q(t - x)]dx \\
& + \int_{t_1}^{t} w(x)[1 - Q(t - x)]dx \\
& +\beta_1(1-\beta_0) \int_0^{t_0} w(x)[Q(t_1 - x) - Q(t - x)]dx \\
& +\beta_1 \int_{t_0}^{t_1} w(x)[Q(t_1 - x) - Q(t - x)]dx \\
= \; & \mathbf{A} + \mathbf{B} + \mathbf{C} + \mathbf{D} + \mathbf{E} + \mathbf{F} + \mathbf{G} + \mathbf{H}
\end{aligned}
$$

Combine $(\mathbf{D} + \mathbf{G})$ and $(\mathbf{E} + \mathbf{H})$:

$$
\begin{aligned}
\mathbf{D} + \mathbf{G} &= (1-\beta_0) \int_0^{t_0} w(x)[Q(t_1 - x) - Q(t - x)]dx. \\
\mathbf{E} + \mathbf{H} &= \int_{t_0}^{t_1} w(x)[Q(t_1 - x) - Q(t - x)]dx.
\end{aligned}
$$

Now combine $\mathbf{A} + (\mathbf{D} + \mathbf{G})$:

$$
\mathbf{A} + (\mathbf{D} + \mathbf{G}) = (1-\beta_0) \int_0^{t_0} w(x)[Q(a_0 - x) - Q(t - x)]dx.
$$

Recall that $t_0 \le a_0 \le t_1$, we combine $\mathbf{B} + (\mathbf{E} + \mathbf{H})$:

$$
\begin{aligned}
& \mathbf{B} + (\mathbf{E} + \mathbf{H}) \\
= \; & \int_{t_0}^{a_0} w(x)[Q(a_0 - x) - Q(t_1 - x)]dx \\
& + \int_{t_0}^{a_0} w(x)[Q(t_1 - x) - Q(t - x)]dx + \int_{a_0}^{t_1} w(x)[Q(t_1 - x) - Q(t - x)]dx \\
= \; & \int_{t_0}^{a_0} w(x)[Q(a_0 - x) - Q(t - x)]dx + \int_{a_0}^{t_1} w(x)[Q(t_1 - x) - Q(t - x)]dx
\end{aligned}
$$

Now combine $\mathbf{B} + (\mathbf{E} + \mathbf{H}) + \mathbf{C}$:

$$
\mathbf{B} + (\mathbf{E} + \mathbf{H}) + \mathbf{C} = \int_{t_0}^{a_0} w(x)[Q(a_0 - x) - Q(t - x)]dx + \int_{a_0}^{t_1} w(x)[1 - Q(t - x)]dx
$$

Recall that $a_0 \leq t_1 < t$, combine $\mathbf{B} + (\mathbf{E} + \mathbf{H}) + \mathbf{C} + \mathbf{F}$:

$$\mathbf{B} + (\mathbf{E} + \mathbf{H}) + \mathbf{C} + \mathbf{F} = \int_{t_0}^{a_0} w(x)[Q(a_0 - x) - Q(t - x)]dx + \int_{a_0}^{t} w(x)[1 - Q(t - x)]dx.$$

Now add $\mathbf{A} + (\mathbf{D} + \mathbf{G})$ and $\mathbf{B} + (\mathbf{E} + \mathbf{H}) + \mathbf{C} + \mathbf{F}$ together and compare with the formula (4.20). That is exactly $P(D = 1, H_1 | T = t)$. We have finished the proof.

5

Evaluating Long-Term Outcomes and Overdiagnosis in Screening

CONTENTS

The US Preventive Services Task Force (USPSTF) examines the risks for potential cancer patients and updates screening recommendations for people at higher risk regularly [17]. There are published screening recommendations and guidelines regarding breast, cervical, colorectal, lung, and prostate cancer. These recommendations usually are built for adults 50 years and older, or for people with high risks, such as heavy smokers. However, there is an urgent need to quantify the *long-term outcomes* of periodic screening, especially

DOI: 10.1201/9781003404125-5

the risk of overdiagnosis, which can cause unnecessary anxiety and treatment. We introduce probability methods for evaluating the long-term outcomes due to regular screening, including overdiagnosis as one outcome in this chapter. We will derive probability formulas under two different situations: for asymptomatic people without any screening history (usually younger people), and for asymptomatic people with a screening history (older people). These formulas are for the case when sensitivity and sojourn time are independent. Then we will expand to the situation when sensitivity is a function of the ratio of time in the preclinical state to the sojourn time.

People who take part in cancer screening can be categorized into four mutually exclusive groups depending on their ultimate disease status and diagnosis status: *symptom-free-life*, *no-early-detection*, *true-early-detection*, and *over-diagnosis*. For each case, we will derive the probability formula for younger age groups *without* any screening history, and the older age group *with* a screening history. Simulation studies were carried out to show the proportions of these four groups, the proportion of no-early-detection, true-early-detection, and overdiagnosis among the diagnosed cases, and the proportion of true-early-detection and overdiagnosis among the screen-detected cases. Human lifetime was treated as a random variable and was derived from the US Social Security Administration (SSA) actuarial life table as in Chapter 4. These probabilities are functions of the three key parameters (the sensitivity, the sojourn time in the preclinical state, and the transition probability density from the disease-free to the preclinical state), a person's current age, screening frequency in the past (if any), and in the future. We applied the methods to the HIP study and the NLST CT data, to evaluate long-term outcomes for breast cancer and lung cancer. The models can provide policymakers and the general public with predictive information regarding the distribution of the four categories (symptom-free-life, no-early-detection, true-early-detection, and over-diagnosis), and the probability of overdiagnosis among the screen-detected cases in the future.

5.1 Introduction

Cancer screenings have been effective in detecting tumors early before symptoms are present. However, a challenge remains as to how to evaluate the long-term outcomes due to continued regular screening. For example, what is the percentage of people that lives a cancer-free life? What is the risk of overdiagnosis among the screen-detected cases? How to estimate the probability of true-early-detection in regular screening? Will continuous screening exams lead to a greater chance of overdiagnosis? How should the probabilities of no-early detection be estimated? What is the percentage of people who will die from other causes rather than a specific cancer (i.e., overdiagnosis)?

Some research has been done in the area of overdiagnosis, the diagnosis of cancer that would never have become symptomatic during a person's lifetime (Davidov and Zelen 2004[13], Zahl et al 2008[41]). Most of the research has been based on observational studies or simple linear regression. The research may be biased due to a lack of probability modeling. The estimated percentage of overdiagnosis varies from 7% (Duffy et al 2008 [52]) to 52% (Jorgensen and Gotzsche 2009 [29]). Hence, there is controversy concerning the benefit of regular screening. Although some findings suggest that regular mammograms may be beneficial to women older than 80 (Badgwell et al 2008 [2]), other reports argue that there will be more harm than benefit related to treatment associated with overdiagnosis (Berry et al 2009 [3]). A recent publication estimated that one in seven screen-detected breast cancers is overdiagnosed (Ryser et al 2022 [45]). Therefore, there is a need for clarification. There were some problems using observational studies as well; for example, a result obtained from one study cannot be extended to other scenarios; and observational studies usually need a long follow-up period to collect incidence data from both the study arm and the control arm.

Instead of dealing with overdiagnosis alone, we want to address the long-term effect attributable to regular screening for the whole cohort undergoing screening exams. Participants in a periodic screening program can be classified into four mutually exclusive groups: *symptom-free-life*, *no-early-detection*, *true-early-detection*, and *overdiagnosis*. depending on whether the individuals would be diagnosed with specific cancer and whether their symptoms would have appeared before death. We have to consider the fact that human life is a random variable: A person might die of a specific cancer or one might die of other causes, such as a heart attack, a stroke, or maybe a car accident, etc. Using breast cancer as an example, we will assume that an individual is asymptomatic at her current age. Based on a woman's diagnosis status and her ultimate lifetime disease status, we will categorize people who take part in periodic screening into four mutually exclusive groups as follows.

- *Group 1:* **Symptom-free-life (SympF)**: A woman who took part in screening exams, but breast cancer was never detected and ultimately she died of other causes.

- *Group 2:* **No-early-detection (NoED)**: A woman who took part in screening exams, but whose disease manifested itself clinically and was not detected by scheduled screening.

- *Group 3:* **True-early-detection (TrueED)**: A woman whose breast cancer was diagnosed at a scheduled screening exam and her clinical symptoms would have appeared before her death.

- *Group 4:* **Overdiagnosis (OverD)**: A woman who was diagnosed with breast cancer at a scheduled screening exam but her clinical symptoms would NOT have appeared before her death.

TABLE 5.1
Definition of long-term outcomes and events in screening.

	no symptom before death	*symptoms before death*
not-screen-detected	symptom-free-life	no-early-detection
screen-detected	overdiagnosis	true-early-detection

Adapted from Table 1 in Wu et al 2014[71].

The more familiar term "interval case" falls in *Group 2*; however, as defined above, *Group 2* includes all possible interval cases, with the lifetime being treated as a random variable. Eventually, every participant falls into one of the four groups, as in Table 5.1.

In the next sections, we will derive the probability of each group under two scenarios: without any screening history, and with a screening history. And human life is treated as a random variable or competing risk in this chapter. We start with the case that sensitivity does not depend on the sojourn time, then we expand to the case when sensitivity is a function of the ratio of time in the preclinical state and the sojourn time. In all cases, it is assumed that the sojourn time and the onset time of the S_p are independent as before.

5.2 Long-term outcomes for people with no screening history

This is the first probability model that we developed for evaluating the long-term effect of continued screening for participants without a screening history. We assume the commonly followed disease progressive model [87]: $S_0 \to S_p \to S_c$. S_0 refers to the disease-free state or the state in which the disease cannot be detected; S_p refers to the preclinical disease state, in which an asymptomatic individual unknowingly has a disease that a screening exam can detect; and S_c refers to the disease state at which the disease manifests itself in clinical symptoms.

Consider a cohort of initially asymptomatic individuals who enroll in a screening program. We let $\beta(t)$ be the sensitivity at age t. We let $q(x)$ be the probability density function (PDF) of the sojourn time in the S_p, and $Q(z) = \int_z^\infty q(x)dx$ is the survival function of the sojourn time. We use $w(t)$ to measure the distribution of time duration in the S_0, a sub-PDF. Throughout this chapter, the time variable t represents an individual's age; the capital letter T represents a person's lifetime, which is a continuous random variable with a probability density function $f_T(t)$. We define an event:

$$A = \{\text{A woman is asymptomatic of breast cancer before and at age } t_0\}.$$

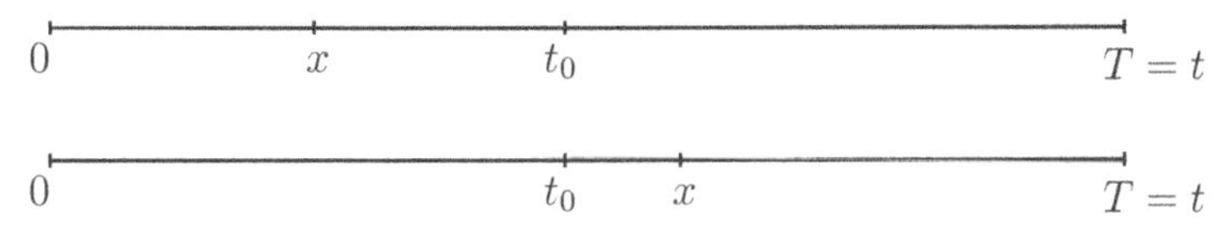

x = the onset of the preclinical state S_p
t_0 = screening time
T = lifetime

FIGURE 5.1
Probability calculation of four cases with one exam at age t_0.

Event A is the requirement to be enrolled in a screening program. We can calculate $P(A|T > t_0)$, the conditional probability that one is asymptomatic before/at age t_0, given that one's lifetime T exceeds t_0. This could only happen in two mutually exclusive events: either (i) she remains in the disease-free state through age t_0, the probability of which is $1 - \int_0^{t_0} w(x)dx$; or (ii) she enters the state S_p before t_0 but remains in the S_p long enough that no symptoms appear before t_0, the probability of which is $\int_0^{t_0} w(x)Q(t_0 - x)dx$. And we add these two to obtain:

$$P(A|T > t_0) = 1 - \int_0^{t_0} w(x)dx + \int_0^{t_0} w(x)Q(t_0 - x)dx. \tag{5.1}$$

We will deal with the problem of long-term outcomes in the following steps: (a) first, we derive the probability of each of the four cases in the simplest situation, when screening number $K = 1$ and lifetime $T = t$ is fixed; then we allow $T \sim f_T(t)$ to be random. (b) next, we derive the probability of each case for any screening number $K > 1$ when the lifetime $T = t$ is fixed, then we allow $T \sim f_T(t)$ to be random, and the screening number K will be a random variable as well.

5.2.1 Probability calculation with one exam

Suppose an asymptomatic woman plans to take one screening exam at her current age t_0, we will derive the conditional probability given her lifetime $T = t(> t_0)$ for each case as follows. See Figure 5.1 for illustrations.

For a Group 1 case of symptom-free-life, a woman who has no breast cancer detected during her lifetime, there are three mutually exclusive events: (i) she stayed in the disease-free state S_0 all her life, the probability of which is $1 - \int_0^t w(x)dx$; (ii) she may have entered the preclinical state S_p before t_0, but was not detected, and her sojourn time was longer than $(t_0 - x)$, so that no clinical symptom appeared before her death, the probability is $(1 - \beta_0) \int_0^{t_0} w(x)Q(t - x)dx$; and (iii) she may have entered the preclinical state S_p after t_0 and with a long sojourn time, so that no symptom appeared before her death, the probability is $\int_{t_0}^{t} w(x)Q(t-x)dx$. In the case of (ii) and (iii), x represents the onset time/age of her preclinical state. Hence,

$$\begin{aligned} & P(\textit{Case 1: SympF, } A|T=t) \qquad (5.2) \\ = & \; 1-\int_0^t w(x)dx + (1-\beta_0)\int_0^{t_0} w(x)Q(t-x)dx + \int_{t_0}^{t} w(x)Q(t-x)dx. \end{aligned}$$

For a Group 2 case, a woman has clinical cancer in $(t_0, T=t)$ (i.e., an interval case), either she entered S_p before t_0 and was missed by the screening exam, of which the probability is $(1-\beta_0)\int_0^{t_0} w(x)[Q(t_0-x)-Q(t-x)]dx$; or she entered the preclinical state after t_0, and the probability is $\int_{t_0}^{t} w(x)[1-Q(t-x)]dx$. In both events, her sojourn time in the S_p must be longer than t_0-x, and shorter than $(t-x)$, where x is her age entering the S_p (i.e. her onset age). Hence the probability is

$$\begin{aligned} & P(\textit{Case 2: NoED, } A|T=t) \qquad (5.3) \\ = & \; (1-\beta_0)\int_0^{t_0} w(x)[Q(t_0-x)-Q(t-x)]dx + \int_{t_0}^{t} w(x)[1-Q(t-x)]dx. \end{aligned}$$

For a Group 3 case, a woman who truly benefited from screening, her cancer was diagnosed at t_0, and her symptoms would have appeared before her death. That is, she must have entered S_p at age x before t_0, and her sojourn time would be between (t_0-x) and $(t-x)$. Hence,

$$P(\textit{Case 3: TrueED, } A|T=t) = \beta_0\int_0^{t_0} w(x)[Q(t_0-x)-Q(t-x)]dx. \quad (5.4)$$

For a Group 4 case, the case of overdiagnosis, she was diagnosed at t_0, but her symptoms would not have appeared before her death. That is, she must have entered S_p at some age x before t_0, but her sojourn time was longer than $(t-x)$. Hence,

$$P(\textit{Case 4: OverD, } A|T=t) = \beta_0\int_0^{t_0} w(x)Q(t-x)dx. \quad (5.5)$$

The probability of each case when the lifetime $T(>t_0)$ is a random variable can be obtained by

$$\begin{aligned} P(\text{Case } i, A|T>t_0) &= \int_{t_0}^{\infty} P(\text{Case } i, A|T=t)f_T(t|T>t_0)dt, \quad (5.6) \\ & \qquad \text{for } i=1,2,3,4. \end{aligned}$$

And the conditional probability density function of the lifetime is

$$f_T(t|T>t_0) = \begin{cases} \frac{f_T(t)}{P(T>t_0)} = \frac{f_T(t)}{1-F_T(t_0)}, & \text{if } t>t_0 \\ 0, & \text{otherwise.} \end{cases} \quad (5.7)$$

Exercise 5.1. Prove that for any $t > t_0$,

$$\begin{aligned}\sum_{i=1}^{4} P(\text{Case } i, A|T=t) &= 1 - \int_0^{t_0} w(x)dx + \int_0^{t_0} w(x)Q(t_0 - x)dx. \\ &= P(A|T > t_0). \end{aligned} \tag{5.8}$$

Since the $P(A|T > t_0)$ does not depend on t, we have

$$\begin{aligned}\sum_{i=1}^{4} P(\text{Case } i, A|T > t_0) &= \int_{t_0}^{\infty} \left[\sum_{i=1}^{4} P(\text{Case } i, A|T=t)\right] f_T(t|T > t_0)dt \\ &= P(A|T > t_0). \end{aligned} \tag{5.9}$$

Which implies

$$\sum_{i=1}^{4} P(\text{Case } i|A, T > t_0) = \sum_{i=1}^{4} \frac{P(\text{Case } i, A|T > t_0)}{P(A|T > t_0)} = 1. \tag{5.10}$$

The derived probability formulas are correct because they add up to 1.

5.2.2 Probability calculation with multiple exams

Now we generalize the idea to any number of screening exams. For an initially asymptomatic individual at current age t_0, assume that she plans to take $K(> 1)$ exams in the future, occurring at her ages $t_0 < t_1 < \cdots < t_{K-1}$. We define $t_{-1} = 0$. The conditional probability of each case given that her lifetime $T = t_K(> t_{K-1})$ can be generalized as follows.

A Group 1 case where clinical breast cancer never occurs in her lifetime, can arise as any one of $(K+2)$ disjoint events: (a) She remains in the disease-free state S_0 throughout her lifetime, the probability of which is $1 - \int_0^{t_K} w(x)dx$. (b) She enters the preclinical state S_p in the screening (age) interval $(t_{j-1}, t_j), j = 0, \ldots, K-1$, is not detected by the following $(K-j)$ exams, and has a long sojourn time, so no symptom appears before her death (K disjoint events). (c) She enters S_p after t_{K-1} and with no symptoms before her death. When we add the probability of these events together, the probability is

$$\begin{aligned}&P(\text{Case } 1, A|T = t_K) \\ =&1 - \int_0^{t_K} w(x)dx + \int_{t_{K-1}}^{t_K} w(x)Q(t_K - x)dx \\ &+ \sum_{j=0}^{K-1} (1-\beta_j)\cdots(1-\beta_{K-1}) \int_{t_{j-1}}^{t_j} w(x)Q(t_K - x)dx. \end{aligned} \tag{5.11}$$

For a Group 2 case, we calculate the probability of no early detection by defining $I_{K,j}$ as the probability of being an interval case in the interval (t_{j-1}, t_j) in a sequence of K screening exams. Thus,

$$P(\text{Case } 2, A|T = t_K) = I_{K,1} + I_{K,2} + \cdots + I_{K,K}, \tag{5.12}$$

where

$$\begin{aligned} I_{K,j} &= \sum_{i=0}^{j-1}(1-\beta_i)\cdots(1-\beta_{j-1})\int_{t_{i-1}}^{t_i} w(x)[Q(t_{j-1}-x) - Q(t_j - x)]dx \\ &+ \int_{t_{j-1}}^{t_j} w(x)[1 - Q(t_j - x)]dx, \qquad \text{for all } j = 1, \cdots, K. \end{aligned} \tag{5.13}$$

A Group 3 case, true-early-detection, can happen as one of K mutually exclusive events, depending on her age at diagnosis by screening, namely, at $t_j, j = 0, 1, \cdots, K-1$. If she is diagnosed at t_j and x is the onset time of her preclinical state, then she must have entered the preclinical state S_p before t_j, was missed by the previous exams and her sojourn time must have been at least $(t_j - x)$ and at most $(t_K - x)$. Therefore,

$$\begin{aligned} &P(\text{Case } 3, A|T = t_K) \\ &= \sum_{j=1}^{K-1}\beta_j\left\{\sum_{i=0}^{j-1}(1-\beta_i)\cdots(1-\beta_{j-1})\int_{t_{i-1}}^{t_i} w(x)[Q(t_j - x) - Q(t_K - x)]dx\right. \\ &\left.+ \int_{t_{j-1}}^{t_j} w(x)[Q(t_j - x) - Q(t_K - x)]dx\right\} \\ &+\beta_0\int_0^{t_0} w(x)[Q(t_0 - x) - Q(t_K - x)]dx. \end{aligned} \tag{5.14}$$

A Group 4 case, overdiagnosis, can also arise as one of K disjoint events. She might have been diagnosed at the j-th exam, but her symptoms would not appear before her death. Hence,

$$\begin{aligned} &P(\text{Case } 4, A|T = t_K) \\ &= \sum_{j=1}^{K-1}\beta_j\left\{\sum_{i=0}^{j-1}(1-\beta_i)\cdots(1-\beta_{j-1})\int_{t_{i-1}}^{t_i} w(x)Q(t_K - x)dx\right. \\ &\left.+ \int_{t_{j-1}}^{t_j} w(x)Q(t_K - x)dx\right\} + \beta_0\int_0^{t_0} w(x)Q(t_K - x)dx. \end{aligned} \tag{5.15}$$

Exercise 5.2. Prove that for any integer $K > 1$, and $T = t_K > t_{K-1}$,

$$\begin{aligned} &\sum_{i=1}^{4} P(\text{Case } i, A|T = t_K) \\ &= 1 - \int_0^{t_0} w(x)dx + \int_0^{t_0} w(x)Q(t_0 - x)dx = P(A|T > t_0). \end{aligned}$$

For an individual currently at age t_0, her life isn't fixed but random, so it is unrealistic to consider the future number of exams K to be a fixed value. However, if she plans to follow a future screening schedule, such as $t_0 < t_1 < \ldots$, then $K = n$ if $t_{n-1} < T \leq t_n$; that is, the screening number $K = K(T)$ is a random variable, changing with the lifetime T. The probability of each case when her lifetime T is longer than t_0 can be obtained by taking the integral (i.e., a weighted average):

$$P(\text{Case } i, A|T > t_0) = \int_{t_0}^{\infty} P(\text{Case } i, A|K = K(T), T = t) f_T(t|T > t_0) dt, \quad i = 1, 2, 3, 4, \qquad (5.16)$$

where the lifetime probability density function $f_T(t|T > t_0)$ was defined in equation (5.7). The probability $P(\text{Case i}, A|K = K(T), T = t)$ was derived in the above equations (5.11)-(5.15).

Exercise 5.3. Prove that for any future screening schedule when the lifetime T is random,

$$\sum_{i=1}^{4} P(\text{Case } i|A, T > t_0) = 1.$$

The probability of overdiagnosis among the screen-detected cases is

$$P(\text{OverD}|\text{Scr. Det.}) = \frac{P(\text{Case 4}, A|T > t_0)}{P(\text{Case 3}, A|T > t_0) + P(\text{Case 4}, A|T > t_0)}. \qquad (5.17)$$

This is the probability causing much debate among researchers regarding overdiagnosis.

5.2.3 Simulation study

Simulation studies to evaluate long-term outcomes in cancer screening were carried out. The probability of each case is a function of the three key parameters (sensitivity, sojourn time, and transition density), the initial age, future screening interval, and the human lifetime, we want to explore the effects of these factors on the probability of each outcome, and also explore how the proportion of true-early-detection and overdiagnosis change among the screen-detected cases due to these factors. Among these factors, the three key parameters are determined by the kinds of cancer and screening modalities; the initial age can be anywhere between 40 and 60 since most people will start their first screening exam during those ages; the future screening frequency can be chosen reasonably between 6 months and 2 years; finally, the human life can be obtained by the published actuarial life table from the US Social Security Administration (SSA). We selected the following scenarios for simulation:

1. Age at initial screening: $t_0 = 40$, 50, or 60 years old
2. Future screening interval: $\Delta = 6, 12, 24$ months

3. Screening sensitivities: $\beta = 0.3$, 0.7, or 0.9
4. Sojourn time PDF: exponential(λ) or log-logistic (κ, ρ)
5. Transition density $w(t)$: log Normal $(\mu, \sigma^2) \times 0.2$

We picked $\beta = 0.3$ assuming some screening test has very low sensitivities, such as prostate-specific antigen test (PSA); see Davidov and Zelen 2004 [13]. The transition probability density was chosen to follow log Normal, with an upper limit of 20%, which is applicable to different sites of cancer. Hence,

$$w(t) = \frac{0.2}{\sqrt{2\pi}\sigma t} \exp\left\{-(\log t - \mu)^2/(2\sigma^2)\right\}.$$

We picked $(\mu, \sigma^2) = (4.2, 0.1)$, so that $w(t)$ has a single mode around 60 years old. The sojourn time distribution was chosen to be either exponential,

$$q(x) = \lambda e^{-\lambda x}, x > 0,$$

or log-logistic,

$$q(x) = \frac{\kappa x^{\kappa-1}\rho^{\kappa}}{1 + (x\rho)^{\kappa}}, x > 0, \kappa > 0, \rho > 0.$$

The parameters were carefully chosen, so that the *mean sojourn time* (MST) is 2, 5, 10, or 20 years. That is, under the exponential PDF, $\lambda = 0.5, 0.2, 0.1, 0.05$; and under the log-logistic PDF, the parameters are $(\kappa, \rho) = (2.5, 0.661), (2.5, 0.264), (2.5, 0.132), (2.5, 0.066)$.

The number of screens $K = K(T) = \lceil (T - t_0)/\Delta \rceil$ is the largest integer that is less than or equal to $(T - t_0)/\Delta$. It is a function of the lifetime T, and therefore it is a variable in the simulation. For the lifetime distribution, we used the actuarial life table from the SSA, which was published online at *http://www.ssa.gov/OACT/STATS/table4c6.html.* The period life table was reviewed and updated every 6 months. It is based on mortality from all US citizens registered for social security benefits and it provides the probability of death within 1 year from age 0 to 119 for males and females separately. We derived the conditional lifetime distribution $f_T(t|T > t_0)$ based on the actuarial life table in 2012 in this simulation. Since the life table barely changes over a long-time frame, our simulation results won't change much if we use the recently updated life table.

The results for different initial age groups are very similar, so we only report the case of $t_0 = 50$. The results have little difference when using male or female lifetime density, so we reported the case of *females* here. However, there are obvious differences when the sojourn time was an exponential or a log-logistic pdf, even if the mean sojourn times were the same, so we report the corresponding results in Tables 5.2 and 5.3.

Exercise 5.4. Numerically reproduce Tables 5.2 and 5.3 using the parameters in the simulation in this section, rounding to two decimal places.

TABLE 5.2
Probability of each outcome (in %): When the sojourn time is log-logistic.

MST	[a]P(SympF)	P(NoED)	P(TrueED)	P(OverD)	[b]P(TrueED$\|D$)	P(OverD$\|D$)
		screening interval $\Delta = 6$ **month,** $\beta = 0.3$				
2	88.47	4.08	7.13	0.29	96.08	3.92
5	87.91	1.58	9.44	1.04	90.06	9.94
10	87.22	0.61	9.71	2.44	79.95	20.05
20	86.52	0.22	8.16	5.08	61.66	38.34
		screening interval $\Delta = 6$ **month,** $\beta = 0.7$				
2	88.34	1.00	10.21	0.42	96.07	3.93
5	87.70	0.20	10.82	1.25	89.66	10.34
10	86.98	0.07	10.25	2.67	79.31	20.69
20	86.27	0.03	8.35	5.33	61.06	38.94
		screening interval $\Delta = 6$ **month,** $\beta = 0.9$				
2	88.31	0.39	10.83	0.45	96.00	4.00
5	87.66	0.06	10.97	1.29	89.49	10.51
10	86.94	0.02	10.30	2.71	79.15	20.85
20	86.23	0.01	8.37	5.37	60.94	39.06
		screening interval $\Delta = 12$ **month,** $\beta = 0.3$				
2	88.56	6.39	4.82	0.20	95.96	4.04
5	88.12	3.45	7.57	0.83	90.08	9.92
10	87.52	1.66	8.66	2.13	80.26	19.74
20	86.88	0.63	7.75	4.71	62.20	37.80
		screening interval $\Delta = 12$ **month,** $\beta = 0.7$				
2	88.42	2.66	8.55	0.34	96.18	3.82
5	87.81	0.72	10.30	1.14	90.03	9.97
10	87.10	0.23	10.09	2.56	79.79	20.21
20	86.39	0.08	8.30	5.21	61.46	38.54
		screening interval $\Delta = 12$ **month,** $\beta = 0.9$				
2	88.37	1.45	9.77	0.39	96.20	3.80
5	87.74	0.25	10.77	1.21	89.88	10.12
10	87.01	0.07	10.26	2.64	79.54	20.46
20	86.30	0.02	8.36	5.29	61.24	38.76
		screening interval $\Delta = 24$ **month,** $\beta = 0.3$				
2	88.64	8.30	2.91	0.13	95.75	4.25
5	88.36	5.72	5.31	0.60	89.85	10.15
10	87.97	3.48	6.85	1.69	80.20	19.80
20	87.54	1.62	6.77	4.06	62.49	37.51
		screening interval $\Delta = 24$ **month,** $\beta = 0.7$				
2	88.52	5.15	6.06	0.24	96.12	3.88
5	87.99	2.05	8.97	0.96	90.33	9.67
10	87.32	0.76	9.56	2.33	80.38	19.62
20	86.63	0.24	8.14	4.97	62.11	37.89
		screening interval $\Delta = 24$ **month,** $\beta = 0.9$				
2	88.47	3.79	7.42	0.29	96.22	3.78
5	87.88	0.99	10.04	1.07	90.34	9.66
10	87.17	0.26	10.06	2.49	80.19	19.81
20	86.46	0.07	8.31	5.14	61.81	38.19

[a]Columns 2 to 5 is the probability of the four outcomes, i.e., $P(\text{Case } i|A, T > t_0)$.
[b]Columns 6 to 7 report the probability of true-early-detection and of overdiagnosis given that it is a screen-detected case.
Adapted from Table 1 in the Supplement of Wu et al 2014 [71].

TABLE 5.3
Probability of each outcome (in %): When the sojourn time is exponential.

MST	[a]P(SympF)	P(NoED)	P(TrueED)	P(OverD)	[b]P(TrueED$\|D$)	P(OverD$\|D$)
		screening interval $\Delta = 6$ month, $\beta = 0.3$				
2	88.45	4.75	6.46	0.32	95.34	4.66
5	87.91	2.62	8.33	1.12	88.16	11.84
10	87.34	1.53	8.51	2.60	76.64	23.36
20	86.81	0.84	7.23	5.09	58.65	41.35
		screening interval $\Delta = 6$ month, $\beta = 0.7$				
2	88.33	2.17	9.04	0.43	95.43	4.57
5	87.73	0.99	9.96	1.30	88.48	11.52
10	87.13	0.53	9.51	2.81	77.22	22.78
20	86.58	0.27	7.79	5.33	59.41	40.59
		screening interval $\Delta = 6$ month, $\beta = 0.9$				
2	88.30	1.53	9.69	0.46	95.45	4.55
5	87.69	0.66	10.30	1.33	88.54	11.46
10	87.09	0.34	9.70	2.84	77.33	22.67
20	86.54	0.17	7.90	5.36	59.54	40.46
		screening interval $\Delta = 12$ month, $\beta = 0.3$				
2	88.54	6.68	4.53	0.22	95.29	4.71
5	88.10	4.23	6.72	0.93	87.88	12.12
10	87.61	2.66	7.38	2.33	76.00	24.00
20	87.14	1.54	6.53	4.77	57.76	42.24
		screening interval $\Delta = 12$ month, $\beta = 0.7$				
2	88.40	3.67	7.54	0.36	95.39	4.61
5	87.82	1.82	9.13	1.20	88.35	11.65
10	87.23	1.00	9.04	2.70	76.99	23.01
20	86.69	0.53	7.54	5.21	59.11	40.89
		screening interval $\Delta = 12$ month, $\beta = 0.9$				
2	88.35	2.74	8.47	0.41	95.43	4.57
5	87.76	1.25	9.70	1.27	88.46	11.54
10	87.16	0.66	9.38	2.77	77.19	22.81
20	86.62	0.34	7.73	5.29	59.37	40.63
		screening interval $\Delta = 24$ month, $\beta = 0.3$				
2	88.62	8.37	2.84	0.14	95.27	4.73
5	88.34	6.10	4.85	0.69	87.58	12.42
10	88.02	4.22	5.82	1.92	75.16	24.84
20	87.71	2.62	5.45	4.21	56.44	43.56
		screening interval $\Delta = 24$ month, $\beta = 0.7$				
2	88.49	5.61	5.60	0.27	95.36	4.65
5	87.98	3.15	7.80	1.05	88.17	11.83
10	87.43	1.84	8.20	2.51	76.59	23.41
20	86.91	1.01	7.06	5.00	58.56	41.44
		screening interval $\Delta = 24$ month, $\beta = 0.9$				
2	88.44	4.53	6.68	0.32	95.40	4.60
5	87.88	2.28	8.67	1.15	88.33	11.67
10	87.30	1.25	8.79	2.64	76.94	23.06
20	86.76	0.65	7.41	5.15	59.03	40.97

[a]Columns 2 to 5 is the probability of the four outcomes, i.e., $P(\text{Case } i|A, T > t_0)$.
[b]Columns 6 to 7 report the probability of true-early-detection and of overdiagnosis given that it is a screen-detected case.
Adapted from Table 2 in the Supplement of Wu et al 2014 [71].

From the simulation, we can see clearly that the mean sojourn time (MST) plays the most important role in the case of overdiagnosis. For example, in the last column of Table 5.2, the proportion of overdiagnosis could be as high as 39% among the screen-diagnosed cases if the mean sojourn time is 20 years; the overdiagnosis percentage is around 20% if the mean sojourn time is 10 years; and it is only about 4-9% when the mean sojourn time changes from 2 to 5 years. In Table 5.3, when the sojourn time is exponentially distributed, this pattern is more dramatic, the probability of overdiagnosis could be as high as 43%.

The screening sensitivity will affect the ratio of the no-early-detection and the true-early-detection: when sensitivity is higher, the probability of true-early-detection is higher, and the probability of no-early-detection is lower. However, the sensitivity only has a small effect on the proportion of true-early-detection and overdiagnosis among the screen-detected cases, when the sojourn time is the same: the percentage of overdiagnosis increases slightly (<0.1%) when the sensitivity increases from 0.3 to 0.9.

The screening interval also plays a role in these probabilities: when the screening interval is longer, the probability of no-early-detection is larger, the probability of the true-early-detection is smaller, and the probability of overdiagnosis is slightly smaller (<0.1% in the fifth column). The probability of the symptom-free-life is pretty stable in all the simulations, it is about 86-89% for the whole population.

The transition probability density $w(t)$ is surely important, but in this simulation, we limit it to the situation where the density has a single peak around age 60. We consider the log-logistic density is a more suitable candidate for the sojourn time distribution compared with the exponential, because the exponential density has its mode at 0 and with a constant hazard rate, which is not appropriate in reality.

5.2.4 Application: Breast cancer long-term outcomes using the HIP

We apply the method to the Health Insurance Plan for the Greater New York (HIP) data [47]. The age-dependent sensitivity $\beta(t)$ and transition density $w(t)$, and the sojourn time distribution $q(x)$ using the HIP data were estimated using a Bayesian approach in Wu et al 2005[79]. The parametric link functions were

$$\begin{aligned} \beta(t) &= [1+\exp(-b_0-b_1(t-m))]^{-1}, \\ w(t) &= \frac{0.2}{\sqrt{2\pi}\sigma t}\exp\left\{-(\log t-\mu)^2/(2\sigma^2)\right\}, \\ Q(x) &= \frac{1}{1+(x\rho)^\kappa}, \quad \kappa>0, \rho>0, \end{aligned} \tag{5.18}$$

where m is the average age of women at the study entry. The 0.2 in the $w(t)$ is the upper limit of making a transition from the disease-free state to the preclinical state. The unknown parameters in the above model are $\theta = (b_0, b_1, \mu, \sigma^2, \kappa, \rho)$. 2000 posterior samples were obtained using Markov Chain Monte Carlo (MCMC) and the posterior distribution [79]. The posterior predictive probability of each case can be estimated as

$$\begin{aligned}
&P(\text{Case } i|T > t_0, A, HIP) \\
&= \int P(\text{Case } i, \theta|T > t_0, A, HIP)d\theta \\
&= \int P(\text{Case } i|T > t_0, A, \theta)f(\theta|HIP)d\theta \\
&\approx \frac{1}{n}\sum_{j=1}^{n} P(\text{Case } i|T > t_0, A, \theta_j^*)
\end{aligned} \tag{5.19}$$

where θ_j^* is a posterior sample drawn from the posterior distribution $f(\theta|HIP)$ and $n = 2000$ is the posterior sample size. The last step is the Monte Carlo simulation.

We conduct Bayesian inference in the case of periodic exams for three hypothetical cohorts of asymptomatic women, with an age of 40, 50, and 60 respectively at the first exam, using (5.19) and the 2000 posterior samples. For each group, we examined screening frequencies, with screening intervals $\Delta = 6$, 12, 18, 24, and 30 months. The number of screens $K = K(T) = \lceil (T - t_0)/\Delta \rceil$ is a function of the lifetime T; therefore, it is a variable in the simulation. For the lifetime distribution, we used the conditional lifetime probability density derived from the actuarial life table from the SSA for females as in the previous chapter. The conditional probabilities of each of the four cases, i.e., $P(\text{Case } i|A, T > t_0, HIP)$, are reported in Table 5.4.

For all three age groups of $t_0 = 40, 50, 60$, the percentage of overdiagnosis is very small. For the 12-month screening interval, it is 0.32%, 0.33%, and 0.33%, respectively, for ages 40, 50, and 60 years old at the first exam. This probability barely changes when the age at the initial screening exam increases. It decreases as the screening time interval (Δ) increases.

The probability of true-early-detection is 7.34%, 6.49%, and 5.03%, respectively for these three cohorts if screening is annual. This probability also decreases as the screening time interval increases. The probability of true-early-detection is slightly lower when the initial screen age is 60; however, there is little difference between the two age groups, 40 and 50.

The probability of no-early-detection is 2.48%, 1.95%, and 1.39% for the 12-month screening schedule if the woman initiates screening at ages 40, 50, and 60. It increases as the screening interval increases; it decreases slightly when the age at the initial screen increases.

The probability of a symptom-free-life is very high. It increases from about 89% to 93% when the initial screening age increases from 40 to 60. It is comparatively stable when the screening interval changes within each age group. Overall, the difference in the corresponding probabilities is smaller

TABLE 5.4
Application: Long-term outcome for breast cancer screening using the HIP data.

$^a\Delta$	^bP(SympF)	P(NoED)	P(TrueED)	P(OverD)
		Age at initial screen $t_0 = 40$		
6 mo.	89.66(1.34)	0.99(0.47)	8.83(1.58)	0.37(0.25)
12 mo.	89.71(1.35)	2.48(0.70)	7.34(1.31)	0.32(0.24)
18 mo.	89.75(1.35)	3.79(0.94)	6.03(1.01)	0.28(0.23)
24 mo.	89.78(1.35)	4.77(1.12)	5.04(0.80)	0.25(0.22)
30 mo.	89.81(1.36)	5.51(1.25)	4.31(0.67)	0.23(0.21)
		Age at initial screen $t_0 = 50$		
6 mo.	91.15(1.28)	0.74(0.47)	7.70(1.46)	0.38(0.25)
12 mo.	91.21(1.28)	1.95(0.71)	6.49(1.25)	0.33(0.24)
18 mo.	91.25(1.29)	3.06(0.91)	5.38(0.99)	0.29(0.23)
24 mo.	91.28(1.29)	3.91(1.07)	4.52(0.81)	0.26(0.22)
30 mo.	91.30(1.29)	4.55(1.18)	3.88(0.69)	0.23(0.21)
		Age at initial screen $t_0 = 60$		
6 mo.	93.15(1.02)	0.52(0.43)	5.90(1.16)	0.39(0.26)
12 mo.	93.21(1.02)	1.39(0.63)	5.03(1.02)	0.33(0.25)
18 mo.	93.25(1.02)	2.21(0.78)	4.21(0.85)	0.29(0.24)
24 mo.	93.28(1.02)	2.86(0.89)	3.57(0.72)	0.26(0.23)
30 mo.	93.30(1.03)	3.34(0.96)	3.08(0.63)	0.24(0.22)

$^a\Delta = t_i - t_{i-1}$ is the time interval between screens.
^{b}The mean probability and its standard error (in parenthesis) are reported as percentages in the table.
Adapted from Table 2 in Wu et al 2014 [71].

between the age groups 40 and 50 than that between the age groups 50 and 60.

Boxplots of the probability of each case when $t_0 = 50$ are presented in Figure 5.2. The boxplots for age groups 40 and 60 are very similar, so we omit them. We can see that the probability of symptom-free-life and that of Overdiagnosis is either stable or barely changes with the screening time interval. The probability of no-early-detection increases monotonically with the screening time interval, while the probability of true-early-detection decreases monotonically with the screening time interval.

If we calculate the conditional probability of cases 2, 3, and 4, given that she is a diagnosed cancer case (either an interval case or a screen-detected case), then the percentage of overdiagnosis is 3.93%, 4.62%, or 6.02% for the 6-month screening group if the starting age is 40, 50, or 60. See Table 5.5 for details. The conditional probability of true-early-detection given it is a diagnosed case dramatically decreases when the screening interval Δ increases; it changes from 86% to 43% in the 40-year-old group, from 87% to 45% in

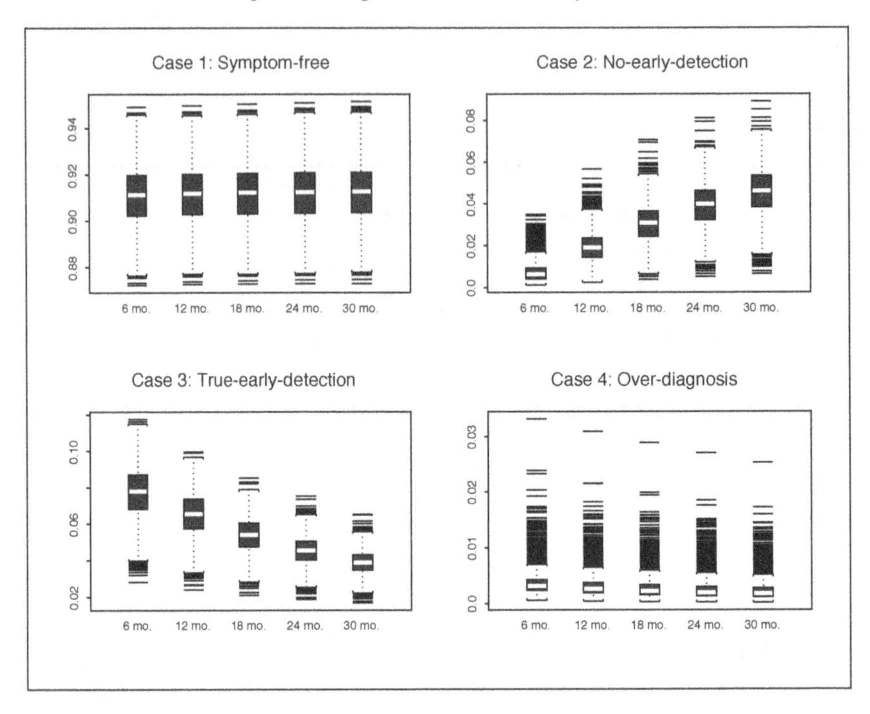

FIGURE 5.2
The boxplot of the estimated probability for each case with $t_0 = 50$. Adapted from Figure 1 in Wu et al 2014 [71].

the 50-year-old group, and from 86% to 46% in the 60-year-old group. See the third column in Table 5.5. For the same screening interval, the probability of true-early-detection slightly increases with the initial screening age. The conditional probability of no-early-detection increases within each age group as the screening interval increases; while the conditional probability of overdiagnosis slightly decreases within each age group.

The probability and the 95% HPD intervals of true-early-detection and overdiagnosis among the screen-detected case are listed in Table 5.6. This is the number that the general public and medical community really want to know. The percentage of overdiagnosis increases from 4.41% to 5.05% in the 40-year-old age group. This percentage increases from 5.09% to 5.69% in the 50-year-old group, and it increases from 6.56% to 7.08% in the 60-year-old group. In summary, the probability of overdiagnosis is lower than we expected; while the probability of true-early-detection is often above 93% and is higher than we expected. The length of the 95% HPD interval for these two probabilities (percentages) increases as the screening interval increases.

TABLE 5.5
Application: Estimated probability given that it is a diagnosed cancer using the HIP study.

Δ	$^{a}P(\text{NoED}\|^{b}D)$	P(TrueED$\|D$)	P(OverD$\|D$)
	Age at initial screen $t_0 = 40$		
6 mo.	9.87	86.20	3.93
12 mo.	24.44	72.12	3.44
18 mo.	37.21	59.73	3.06
24 mo.	46.97	50.27	2.76
30 mo.	54.29	43.18	2.53
	Age at initial screen $t_0 = 50$		
6 mo.	8.49	86.89	4.62
12 mo.	22.17	73.78	4.05
18 mo.	34.72	61.67	3.61
24 mo.	44.48	52.25	3.27
30 mo.	51.88	45.11	3.00
	Age at initial screen $t_0 = 60$		
6 mo.	7.73	86.24	6.02
12 mo.	20.48	74.22	5.29
18 mo.	32.60	62.68	4.72
24 mo.	42.20	53.52	4.27
30 mo.	49.55	46.53	3.92

[a]The estimated conditional probability was calculated by $p_i^*/(p_2^* + p_3^* + p_4^*), i = 2, 3, 4$, for each of the 2000 posterior samples, then take the average. It is in percentage.
[b]The event $D = \{$Diagnosed cases: including both interval and screen-detected cases$\}$.
Adapted from Table 3 in Wu et al 2014 [71].

5.2.5 Application: Colorectal cancer outcomes using MCCCS

We have introduced the Minnesota Colorectal Cancer Study in Chapter 1, and we have obtained 1000 Bayesian posterior samples of the six parameters $\theta = (b_0, b_1, \mu, \sigma^2, \kappa, \rho)$ for each gender using the Markov Chain Monte Carlo (MCMC) from the posterior distribution, see Chapter 2 section 2.4.4. We apply the method to the 1000 posterior samples of each gender, to estimate the long-term outcomes. The posterior predictive probability of each of the four cases can be estimated by

$$P(\text{Case i}|T > t_0, A, MCCCS) \approx \frac{1}{n}\sum_j P(\text{Case i}|T > t_0, A, \theta_j^*).$$

where $\theta_j^*, j = 1, 2, \ldots, 1000$ is the posterior random samples and $n = 1000$ is the posterior sample size.

We assumed there are six hypothetical cohorts with initial screening age at 40, 50, and 60 years for each gender. For each cohort, we examined various

TABLE 5.6
Application: The estimated probability of overdiagnosis among the screen-detected cases (with 95% HPD interval) using the HIP.

Δ	^aP(TrueED|^{b}ScrD)	P(OverD|ScrD)
	Age at initial screen $t_0 = 40$	
6 mo.	95.59 (82.78, 98.62)	4.41 (1.38, 17.22)
12 mo.	95.47 (81.49, 98.76)	4.53 (1.24, 18.51)
18 mo.	95.29 (80.75, 98.79)	4.71 (1.21, 19.25)
24 mo.	95.12 (79.91, 98.79)	4.88 (1.21, 20.09)
30 mo.	94.95 (79.46, 98.78)	5.05 (1.22, 20.54)
	Age at initial screen $t_0 = 50$	
6 mo.	94.91 (80.76, 98.34)	5.09 (1.66, 19.24)
12 mo.	94.84 (79.38, 98.53)	5.16 (1.47, 20.62)
18 mo.	94.68 (78.97, 98.57)	5.32 (1.43, 21.03)
24 mo.	94.50 (78.16, 98.55)	5.50 (1.45, 21.84)
30 mo.	94.31 (77.65, 98.52)	5.69 (1.48, 22.35)
	Age at initial screen $t_0 = 60$	
6 mo.	93.44 (76.44, 97.74)	6.56 (2.26, 23.56)
12 mo.	93.43 (75.37, 97.97)	6.57 (2.03, 24.63)
18 mo.	93.28 (75.04, 98.04)	6.72 (1.96, 24.96)
24 mo.	93.10 (74.44, 98.05)	6.90 (1.95, 25.56)
30 mo.	92.92 (73.81, 98.04)	7.08 (1.96, 26.19)

[a]The estimated conditional probability was calculated by $p_i^*/(p_3^* + p_4^*), i = 3, 4$, for each of the 2000 posterior samples, then take the average. It is a percentage.
[b]The event ScrD= {Screen-detected case}. Adapted from Table 4 in Wu et al 2014 [71].

screening frequencies, with screening interval $\Delta = 12$, 18, and 24 months. The results are summarized in Tables 5.7 and 5.8.

Based on the MCCCS data, we found that the probability of symptom-free-life is large and stable for both genders. It is over 95% for all age groups, which means the majority of the general population will live a life free from colorectal cancer. We checked the NIH SEER database [4], and based on the report from 2005 to 2007, the lifetime risk of colorectal cancer for both genders is 5.12%. This number can also be expressed as 1 in 20 men and women will be diagnosed with colorectal cancer during their lifetime. Our estimated probability of symptom-free-life for both genders (95.37% for females and 95.44% for males at age 40) is close to one minus the lifetime risk, which shows that the model is reliable to provide an accurate estimate of the probability. This could be good news for people who have no family history of colorectal cancer, or who perceive themselves as low-risk people.

TABLE 5.7
Application: Long-term outcome of colorectal cancer screening using the MC-CCS data.

[a]Δ	[b]P(SympF)	P(NoED)	P(TrueED)	P(OverD)
	Female with first screen age $t_0 = 40$			
12 mo	95.37 (0.63)	0.44 (0.25)	3.76 (0.66)	0.27 (0.19)
18 mo	95.40 (0.63)	0.89 (0.40)	3.31 (0.57)	0.24 (0.18)
24 mo	95.43 (0.63)	1.34 (0.53)	2.85 (0.50)	0.21 (0.17)
	Female with first screen age $t_0 = 50$			
12 mo	95.52 (0.66)	0.38 (0.21)	3.79 (0.68)	0.28 (0.19)
18 mo	95.56 (0.66)	0.83 (0.38)	3.34 (0.59)	0.24 (0.18)
24 mo	95.59 (0.66)	1.28 (0.51)	2.89 (0.51)	0.21 (0.17)
	Female with first screen age $t_0 = 60$			
12 mo	95.81 (0.71)	0.29 (0.19)	3.57 (0.70)	0.29 (0.20)
18 mo	95.85 (0.71)	0.69 (0.35)	3.17 (0.61)	0.25 (0.19)
24 mo	95.88 (0.70)	1.11 (0.48)	2.75 (0.54)	0.22 (0.18)
	Male with first screen age $t_0 = 40$			
12 mo	95.44 (0.73)	0.94 (0.41)	3.28 (0.73)	0.22 (0.19)
18 mo	95.47 (0.74)	1.50 (0.53)	2.73 (0.59)	0.19 (0.18)
24 mo	95.50 (0.74)	1.95 (0.62)	2.28 (0.48)	0.16 (0.16)
	Male with first screen age $t_0 = 50$			
12 mo	95.84 (0.73)	0.75 (0.29)	3.17 (0.73)	0.22 (0.20)
18 mo	95.87 (0.74)	1.27 (0.44)	2.64 (0.59)	0.19 (0.18)
24 mo	95.90 (0.74)	1.70 (0.55)	2.22 (0.48)	0.17 (0.17)
	Male with first screen age $t_0 = 60$			
12 mo	96.53 (0.71)	0.53 (0.25)	2.69 (0.70)	0.23 (0.20)
18 mo	96.57 (0.71)	0.96 (0.38)	2.26 (0.58)	0.20 (0.19)
24 mo	96.59 (0.71)	1.31 (0.48)	1.91 (0.48)	0.18 (0.17)

[a]$\Delta = t_i - t_{i-1}$ is the time interval between two consequtive exams.
[b]The mean probabilities (with standard error) are in percentage (%).
Adapted from Tables 1a and 1b from Luo et al 2012 [35].

Among the screen-detected cases (Tables 5.8), the probability of overdiagnosis is lower than expected (about 6–9%), while the probability of true-early-detection is about 91–94%. This means that the proportion of overdiagnosis among the screen-detected cases is very small; most of those diagnosed with colorectal cancer by screening are true early detections, and if they are left untreated, colorectal cancer will appear before death. Therefore, overdiagnosis is not a big issue in colorectal cancer, and those diagnosed by screening should be treated immediately.

TABLE 5.8
Application: Estimated probability of true-early-detection and overdiagnosis among the screen-detected cases using the MCCCS data.

Δ	${}^{a}P(\text{TrueED}\mid{}^{b}\text{D})$	P(OverD|D)
	Female with first screen age $t_0 = 40$	
12 mo	92.88 (80.09, 97.24)	7.12 (2.76, 19.91)
18 mo	93.13 (80.63, 97.39)	6.87 (2.61, 19.37)
24 mo	93.25 (80.72, 97.44)	6.75 (2.56, 19.27)
	Female with first screen age $t_0 = 50$	
12 mo	92.79 (80.01, 97.16)	7.21 (2.84, 19.99)
18 mo	93.07 (80.52, 97.32)	6.93 (2.68, 19.48)
24 mo	93.16 (80.59, 97.36)	6.84 (2.64, 19.41)
	Female with first screen age $t_0 = 60$	
12 mo	92.17 (78.72, 96.79)	7.83 (3.21, 21.28)
18 mo	92.50 (79.51, 96.95)	7.50 (3.04, 20.49)
24 mo	92.65 (79.53, 97.03)	7.35 (2.97, 20.47)
	Male with first screen age $t_0 = 40$	
12 mo	93.03 (65.52, 98.01)	6.97 (1.99, 34.48)
18 mo	93.00 (64.09, 98.06)	7.00 (1.94, 35.91)
24 mo	92.93 (63.62, 98.08)	7.07 (1.92, 36.38)
	Male with first screen age $t_0 = 50$	
12 mo	92.59 (61.56, 97.80)	7.41 (2.20, 38.44)
18 mo	92.63 (61.29, 97.92)	7.38 (2.08, 38.71)
24 mo	92.51 (60.47, 97.95)	7.49 (2.05, 39.53)
	Male with first screen age $t_0 = 60$	
12 mo	91.22 (55.83, 97.23)	8.78 (2.77, 44.17)
18 mo	91.28 (55.41, 97.37)	8.72 (2.63, 44.59)
24 mo	91.23 (55.31, 97.38)	8.77 (2.62, 44.69)

[a]The estimated conditional probability is $P_i/(P_3 + P_4), i = 3, 4$ in Table 5.7 for the 1000 posterior samples, then taking the average.
[b]Event D ={screen-detected cancer case}.
Adapted from Tables 3a and 3b from Luo et al 2012 [35].

5.3 Long-term outcomes for people with a screening history

We have developed a probability model to evaluate the long-term effects, including overdiagnosis, for asymptomatic individuals who have no history of screening (Wu et al 2014 [71]). However, many old people may have had at least one screening exam already, the question is: how to evaluate their future screening outcomes? Given, say, K_1 previous exams with negative results, how much benefit will be derived by undergoing additional screens? If there is some benefit, how many additional screens should be taken, and at what frequency? Previous models do not address this issue, which has become critical for both public health and policy decision-makers (Badgwell et al 2008 [2]). In this section, we develop a model that incorporates various characteristics of a potential screening participant, including one's current age, previous screening history (number of previous negative screens), and the three key parameters.

We will use women's breast cancer as an example, assuming that a woman has undergone breast cancer screening exams, all of which were negative, and currently, she is asymptomatic. If she continues to undergo screening exams in the future, then eventually, she will fall into one of the four outcomes: *symptom-free-life, no-early-detection, true-early-detection*, and *over-diagnosis*. We develop a probability model to estimate the probability of each case. Because individuals in the true-early-detection group derive the greatest benefit from screening, it is important to have estimates of the proportion of screened individuals who are likely to benefit from screening.

Consider a currently asymptomatic individual with a screening history who has had no previous cancer diagnosis. We assume the commonly followed disease progressive model in which the disease develops through three states, $S_0 \rightarrow S_p \rightarrow S_c$ [87], where S_0 refers to the disease-free state or the state in which the disease cannot be detected; S_p refers to the preclinical disease state, in which an asymptomatic individual unknowingly has the disease that a screening exam can detect; and S_c refers to the clinical state in which the disease manifests itself in clinical symptoms.

Assume that an individual at current age t_{K_1} has gone through a sequence of screenings at ages $t_0 < t_1 < \cdots < t_{K_1-1}$, all were negative results and with plans for K more exams at ages $t_{K_1} < t_{K_1+1} < t_{K_1+2} < \cdots < t_{K_1+K-1}$, and her lifetime $T > t_{K_1+K-1}$, see Figure 5.3.

We let $\beta_i = \beta(t_i)$ be the sensitivity of the screening test at age t_i. We let X and Y represent the time duration in the S_0 and the S_p respectively, $w(t)$ and $q(y)$ are the corresponding probability density functions (PDF) of X and Y, and $Q(z) = \int_z^\infty q(y)dy$ is the survival function of the sojourn time Y. We assume that X and Y are independent. We use the time variable t to represent an individual's age at the time of screening, and T represents a person's

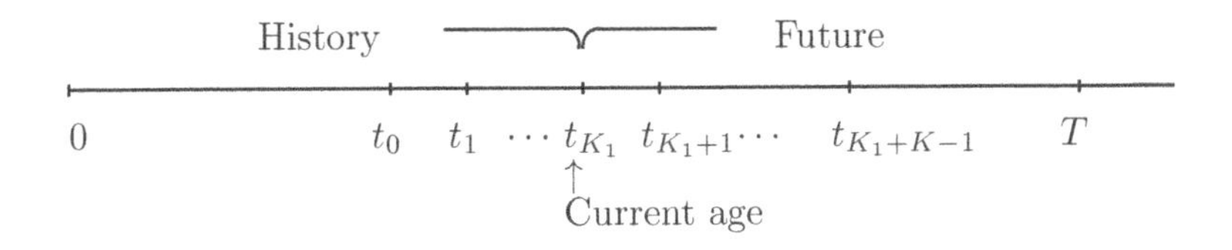

FIGURE 5.3
Illustration of a course of screening examinations (history and future).

lifetime, a continuous random variable with a probability density function $f_T(t)$. To derive the probability of each case, we proceed in the following steps:

1. We derive the probability in the simplest case when $K_1 = K = 1$ (single previous and single future exam) with the lifetime T fixed. Then we allow the lifetime T to be random.
2. We generalize the result to any fixed positive integers K_1 and K when the lifetime T is fixed. Then we allow the lifetime T to be random; hence, the number of future screening exams K is random as well.

5.3.1 Probability calculation when $K_1 = K = 1$

Suppose an asymptomatic woman at current age t_1 had taken only one screening exam at her age $t_0(< t_1)$, which was negative; and she plans to take one more exam at her age t_1. We derive the probability of each of the four possible outcomes, assuming a fixed lifetime $T = t(> t_1)$; then we extend to the case when her lifetime is a random variable, $T \sim f_T(t)$. See Figure 5.4.

We define the event H_1:

$$H_1 = \left\{ \begin{array}{l} \text{A woman had a screening at age } t_0\text{, no breast cancer was found,} \\ \text{and she is asymptomatic at her current age } t_1 \end{array} \right\}.$$

To calculate the probability of H_1, that is, the conditional probability that *no* breast cancer was found before/at her age t_1 when one's lifetime T exceeds t_1, this outcome could arise as one of three mutually exclusive events: (i) she remains in the disease-free state through age t_1, the probability of which is $1 - \int_0^{t_1} w(x)dx$; or (ii) she enters the state S_p at $x \in (0, t_0)$, not detected at t_0, and remains in S_p without symptoms before $t_1(> t_0)$, the probability is $(1 - \beta_0) \int_0^{t_0} w(x)Q(t_1 - x)dx$; or (iii) she enters the state S_p at $x \in (t_0, t_1)$,

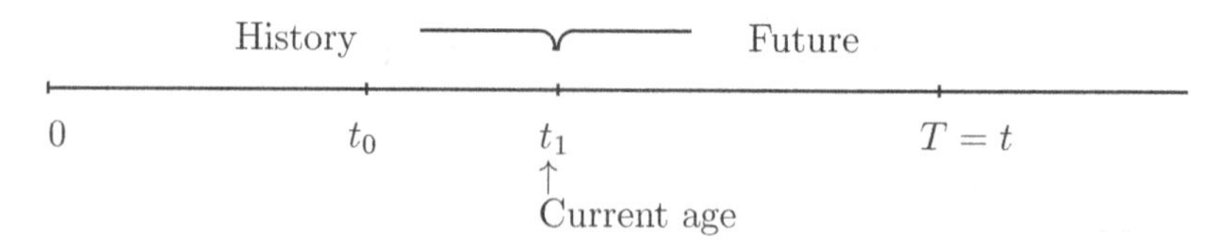

FIGURE 5.4
Screening history and future schedule when $K_1 = K = 1$.

and no symptom presents before t_1, with probability $\int_{t_0}^{t_1} w(x)Q(t_1-x)dx$. We add the three probabilities to obtain:

$$\begin{aligned} & P(H_1|T>t_1) \\ = & \ 1-\int_0^{t_1} w(x)dx+(1-\beta_0)\int_0^{t_0} w(x)Q(t_1-x)dx \\ & +\int_{t_0}^{t_1} w(x)Q(t_1-x)dx. \end{aligned} \tag{5.20}$$

For a Group 1 case, a woman who never has detectable breast cancer during her lifetime $(0,T)$ can follow one of four possible trajectories: (a) she remains in the disease-free state S_0 throughout her lifetime $(0,T)$; (b) she enters the preclinical state S_p before t_0, her cancer is not detected at t_0 nor at t_1, and no clinical symptoms appear before her death at her age T; (c) she enters the preclinical state S_p in (t_0,t_1), her cancer is not detected at t_1, and no symptoms appear before her death; (d) she enters the preclinical state S_p in (t_1,t), and no symptoms appear before her death; Hence the conditional probability given her lifetime $T=t(>t_1)$ is

$$\begin{aligned} & P(\textit{Case 1}\text{: SympF}, H_1|T=t) \\ = & \ 1-\int_0^{t} w(x)dx+(1-\beta_1)(1-\beta_0)\int_0^{t_0} w(x)Q(t-x)dx \\ & +(1-\beta_1)\int_{t_0}^{t_1} w(x)Q(t-x)dx+\int_{t_1}^{t} w(x)Q(t-x)dx. \end{aligned} \tag{5.21}$$

For a Group 2 case, a woman whose cancer became symptomatic in (t_1,T), there are three mutually exclusive events that could happen: (i) she enters the S_p before t_0 and is not detected by the two exams at t_0,t_1, or (ii) she enters the preclinical state in (t_0,t_1) and is missed by the exam at t_1, or (iii) she enters the preclinical state after t_1. In all situations, her sojourn time in the S_p is shorter than $(t-x)$, where x is her age entering S_p. Hence the probability is

$$\begin{aligned} & P(\textit{Case 2}\text{: NoED}, H_1|T=t) \\ = & \ (1-\beta_1)(1-\beta_0)\int_0^{t_0} w(x)[Q(t_1-x)-Q(t-x)]dx \\ & +(1-\beta_1)\int_{t_0}^{t_1} w(x)[Q(t_1-x)-Q(t-x)]dx \\ & +\int_{t_1}^{t} w(x)[1-Q(t-x)]dx. \end{aligned} \tag{5.22}$$

For a Group 3 case, a woman is detected early at t_1, and her symptoms would have appeared before death. She must have entered the S_p at some age x before t_1, and her sojourn time would have been between $(t_1 - x)$ and $(T - x)$. Hence,

$$\begin{aligned} & P(\textit{Case 3}\text{: TrueED}, H_1|T = t) \\ = & \ \beta_1(1-\beta_0)\int_0^{t_0} w(x)[Q(t_1 - x) - Q(t - x)]dx \\ & +\beta_1 \int_{t_0}^{t_1} w(x)[Q(t_1 - x) - Q(t - x)]dx. \end{aligned} \tag{5.23}$$

For a Group 4 case, the case of overdiagnosis, she is to be diagnosed at t_1 but her symptoms would not have appeared before death. That is, she must have entered S_p at some age $x(< t_1)$, but her sojourn time would have extended to beyond time $(T - x)$. Hence,

$$\begin{aligned} & P(\textit{Case 4}\text{: OverD}, H_1|T = t) \\ & = \beta_1(1-\beta_0)\int_0^{t_0} w(x)Q(t - x)dx + \beta_1 \int_{t_0}^{t_1} w(x)Q(t - x)dx. \end{aligned} \tag{5.24}$$

The probability of each case when the lifetime $T(> t_1)$ is a random variable can be obtained by

$$\begin{aligned} P(\text{Case } i, H_1|T > t_1) &= \int_{t_1}^{\infty} P(\text{Case } i, H_1|T = t) f_T(t|T > t_1)dt, \\ & \qquad i = 1, 2, 3, 4. \end{aligned} \tag{5.25}$$

where the conditional pdf $f_T(t|T > t_1)$ is

$$f_T(t|T > t_1) = \begin{cases} \frac{f_T(t)}{P(T>t_1)} = \frac{f_T(t)}{1-F_T(t_1)}, & \text{if } t > t_1; \\ 0, & \text{otherwise.} \end{cases} \tag{5.26}$$

Exercise 5.5. Prove that for any $t > t_1$,

$$\sum_{i=1}^{4} P(\text{Case } i, H_1|T = t) = P(H_1|T > t_1).$$

Since the $P(H_1|T > t_1)$ does not depend on T, we have

$$\begin{aligned} \sum_{i=1}^{4} P(\text{Case } i, H_1|T > t_1) &= \int_{t_1}^{\infty} [\sum_{i=1}^{4} P(\text{Case } i, H_1|T = t)] f_T(t|T > t_1)dt \\ &= P(H_1|T > t_1). \end{aligned}$$

This implies

$$\sum_{i=1}^{4} P(\text{Case } i|H_1, T > t_1) = \sum_{i=1}^{4} \frac{P(\text{Case } i, H_1|T > t_1)}{P(H_1|T > t_1)} = 1.$$

Therefore, the derived probability of each case is correct.

5.3.2 Probability calculation for positive integers K_1 and K

We generalize this idea to an individual with a history of any number of screenings. To derive the probability of each outcome, we assume that an initially asymptomatic individual has gone through $K_1(>1)$ screening exams, which occurred at her ages $t_0 < t_1 < \cdots < t_{K_1-1}$, and her current age is $t_{K_1}(> t_{K_1-1})$ without any symptom. see Figure 5.3. We let $t_{-1} = 0$. Define the event of screening history:

$$H_{K_1} = \left\{ \begin{array}{l} \text{A woman had screenings at her ages } t_0 < t_1 < \cdots < t_{K_1-1}, \\ \text{no breast cancer was found,} \\ \text{and she is asymptomatic at her current age } t_{K_1}. \end{array} \right\}.$$

We first calculate $P(H_{K_1}|T > t_{K_1})$, the conditional probability that no breast cancer was found before/at her age t_{K_1} given that her lifetime T exceeds t_{K_1}. There are $(K_1 + 2)$ mutually exclusive events for H_{K_1} to happen: (i) she never progressed out of the disease-free state S_0 throughout her lifetime, the probability of which is $1 - \int_0^{t_{K_1}} w(x)dx$; or (ii) she entered state S_p in age interval $(t_{j-1}, t_j), j = 0, \ldots, K_1 - 1$, but remains in S_p long enough that no symptom presents before t_{K_1}, and she was missed by the following $(K_1 - j)$ exams; or (iii) she entered the S_p after t_{K_1-1}, and with no symptoms before t_{K_1}. And the probability of H_{K_1} is the sum of these probabilities:

$$\begin{aligned} & P(H_{K_1}|T > t_{K_1}) \\ = \;& 1 - \int_0^{t_{K_1}} w(x)dx + \int_{t_{K_1-1}}^{t_{K_1}} w(x)Q(t_{K_1} - x)dx \qquad (5.27) \\ & + \sum_{j=0}^{K_1-1} (1 - \beta_j) \cdots (1 - \beta_{K_1-1}) \int_{t_{j-1}}^{t_j} w(x)Q(t_{K_1} - x)dx. \end{aligned}$$

Now if she plans to undergo K screening exams in the future, occurring at her age $t_{K_1} < t_{K_1+1} < \cdots < t_{K_1+K-1}$, we first derive the conditional probability for each outcome when her lifetime T is fixed, then we allow her lifetime to be random.

Given that her lifetime is $T = t_{K_1+K}(> t_{K_1+K-1})$, a Group 1 case where clinical breast cancer never occurs in her lifetime, can arise as any one of $(K_1 + K + 2)$ mutually exclusive events: (a) she remained in the disease-free state S_0 throughout her lifetime, the probability of which is $1 - \int_0^{t_{K_1+K}} w(x)dx$; (b) she entered the preclinical state S_p in the age interval (t_{j-1}, t_j), $j = 0, \ldots, K_1 + K - 1$, and she was not detected by the following $(K_1 + K - j)$ exams, and she had a long sojourn time, so no clinical symptom appeared before her death (these are $K_1 + K$ disjoint events); (c) she entered S_p after t_{K_1+K-1} and without clinical symptoms before her death. Summing these probabilities:

$$
\begin{aligned}
&P(\text{Case } 1, H_{K_1}|T = t_{K_1+K}) \\
&= 1 - \int_0^{t_{K_1+K}} w(x)dx + \int_{t_{K_1+K-1}}^{t_{K_1+K}} w(x)Q(t_{K_1+K} - x)dx \\
&\quad + \sum_{j=0}^{K_1+K-1} (1-\beta_j)\cdots(1-\beta_{K_1+K-1}) \int_{t_{j-1}}^{t_j} w(x)Q(t_{K_1+K} - x)dx.
\end{aligned} \tag{5.28}
$$

For a Group 2 case, we calculate the probability of no early detection by defining $I_{K_1+K,j}$ as the probability of being an interval case in the interval $(t_{j-1}, t_j), j = (K_1+1), (K_1+2), \cdots, (K_1+K)$, in a sequence of K screening exams in the future. Thus

$$
P(\text{Case } 2, H_{K_1}|T = t_{K_1+K}) = \sum_{j=K_1+1}^{K_1+K} I_{K_1+K,j} \tag{5.29}
$$

where

$$
\begin{aligned}
&I_{K_1+K,j} \\
&= \sum_{i=0}^{j-1}(1-\beta_i)\cdots(1-\beta_{j-1}) \int_{t_{i-1}}^{t_i} w(x)[Q(t_{j-1} - x) - Q(t_j - x)]dx \\
&\quad + \int_{t_{j-1}}^{t_j} w(x)[1 - Q(t_j - x)]dx, \text{ for } j = K_1+1, \cdots, K_1+K.
\end{aligned} \tag{5.30}
$$

A Group 3 case, true early detection, can arise as one of K disjoint events depending on her age at diagnosis by screening, namely, at $t_j, j = K_1, (K_1+1), \cdots, (K_1+K-1)$. If she is diagnosed at t_j, then she must have entered the preclinical state S_p before t_j, was not detected by the previous j exams and her sojourn time must have been in the interval $(t_j - x, t_{K_1+K} - x)$, where x represents the onset time of the preclinical state. Therefore,

$$
\begin{aligned}
&P(\text{Case } 3, H_{K_1}|T = t_{K_1+K}) \\
&= \sum_{j=K_1}^{K_1+K-1} \beta_j \left\{ \sum_{i=0}^{j-1}(1-\beta_i)\cdots(1-\beta_{j-1}) \right. \\
&\quad \times \int_{t_{i-1}}^{t_i} w(x)[Q(t_j - x) - Q(t_{K_1+K} - x)]dx \\
&\quad \left. + \int_{t_{j-1}}^{t_j} w(x)[Q(t_j - x) - Q(t_{K_1+K} - x)]dx \right\}
\end{aligned} \tag{5.31}
$$

A Group 4 case, overdiagnosis, also can arise as one of K disjoint events. She might have been diagnosed at the j-th exam, $j = K_1, (K_1+1), \cdots, (K_1+K-1)$, but her sojourn time would have been longer than $(t_{K_1+K} - x)$; thus, her symptoms would not appear before her death:

$$\begin{aligned} &P(\text{Case } 4, H_{K_1} | T = t_{K_1+K}) \\ &= \sum_{j=K_1}^{K_1+K-1} \beta_j \left\{ \sum_{i=0}^{j-1} (1-\beta_i)\cdots(1-\beta_{j-1}) \int_{t_{i-1}}^{t_i} w(x) Q(t_{K_1+K} - x) dx \right. \\ &\left. + \int_{t_{j-1}}^{t_j} w(x) Q(t_{K_1+K} - x) dx \right\}. \end{aligned} \tag{5.32}$$

Exercise 5.6. Prove that for any screening number $K_1 > 1$ and $K > 1$,

$$\sum_{i=1}^{4} P(\text{Case } i, H_{K_1} | T = t_{K_1+K}) = P(H_{K_1} | T > t_{K_1}).$$

For an individual currently at age t_{K_1}, her life is not fixed but is a random variable, so it may not be realistic to consider the future number of exams K to be a fixed value. However, if she plans to follow a future screening schedule $t_{K_1} < t_{K_1+1} < \ldots$, then $K = n$ if $t_{K_1+n-1} < T < t_{K_1+n}$, the screening number $K = K(T)$ is a random variable, changing with the lifetime T. The probability of each case ($i = 1, 2, 3, 4$) when her lifetime T is longer than her current age t_{K_1} can be obtained by the integration (i.e., a weighted average):

$$\begin{aligned} &P(\text{Case } i, H_{K_1} | T > t_{K_1}) \\ &= \int_{t_{K_1}}^{\infty} P(\text{Case } i, H_{K_1} | K = K(T), T = t) f_T(t | T > t_{K_1}) dt. \end{aligned} \tag{5.33}$$

Where the conditional PDF of the lifetime is

$$f_T(t|T > t_{K_1}) = \begin{cases} \frac{f_T(t)}{P(T > t_{K_1})} = \frac{f_T(t)}{1 - F_T(t_{K_1})}, & \text{if } t > t_{K_1}; \\ 0, & \text{otherwise.} \end{cases}$$

And the probability inside the integration, $P(\text{Case i}, H_{K_1} | K = K(T), T = t)$, was derived in equations (5.28) to (5.32).

Exercise 5.7. Prove that for any future screening schedule, when the lifetime T is random,

$$\sum_{i=1}^{4} P(\text{Case } i | H_{K_1}, T > t_{K_1}) = 1.$$

The probability of overdiagnosis among the screen-detected cases is

$$\begin{aligned} &P(\text{OverD}|\text{screen-detected}) \\ &= \frac{P(\text{Case } 4, H_{K_1} | T > t_{K_1})}{P(\text{Case } 3, H_{K_1} | T > t_{K_1}) + P(\text{Case } 4, H_{K_1} | T > t_{K_1})}. \end{aligned}$$

This is the probability that the general public is really interested.

5.3.3 Simulations

Extensive simulation studies were carried out using the method in this section. Since the probability of each case is a function of one's initial screening age, current age, past and future screening interval, the three key parameters, and the human lifetime, we want to explore the effects of these factors on the probability of each outcome, and also explore how the proportion of true-early-detection and overdiagnosis change among the screen-detected cases due to these factors. We selected the following scenarios for simulation:

1. age at initial screening $t_0 = 50$ years old;
2. current age $t_{K_1} = 70$ years old;
3. past and future screening interval:
$$(\Delta_1, \Delta_2) = (1,1), (2,1), (1,2), (2,2) \text{ years;}$$
4. screening sensitivity: $\beta = 0.7, 0.9$;
5. transition density $w(t)$: log Normal $(\mu = 4.2, \sigma^2 = 0.1)$ times 20%;
6. sojourn time: log-logistic (κ, ρ) $Q(x) = \frac{1}{1+(x\rho)^\kappa}$,
with mean sojourn time (MST) 2, 5, 10, or 15 years.

The parameter of the $w(t)$ was chosen so that it has a single mode at around 60 years old, and with an upper limit of 20%, which is applicable to different kinds of cancer, including breast cancer. The sojourn time distribution was chosen to be a log-logistic pdf, with parameters $\kappa = 2.5$ and $\rho = 0.6607, 0.2643, 0.1321, 0.0881$, and the corresponding mean sojourn time (MST) is 2, 5, 10, and 15 years. The number of screens $K = K(T) = \lceil (T - t_0)/\Delta \rceil$ is a function of the lifetime T; therefore, it is changing with T in the simulation. We used female lifetime distribution in this simulation. We report the results in Table 5.9.

In Table 5.9, the first column (Δ_1, Δ_2) are the past and future screening intervals in the simulation. The next 4 columns present the probabilities of each of the four cases, that is, $P(\text{Case } i|A, T > t_{K_1}), i = 1, 2, 3, 4$, corresponding to the probability of symptom-free-life, no-early-detection, true-early-detection, and overdiagnosis. The last two columns are the conditional probability of true-early-detection and overdiagnosis among the screen-detected cases, and it is calculated by

$$P(\text{Case i}|A, T > t_{K_1})/[P(\text{Case 3}|A, T > t_{K_1}) + P(\text{Case 4}|A, T > t_{K_1})], i = 3, 4.$$

The probabilities are reported as percentages in the table.

The probability of symptom-free-life is very stable, around 95% for all cases. The probability of no-early-detection is influenced more by the future screening intervals; it is larger when the future screening interval is longer. The probability of true-early-detection behaves the other way around: it is smaller when the future screening interval is longer. The probability of overdiagnosis

TABLE 5.9
Simulation: Probability of each outcome (in %) with a screening history when $t_0 = 50$, and the current age is 70.

(Δ_1, Δ_2)	[a]P(SympF)	P(NoED)	P(TrueED)	P(OverD)	[b]P(TrueED$\|D$)	P(OverD$\|D$)
			$\beta = 0.7$, $MST = 2$ **yrs**			
(1,1)	95.27	1.16	3.23	0.32	90.97	9.03
(2,1)	95.10	1.20	3.37	0.33	91.14	8.86
(1,2)	95.37	2.15	2.25	0.22	90.95	9.05
(2,2)	95.20	2.19	2.37	0.23	91.16	8.84
			$\beta = 0.7$, $MST = 5$ **yrs**			
(1,1)	95.21	0.31	3.47	1.01	77.48	22.52
(2,1)	94.81	0.35	3.79	1.05	78.37	21.63
(1,2)	95.40	0.84	2.93	0.82	78.17	21.83
(2,2)	95.00	0.91	3.22	0.85	79.06	20.94
			$\beta = 0.7$, $MST = 10$ **yrs**			
(1,1)	95.19	0.08	2.72	2.01	57.55	42.45
(2,1)	94.67	0.10	3.11	2.12	59.45	40.55
(1,2)	95.43	0.28	2.52	1.77	58.78	41.22
(2,2)	94.91	0.32	2.88	1.87	60.61	39.39
			$\beta = 0.7$, $MST = 15$ **yrs**			
(1,1)	95.19	0.03	2.02	2.76	42.30	57.70
(2,1)	94.63	0.04	2.37	2.95	44.59	55.41
(1,2)	95.44	0.12	1.93	2.50	43.53	56.47
(2,2)	94.89	0.15	2.27	2.69	45.75	54.25
			$\beta = 0.9$, $MST = 2$ **yrs**			
(1,1)	95.27	1.04	3.35	0.33	90.97	9.03
(2,1)	95.10	1.07	3.49	0.34	91.15	8.85
(1,2)	95.37	2.02	2.36	0.23	90.98	9.02
(2,2)	95.19	2.06	2.49	0.24	91.21	8.79
			$\beta = 0.9$, $MST = 5$ **yrs**			
(1,1)	95.21	0.25	3.50	1.03	77.33	22.67
(2,1)	94.82	0.29	3.82	1.06	78.24	21.76
(1,2)	95.39	0.74	3.01	0.84	78.10	21.90
(2,2)	95.00	0.80	3.31	0.88	79.01	20.99
			$\beta = 0.9$, $MST = 10$ **yrs**			
(1,1)	95.20	0.06	2.71	2.02	57.27	42.73
(2,1)	94.70	0.07	3.08	2.13	59.13	40.87
(1,2)	95.42	0.23	2.54	1.80	58.55	41.45
(2,2)	94.93	0.26	2.90	1.91	60.33	39.67
			$\beta = 0.9$, $MST = 15$ **yrs**			
(1,1)	95.20	0.02	2.00	2.77	42.01	57.99
(2,1)	94.67	0.03	2.34	2.95	44.20	55.80
(1,2)	95.43	0.10	1.93	2.53	43.24	56.76
(2,2)	94.91	0.12	2.25	2.71	45.36	54.64

[a]Columns 2 to 5 is the probability of each outcome, i.e., $P(\text{Case } i|A, T > t_{K_1})$.
[b]Columns 6 and 7 is the conditional probability of true-early-detection and of overdiagnosis given that it is a screen-detected case.
Adapted from Table 3 in Wu et al 2018 [70].

is slightly smaller when the future screening interval is longer. The historic screening interval seems to have little influence on the result, it only slightly changes the proportion of these groups.

We can see clearly that the sojourn time plays the most important role in the proportion of overdiagnosis and true-early-detection among those detected by screening. For example, in the last column of Table 5.9, the proportion of overdiagnosis could be as high as 58% among the screen-detected cases if the mean sojourn time is 15 years; it is around 40% if the mean sojourn time is

10 years; it is about 21% if the mean sojourn time is 5 years; and it is only about 9% if the mean sojourn time is 2 years.

The screening sensitivity will slightly affect the ratio of the no-early-detection and the true-early-detection: when sensitivity is higher, the probability of true-early-detection is higher, and the probability of no-early-detection is lower. Compared with the sojourn time, the screening sensitivity does not change the ratio of overdiagnosis and true-early-detection among the screen-detected cases.

The transition probability density $w(t)$ surely is important but in this simulation, we limit it to the situation where the density has a single peak around age 60 based on our previous results in breast cancer screening.

5.3.4 Application: Breast cancer outcomes with a screening history using the HIP

We applied our method to the Health Insurance Plan of the Greater New York (HIP) breast cancer screening data [47]. Using this data, the posterior predictive probability of each case can be estimated by

$$\begin{aligned}
&P(\text{Case } i|T > t_{K_1}, H_{K_1}, HIP) \\
&= \int P(\text{Case } i, \theta|T > t_{K_1}, H_{K_1}, HIP)d\theta \\
&= \int P(\text{Case } i|T > t_{K_1}, H_{K_1}, \theta) f(\theta|HIP)d\theta \qquad (5.34) \\
&\approx \frac{1}{n}\sum_{j=1}^{n} P(\text{Case } i|T > t_{K_1}, H_{K_1}, \theta_j^*)
\end{aligned}$$

where θ_j^* is the random sample drawn from the posterior distribution $f(\theta|HIP)$ and $n = 2000$ is the posterior sample size (Wu et al 2005).

We used the same parametric functions (5.18) for the three key parameters. We applied (5.34) to the 2000 MCMC posterior samples, to conduct Bayesian inference on three hypothetical cohorts of women currently at ages 60, 70, and 80, assuming that they have started their first screening at age 50, with annual, biennial screening, or without any screening until their present age (i.e., 10, 20, or 30 years later). For each group, it is assumed that they look healthy at their current age with no cancer previously found, and we have examined annual or biennial screening intervals in the future ($\Delta_2 = 1, 2$ years). The number of screens $K = \lceil (T - t_{K_1})/\Delta_2 \rceil$ is a function of the lifetime T; therefore, it is changing in the simulation.

For the lifetime distribution, we used the conditional lifetime density for females at current ages 60, 70, and 80 derived from the actuarial life table from the Social Security Administration (SSA) website, and the corresponding PDF curves were plotted in Figure 5.5. The probabilities of each of the four cases $P(\text{Case } i|H_{K_1}, T > t_{K_1}, HIP)$ with standard errors were reported in Table 5.10.

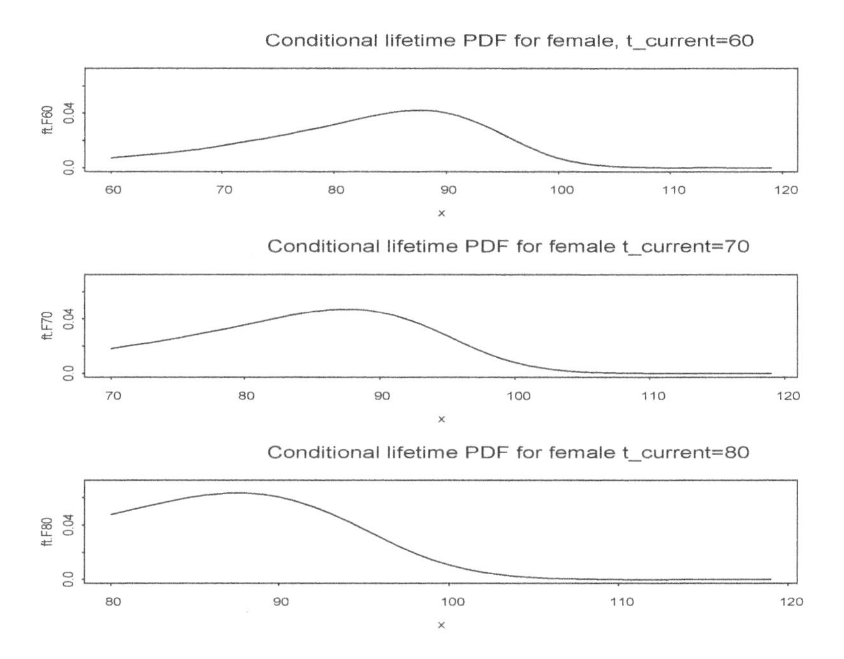

FIGURE 5.5
Conditional PDF of the female lifetime in the United States at current age 60, 70, and 80.

The probability of overdiagnosis for all age groups is very small, between 0.20% and 0.34% from Table 5.10. This probability decreases when a woman's current age increases, and it decreases as the future screening time interval (Δ_2) increases. It depends more on the future screening interval Δ_2, and less on the past screening interval Δ_1.

The probability of true-early-detection is higher for the annual screening group in the future than that for biennial screening within each age group. That is, this probability decreases as the future screening time interval increases. The probability is also lower when the current age increases from 60 to 80. Similar to the probability of overdiagnosis, the past screening interval causes little change in the probability of true-early-detection. Under this model, the probability of no-early-detection is between 0.45% and 2.86%; it increases as the future screening interval length increases and decreases when the current age increases. The probability of symptom-free-life is very high. It increases from about 93% to 98% when the current age increases from 60 to 80, and changes only slightly with the past or future screening intervals. This implies that the majority of women will live a life free of breast cancer.

Figure 5.6 shows how the trends change with screening history for women currently aged $t_{K_1} = 70$ using the boxplots. Other age groups follow a similar pattern, and we omitted here. When other parameters are the same, the probabilities of true-early-detection, overdiagnosis, and no-early-detection slightly

TABLE 5.10
Application: Projection of breast cancer screening outcomes using the HIP data.

[a](Δ_1, Δ_2)	[b]P(SympF)	P(NoED)	P(TrueED)	P(OverD)
	Initial screen age $t_0 = 50$, current age $t_{K_1} = 60$			
(1 yr, 1 yr)	93.62(1.07)	1.34(0.63)	4.69(1.04)	0.32(0.22)
(2 yr, 1 yr)	93.52(1.06)	1.34(0.62)	4.78(1.04)	0.32(0.22)
(–, 1 yr)	93.21(1.02)	1.39(0.63)	5.03(1.02)	0.33(0.25)
(1 yr, 2 yr)	93.69(1.08)	2.75(0.89)	3.28(0.71)	0.25(0.19)
(2 yr, 2 yr)	93.59(1.06)	2.76(0.88)	3.36(0.72)	0.25(0.20)
(–, 2 yr)	93.28(1.02)	2.86(0.89)	3.57(0.72)	0.26(0.23)
	Initial screen age $t_0 = 50$, current age $t_{K_1} = 70$			
(1 yr, 1 yr)	95.84(0.69)	0.84(0.48)	3.00(0.72)	0.30(0.19)
(2 yr, 1 yr)	95.73(0.68)	0.85(0.48)	3.09(0.72)	0.31(0.20)
(–, 1 yr)	95.57(0.63)	0.86(0.47)	3.21(0.68)	0.34(0.26)
(1 yr, 2 yr)	95.91(0.69)	1.73(0.62)	2.11(0.50)	0.23(0.17)
(2 yr, 2 yr)	95.81(0.68)	1.74(0.62)	2.20(0.52)	0.24(0.18)
(–, 2 yr)	95.65(0.63)	1.75(0.60)	2.32(0.52)	0.27(0.23)
	Initial screen age $t_0 = 50$, current age $t_{K_1} = 80$			
(1 yr, 1 yr)	97.74(0.34)	0.45(0.31)	1.55(0.40)	0.27(0.16)
(2 yr, 1 yr)	97.64(0.34)	0.45(0.31)	1.63(0.41)	0.28(0.17)
(–, 1 yr)	97.47(0.35)	0.46(0.31)	1.74(0.38)	0.34(0.26)
(1 yr, 2 yr)	97.80(0.34)	0.90(0.35)	1.09(0.28)	0.20(0.14)
(2 yr, 2 yr)	97.70(0.34)	0.91(0.35)	1.17(0.31)	0.21(0.15)
(–, 2 yr)	97.54(0.33)	0.92(0.34)	1.28(0.31)	0.27(0.24)

[a](Δ_1, Δ_2) are screening intervals (in years) of the past and the future respectively. when Δ_1 is "–", it refers to those who never take any screening exam until the current age; that is, those without a screening history.
[b]Entries are percentages %; i.e., 100 times the mean probability (with standard error).
Adapted from Table 1 in Wu et al 2018 [70].

increase as the historic screening interval increases. However, the probability of symptom-free-life shows a reversed pattern: when the past screening interval increases, this probability decreases.

The general public and the medical community are more concerned with the percentage of overdiagnosis among the screen-detected cases. The estimated probabilities and the 95% highest posterior density (HPD) intervals of overdiagnosis and true-early-detection among the screen-detected cases are listed in Table 5.11. The percentage of overdiagnosis among the screen-detected is about 7%, 10% and 15% for current age groups 60, 70, and 80 respectively, so this probability increases significantly with a person's current age. However, it changes little with future or past screening intervals. The 95% highest posterior density (HPD) interval of this percentage is wide also.

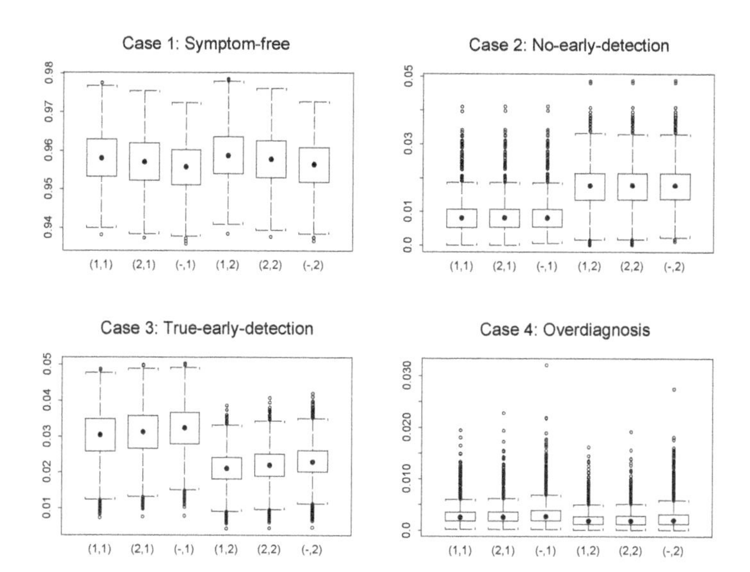

FIGURE 5.6
Boxplot of the estimated probability when $t_0 = 50, t_{K_1} = 70$.
Adapted from Figure 3 in Wu et al 2018 [70].

Since the probability of true-early-detection is one minus the probability of overdiagnosis given that it is a screen-detected case, the changing pattern of this probability is contrary to that of overdiagnosis: it decreases with a person's current age and remains stable with different future and past screening intervals. The lengths of the 95% HPD intervals for these two probabilities (as percentages) increases as a person's current age increases, showing large variations with advanced ages.

5.3.5 Application: Lung cancer outcomes with a screening history using the NLST-CT data

We applied the method to the National Lung Screening Trial (NLST) low-dose helical computed tomography (CT) data, The result was published in Wu et al 2016 [73]. The following link functions were used to estimate the three key parameters for the NLST-CT data (Liu et al 2015 [32]):

$$\begin{aligned}
\beta(t) &= [1 + \exp(-b_0 - b_1(t - m))]^{-1}, \\
w(t) &= \frac{0.3}{\sqrt{2\pi}\sigma t} \exp\left\{-(\log t - \mu)^2/(2\sigma^2)\right\}, \\
Q(x) &= \exp(-\lambda x^\alpha), \quad \lambda > 0, \alpha > 0,
\end{aligned}$$

where $m = 64.5$ is the average age at the study entry in the NLST-CT study. The six unknown parameters $\theta = (b_0, b_1, \mu, \sigma^2, \lambda, \alpha)$ were estimated when both

TABLE 5.11
Application: Estimated mean probability of true-early-detection and overdiagnosis in screen-detected cases with 95% HPD intervals (in %).

(Δ_1, Δ_2)	${}^aP$(TrueED|ScrD)	P(OverD|ScrD)
Initial screen age $t_0 = 50$, current age $t_{K_1} = 60$		
(1 yr, 1 yr)	93.15 (74.55, 97.87)	6.85 (2.13, 25.45)
(2 yrs, 1 yr)	93.24 (74.84, 97.88)	6.76 (2.12, 25.16)
(–, 1 yr)	93.43 (75.37, 97.97)	6.57 (2.03, 24.63)
(1 yr, 2 yrs)	92.81 (73.18, 97.94)	7.19 (2.06, 26.82)
(2 yrs, 2 yr)	92.93 (73.44, 97.96)	7.07 (2.04, 26.56)
(–, 2 yr)	93.10 (74.44, 98.05)	6.90 (1.95, 25.56)
Initial screen age $t_0 = 50$, current age $t_{K_1} = 70$		
(1 yr, 1 yr)	90.32 (67.38, 96.70)	9.68 (3.30, 32.62)
(2 yrs, 1 yr)	90.49 (67.98, 96.73)	9.51 (3.27, 32.02)
(–, 1 yr)	90.22 (67.09, 96.73)	9.78 (3.37, 32.91)
(1 yr, 2 yrs)	90.00 (66.09, 96.80)	10.00 (3.20, 33.91)
(2 yrs, 2 yrs)	90.21 (67.18, 96.84)	9.79 (3.16, 32.82)
(–, 2 yrs)	89.87 (66.11, 96.85)	10.13 (3.15, 33.89)
Initial screen age $t_0 = 50$, current age $t_{K_1} = 80$		
(1 yr, 1 yr)	84.89 (56.66, 94.22)	15.11 (5.78, 43.34)
(2 yrs, 1 yr)	85.16 (57.19, 94.27)	14.84 (5.73, 42.81)
(–, 1 yr)	84.32 (54.22, 94.21)	15.68 (5.79, 45.78)
(1 yr, 2 yrs)	84.56 (55.40, 94.36)	15.44 (5.64, 44.60)
(2 yrs, 2 yrs)	84.92 (55.76, 94.38)	15.08 (5.62, 44.24)
(–, 2 yrs)	83.88 (53.42, 94.36)	16.12 (5.64, 46.58)

[a]The event ScrD = {Screen-detected case}.
The probability was calculated by $p_i^*/(p_3^* + p_4^*), i = 3, 4$, for each of the 2000 posterior samples, then take the average. It is in percentage.
Adapted from Table 2 in Wu et al 2018 [70].

gender's data were pooled together as a group, using Markov Chain Monte Carlo (MCMC) to generate 1000 posterior samples [32]. See Liu et al 2015 for details. We used the 1000 posterior samples θ_j^* to estimate the probability of each outcome:

$$P(\text{Case } i|T > t_{K_1}, H_{K_1}, NLST - CT) \approx \frac{1}{n}\sum_{j=1}^{n} P(\text{Case } i|T > t_{K_1}, H_{K_1}, \theta_j^*).$$

what we presented here is the probability of future outcomes for both genders combined. Hence we let the PDF of the lifetime be the average of that from both males and females.

We applied the method to make Bayesian inference on three hypothetical cohorts of asymptomatic heavy smokers with current age t_{K_1} equals 60, 70,

TABLE 5.12
Application: Lung cancer scr. outcomes for heavy smokers using the NLST-CT data.

$^a(\Delta_1, \Delta_2)$	^bP(SympF)	P(NoED)	P(TrueED)	P(OverD)
	Initial screen age $t_0 = 50$**, current age** $t_{K_1} = 60$			
(1 yr, 1 yr)	80.26(0.57)	1.86(0.28)	17.19(0.60)	0.66(0.09)
(2 yr, 1 yr)	80.05(0.56)	1.86(0.27)	17.40(0.60)	0.66(0.09)
(∞, 1 yr)	80.01(0.56)	1.86(0.27)	17.44(0.59)	0.66(0.09)
(1 yr, 2 yr)	80.50(0.57)	6.31(0.63)	12.74(0.55)	0.42(0.08)
(2 yr, 2 yr)	80.29(0.57)	6.30(0.63)	12.96(0.56)	0.43(0.08)
(∞, 2 yr)	80.25(0.56)	6.30(0.63)	13.00 (0.57)	0.43(0.08)
	Initial screen age $t_0 = 50$**, current age** $t_{K_1} = 70$			
(1 yr, 1 yr)	86.13(0.39)	1.30(0.24)	11.90(0.42)	0.67(0.09)
(2 yr, 1 yr)	85.64(0.42)	1.31(0.24)	12.38(0.44)	0.67(0.09)
(∞, 1 yr)	85.53(0.43)	1.31(0.24)	12.49(0.44)	0.67(0.09)
(1 yr, 2 yr)	86.38(0.39)	4.33(0.44)	8.86(0.45)	0.42(0.08)
(2 yr, 2 yr)	85.88(0.41)	4.33(0.44)	9.36(0.50)	0.43(0.08)
(∞, 2 yr)	85.78(0.43)	4.32(0.44)	9.47(0.53)	0.43(0.08)
	Initial screen age $t_0 = 50$**, current age** $t_{K_1} = 80$			
(1 yr, 1 yr)	94.20(0.26)	0.55(0.16)	4.73(0.23)	0.52(0.08)
(2 yr, 1 yr)	93.75(0.30)	0.57(0.17)	5.16(0.27)	0.53(0.09)
(∞, 1 yr)	93.65(0.35)	0.57(0.17)	5.27(0.30)	0.53(0.09)
(1 yr, 2 yr)	94.38(0.25)	1.75(0.21)	3.54(0.26)	0.34(0.07)
(2 yr, 2 yr)	93.92(0.28)	1.76(0.23)	3.97(0.31)	0.36(0.07)
(∞, 2 yr)	93.84(0.33)	1.76(0.23)	4.08(0.35)	0.36(0.08)

[a] Δ_1, Δ_2 are scr. interval in history and in the future correspondingly.
[b] The mean probability (with standard error) are in percentage.
Adapted from Table 1 in Wu et al 2016 [73].

and 80, assuming that either they started their initial CT screening at the age of 50, or they have never taken any screening exam until their current age now. That is, within each cohort, there are three scenarios in the participants' past: annual screening, biennial screening, or no screening at all, correspondingly represented by $\Delta_1 = 1$, 2, or ∞ years; where ∞ means one has never been screened until the current age. In any case, they would share the same θ_j^* as those participants in the NLST-CT study. For future planning, both annual and biennial screenings in the future were considered, that is, $\Delta_2 = 1$ or 2 years. The results were summarized in Tables 5.12 and 5.13.

From Table 5.12 the probability of symptom-free-life is stable within each age group; it is about 80% for the current 60 years old, about 86% for the 70 years old, and about 94% for the 80 years old. It is not affected by past or future screening intervals but mainly affected by a heavy smoker's current age.

The probability of no-early-detection is mainly determined by the future screening interval Δ_2 and an individual's current age, ranging from 0.55% to 6.31%. For those who have no screening history, the probability of no-early-detection is about the same as those who have annual or biennial screenings if their future screening schedules are the same. If we consider the ratio of this probability as a measure of relative risk when future screening interval Δ_2 changes from 1 to 2 years, the ratio is 3.39, 3.31, 3.09 for the current ages 60, 70, and 80 correspondingly, showing that doubling the future screening intervals will cause the probability of no-early-detection to increase about 3 times.

The probability of true-early-detection depends more on the future screening interval Δ_2 and the current age, ranging from 3.54% to 17.44%. It increases when future screening interval decreases (i.e., more frequent screening), and it decreases as the current age increases. The ratio of this probability between the biennial and annual future screening interval Δ_2 is close to 75% for all three age groups, showing that the probability of true-early-detection would decrease to about 75% of what it was, if the future screening interval changes from annual to biennial.

The probability of overdiagnosis in the whole population is very low, about 0.34-0.67%. It decreases slightly as age advances and as screen interval increases. Each row in Table 5.12 should add to 100%; however, due to simulation accuracy, it is not exactly 100% sometimes. The standard deviations (in percentage) were reported in parenthesis as well.

Table 5.13 summarizes the probability of overdiagnosis among the screen-detected cases. These are the probabilities that most researchers are eager to explore and the general public wants to know. It is increasing when people are aging: about 3% for the 60, about 5% for the 70, and about 9% for the 80 years old. It is slightly decreasing when the historic screening interval increases. Combining all cohorts, there are fewer than 10% of overdiagnosis among the screen-detected cases, while more than 90% are true-early-detection. This means if left untreated, about 3% to 10% of patients may die of other causes before clinical symptoms of lung cancer comes up, while more than 90% of the screen-detected cases are true-early-detection that needs treatment and intervention immediately. The 95% credible intervals (C.I.) are reported in Table 5.13 as well, ranging from 87% to 97% for the probability of true-early-detection; and 2% to 13% for overdiagnosis.

5.4 Model extension: When sensitivity is a function of sojourn time

The methods in sections 5.2 and 5.3 assume that the sensitivity depends on the age and does not relate to the sojourn time. The first model (in section

TABLE 5.13
Application: The estimated probability of true-early-detection and overdiagnosis in screen-detected cases (with 95% HPD interval) using the NLST-CT data.

($^a\Delta_1, \Delta_2$)	P(TrueED|^{b}Diag)	P(OverD|Diag)
Initial screen age $t_0 = 50$, current age $t_{K_1} = 60$		
(1 yr, 1 yr)	96.31 (95.10, 97.12)	3.69 (2.88, 4.90)
(2 yrs, 1 yr)	96.35 (95.17, 97.15)	3.65 (2.85, 4.83)
(∞, 1 yr)	96.36 (95.20, 97.15)	3.64 (2.85, 4.80)
(1 yr, 2 yrs)	96.78 (95.62, 97.51)	3.22 (2.49, 4.38)
(2 yrs, 2 yrs)	96.83 (95.70, 97.54)	3.17 (2.46, 4.30)
(∞, 2 yrs)	96.84 (95.74, 97.55)	3.16 (2.45, 4.26)
Initial screen age $t_0 = 50$, current age $t_{K_1} = 70$		
(1 yr, 1 yr)	94.68 (93.01, 95.79)	5.32 (4.21, 6.99)
(2 yrs, 1 yr)	94.85 (93.26, 95.90)	5.15 (4.10, 6.74)
(∞, 1 yr)	94.89 (93.39, 95.92)	5.11 (4.08, 6.61)
(1 yr, 2 yrs)	95.45 (93.87, 96.46)	4.55 (3.54, 6.13)
(2 yrs, 2 yrs)	95.62 (94.12, 96.58)	4.38 (3.42, 5.88)
(∞, 2 yrs)	95.67 (94.26, 96.60)	4.33 (3.40, 5.74)
Initial screen age $t_0 = 50$, current age $t_{K_1} = 80$		
(1 yr, 1 yr)	90.21 (87.32, 92.16)	9.79 (7.84, 12.68)
(2 yrs, 1 yr)	90.71 (87.98, 92.51)	9.29 (7.49, 12.02)
(∞, 1 yr)	90.86 (88.43, 92.54)	9.14 (7.46, 11.57)
(1 yr, 2 yrs)	91.29 (88.55, 93.06)	8.71 (6.94, 11.45)
(2 yrs, 2 yrs)	91.82 (89.26, 93.44)	8.18 (6.56, 10.74)
(∞, 2 yrs)	91.99 (89.69, 93.49)	8.01 (6.51, 10.31)

[a] $\Delta_1 = \infty$ means one has no screening history.
[b] Event Diag= {cancer is screen-detected}.
Adapted from Table 2 in Wu et al 2016 [73].

5.2) without a screening history can be considered a special case of the second one (in section 5.3) with a screening history when the previous exam number $K_1 = 0$ [70]. We will expand the two models by allowing the sensitivity to be a function of the time spent in the preclinical state and the sojourn time.

5.4.1 Long-term outcome without screening history when sensitivity depends on sojourn time

As we have pointed out, in practice, when the tumor cell is just formed, the sensitivity is fairly small, but as a patient is at the end of the preclinical state, the sensitivity is much higher and tumors could be easily caught by screening. We let the sensitivity be a function of the ratio of time one has stayed in the preclinical state and the sojourn time. That is, we let the sensitivity be $\beta(s|Y), 0 \leq s \leq Y$, where s is the time one has stayed in the S_p, and Y is the sojourn time in the S_p. We define event A as in section 5.2:

$$A = \{\text{A woman is asymptomatic of cancer before and at her age } t_0\}.$$

And we have derived the probability in equation (5.1):

$$P(A|T > t_0) = 1 - \int_0^{t_0} w(x)dx + \int_0^{t_0} w(x)Q(t_0 - x)dx.$$

Now if she plans to take $K(> 1)$ screening exams in the future, occurring at her age $t_0 < t_1 < \cdots < t_{K-1}$, given that her lifetime $T = t_K > t_{K-1}$, the probability of each outcome would be changed since the sensitivity depends on the time in the preclinical state and the sojourn time.

For case 1, a woman who never had detective cancer in her lifetime, there are $(K+2)$ mutually exclusive events: (i) she remained in the disease-free state S_0 all her lifetime; (ii) she entered the preclinical state S_p after t_{K-1} and no symptom appears before her lifetime $T = t_K$; and (iii) she entered the S_p at age $x \in (t_{j-1}, t_j), j = 0, \ldots, K-1$, her sojourn time is longer than $(t_K - x)$, and at the next few exams at her age $t_i, i = j, \ldots, K-1$, the sensitivity would be $\beta(t_i - x|t)$, where t is her sojourn time, $(t_i - x)$ is her time stayed in the S_p at t_i, and she was not detected in these exams. Hence the probability would be

$$\begin{aligned}
&P(\text{Case 1: SympF}, A|T = t_K) \\
=&1 - \int_0^{t_K} w(x)dx + \int_{t_{K-1}}^{t_K} w(x)Q(t_K - x)dx \\
&+ \sum_{j=0}^{K-1} \int_{t_{j-1}}^{t_j} w(x) \int_{t_K - x}^{\infty} q(t) \prod_{i=j}^{K-1} [1 - \beta(t_i - x|t)]dtdx.
\end{aligned} \tag{5.35}$$

For case 2, no early detection, the probability is just the summation of all possible interval cases:

$$P(\text{Case 2: NoED}, A|T = t_K) = I_{K,1} + I_{K,2} + \cdots + I_{K,K}, \tag{5.36}$$

where

$$\begin{aligned}
I_{K,j} =& \sum_{i=0}^{j-1} \int_{t_{i-1}}^{t_i} w(x) \int_{t_{j-1}-x}^{t_j - x} q(t) \prod_{r=i}^{j-1} [1 - \beta(t_r - x|t)]dtdx \\
&+ \int_{t_{j-1}}^{t_j} w(x)[1 - Q(t_j - x)]dx.
\end{aligned} \tag{5.37}$$

Similarly, for cases 3 and 4, we use the same logic to obtain:

$$\begin{aligned}
&P(\text{Case 3: TrueED}, A|T = t_K) \\
&= \sum_{j=1}^{K-1} \left\{ \sum_{i=0}^{j-1} \int_{t_{i-1}}^{t_i} w(x) \int_{t_j - x}^{T-x} q(t)\beta(t_j - x|t) \prod_{r=i}^{j-1} [1 - \beta(t_r - x|t)] dt dx \right. \\
&\left. + \int_{t_{j-1}}^{t_j} w(x) \int_{t_j - x}^{T-x} q(t)\beta(t_j - x|t) dt dx \right\} \\
&+ \int_0^{t_0} w(x) \int_{t_0 - x}^{T-x} q(t)\beta(t_0 - x|t) dt dx.
\end{aligned} \tag{5.38}$$

$$\begin{aligned}
&P(\text{Case 4: OverD}, A|T = t_K) \\
&= \sum_{j=1}^{K-1} \left\{ \sum_{i=0}^{j-1} \int_{t_{i-1}}^{t_i} w(x) \int_{T-x}^{\infty} q(t)\beta(t_j - x|t) \prod_{r=i}^{j-1} [1 - \beta(t_r - x|t)] dt dx \right. \\
&\left. + \int_{t_{j-1}}^{t_j} w(x) \int_{T-x}^{\infty} q(t)\beta(t_j - x|t) dt dx \right\} \\
&+ \int_0^{t_0} w(x) \int_{T-x}^{\infty} q(t)\beta(t_0 - x|t) dt dx.
\end{aligned} \tag{5.39}$$

Exercise 5.8. Prove that for any integer $K \geq 1$,

$$\sum_{i=1}^{4} P(\text{Case } i, A|T = t_K) = P(A|T > t_0).$$

For an individual with a future screening plan, the probability of each case when her lifetime T is longer than t_0 can be obtained by

$$P(\text{Case } i, A|T > t_0) = \int_{t_0}^{\infty} P(\text{Case } i, A|K = K(t), T = t) f_T(t|T > t_0) dt,$$

where the lifetime probability density function $f_T(t|T > t_0)$ was defined in equation (5.7).

Exercise 5.9. Prove that for any future screening schedule when the lifetime T is random,

$$\sum_{i=1}^{4} P(\text{Case } i|A, T > t_0) = 1.$$

5.4.2 Application: NLST-CT

We apply the method to the NLST-CT study, using the link functions for the three modeling parameters $\beta(s|Y), w(t), q(x)$ as that in section 2.5.2, where s is the time that one has stayed in the state S_p and Y is the sojourn time:

$$\begin{aligned}
\beta(s|Y) &= [1+\exp(-b_0 - b_1 \times \frac{s}{Y})]^{-1},\ 0 \leq s \leq Y,\ b_0 > 0,\ b_1 > 0. \\
w(t) &= \frac{0.3}{\sqrt{2\pi}\sigma t}\exp\{-(\log t - \mu)^2/(2\sigma^2)\},\ \sigma > 0. \\
Q(x) &= \exp(-\lambda x^{\alpha}), \quad q(x) = \lambda\alpha x^{\alpha-1}Q(x),\ \lambda > 0, \alpha > 0.
\end{aligned}$$

We have obtained 800 posterior samples for each gender using the NLST-CT data (Wu et al 2022 [76]; see section 2.5.2 for details). The posterior predictive probability of each case can be estimated by

$$P(\text{Case i}|T > t_0, NLST) \approx \frac{1}{n}\sum_j P(\text{Case i}|T > t_0, \theta_j^*).$$

where $\theta_j^*, j = 1, 2, \ldots, 800$ is the posterior random samples and $n = 800$ is the posterior sample size for each gender.

Three age cohorts with current age $t_0 = 60, 70, 80$ for each gender were used. However, since the double integrals in the probability calculation take a much longer time and due to limited computing power, some cases (especially when $\Delta = 1\,years$) cannot be finished within one week, so the sample size used in the simulation was less than 800 (it's just over 200 when $t_0 = 60, \Delta = 1$). We summarized the results in Tables 5.14 and 5.15.

Comparing Table 5.14 with the corresponding row of $(\infty, 1$ yr$)$ and $(\infty, 2$ yr$)$ in Table 5.12, the probability of symptom-free-life using the new model is lower when t_0 is 60 or 70 for both genders. The probability of no-early-detection is close to each other using either method; however, it is lower for females than males using the new method. The probability of true-early-detection is higher using the new model, and it is higher for females than males in Table 5.14. The probability of overdiagnosis is lower using the new model.

In summary, the probability of true-early-detection is much higher when the sensitivity depends on the sojourn time. And this is more obvious when comparing the results in Table 5.15 with that in Table 5.13. The probability of overdiagnosis is smaller in the new model: It is less than 7% (6%) for male (female) heavy smokers in Table 5.15.

5.4.3 Long-term outcome with a screening history when sensitivity depends on sojourn time

The *three* key parameters $(\beta(s|Y), w(t), q(x))$ are defined as before. Specifically, $\beta = \beta(s|Y), 0 \leq s \leq Y$ is the sensitivity function, where s is the time in

TABLE 5.14
Application: Long-term outcomes with no screening history when sensitivity depends on the sojourn time using the NLST-CT data.

[a]Δ	[b]P(SympF)	P(NoED)	P(TrueED)	P(OverD)
		Female with first screen age $t_0 = 60$		
1 yr	77.84 (76.17, 79.28)	1.25 (0.80, 1.81)	19.20 (17.62, 20.73)	0.43 (0.19, 0.69)
2 yr	78.04 (76.36, 79.65)	6.87 (4.22, 10.55)	14.58 (11.31, 16.92)	0.29 (0.09, 0.52)
		Female with first screen age $t_0 = 70$		
1 yr	84.63 (83.25, 85.87)	0.83 (0.48, 1.18)	14.42 (13.07, 16.12)	0.46 (0.20, 0.76)
2 yr	84.87 (83.51, 86.26)	4.44 (2.93, 6.43)	11.36 (8.38, 14.12)	0.31 (0.10, 0.57)
		Female with first screen age $t_0 = 80$		
1 yr	93.74 (92.27, 95.37)	0.31 (0.17, 0.48)	6.14 (4.61, 7.87)	0.39 (0.10, 0.69)
2 yr	93.91 (92.45, 95.46)	1.57 (1.07, 2.10)	5.04 (2.99, 6.84)	0.27 (0.07, 0.52)
		Male with first screen age $t_0 = 60$		
1 yr	78.61 (77.53, 80.11)	2.06 (1.49, 2.77)	17.54 (16.12, 18.74)	0.51 (0.29, 0.74)
2 yr	78.91 (77.66, 80.29)	7.42 (5.55, 9.80)	13.03 (11.22, 14.80)	0.33 (0.12, 0.55)
		Male with first screen age $t_0 = 70$		
1 yr	84.92 (83.78, 85.67)	1.36 (0.95, 1.77)	13.63 (12.48, 14.72)	0.53 (0.29, 0.85)
2 yr	85.15 (84.17, 86.05)	4.86 (3.70, 6.25)	10.68 (8.81, 12.69)	0.36 (0.14, 0.64)
		Male with first screen age $t_0 = 80$		
1 yr	94.41 (93.20, 95.75)	0.44 (0.28, 0.62)	5.28 (3.94, 6.44)	0.40 (0.18, 0.71)
2 yr	94.53 (93.21, 95.75)	1.53 (1.18, 1.90)	4.37 (2.95, 5.82)	0.30 (0.11, 0.58)

[a]Δ is the time interval between two consecutive exams in the future.
[b]The probability and the 95% credible interval are in percentage (%).

the preclinical state and Y is the sojourn time, a random variable. See Figure 5.3. For a woman at her current age t_{K_1} who has gone through K_1 exams, occurring at her ages $t_0 < t_1 < \cdots < t_{K_1-1}$, and she has never been diagnosed with cancer, we define event H_{K_1} as before:

$$H_{K_1} = \left\{ \begin{array}{l} \text{A woman had screening exams at her ages } t_0 < t_1 < \cdots < t_{K_1-1}, \\ \text{no cancer has been diagnosed,} \\ \text{and she is asymptomatic at her current age } t_{K_1} (> t_{K-1}). \end{array} \right\}.$$

Given that the lifetime T exceeds her current age t_{K_1}, the probability of the event H_{K_1}:

$$\begin{aligned} & P(H_{K_1} | T > t_{K_1}) \\ = & \ 1 - \int_0^{t_{K_1}} w(x)dx + \int_{t_{K_1-1}}^{t_{K_1}} w(x)Q(t_{K_1} - x)dx \\ & + \sum_{j=0}^{K_1-1} \int_{t_{j-1}}^{t_j} w(x) \int_{t_{K_1}-x}^{\infty} q(t) \prod_{i=j}^{K_1-1} [1 - \beta(t_i - x|t)]dtdx. \end{aligned} \tag{5.40}$$

We first let her lifetime T be a fixed value, and assume that she would take K exams at her (future) ages $t_{K_1} < t_{K_1+1} < \cdots < t_{K_1+K-1}$, with $T = t_{K_1+K} >$

TABLE 5.15

Application: Probability of true-early-detection and overdiagnosis among the screen-detected cases with no screening history when sensitivity depends on the sojourn time using the NLST-CT data.

Δ	P(TrueED|D)	P(OverD|D)
	Female with first screen age $t_0 = 60$	
1 yr	97.79 (96.44, 99.05)	2.21 (0.95, 3.56)
2 yr	98.13 (96.82, 99.09)	1.87 (0.91, 3.18)
	Female with first screen age $t_0 = 70$	
1 yr	96.92 (95.11, 98.44)	3.08 (1.56, 4.89)
2 yr	97.44 (95.79, 98.68)	2.56 (1.32, 4.21)
	Female with first screen age $t_0 = 80$	
1 yr	94.21 (91.15, 96.83)	5.79 (3.17, 8.85)
2 yr	95.11 (92.55, 97.23)	4.89 (2.77, 7.45)
	Male with first screen age $t_0 = 60$	
1 yr	97.19 (95.73, 98.42)	2.81 (1.58, 4.27)
2 yr	97.58 (96.08, 98.70)	2.42 (1.30, 3.92)
	Male with first screen age $t_0 = 70$	
1 yr	96.26 (94.05, 97.75)	3.74 (2.25, 5.95)
2 yr	96.78 (94.76, 98.19)	3.22 (1.81, 5.24)
	Male with first screen age $t_0 = 80$	
1 yr	93.09 (89.86, 95.79)	6.91 (4.21, 10.14)
2 yr	93.90 (90.71, 96.42)	6.10 (3.58, 9.29)

[c]Event D ={cancer was diagnosed at regular scheduled exam}.
[d]The estimated conditional probability is $P_i/(P_3 + P_4), i = 3, 4$ in Table 5.7 for the 1000 posterior samples, then taking the average.

t_{K_1+K-1}, then the probability of each outcome is

$$
\begin{aligned}
&P(\text{Case } 1, H_{K_1}|T = t_{K_1+K}) \\
&= 1 - \int_0^{t_{K_1+K}} w(x)dx + \int_{t_{K_1+K-1}}^{t_{K_1+K}} w(x)Q(t_{K_1+K} - x)dx \qquad (5.41) \\
&\quad + \sum_{j=0}^{K_1+K-1} \int_{t_{j-1}}^{t_j} w(x) \int_{t_{K_1+K}-x}^{\infty} q(t) \prod_{i=j}^{K_1+K-1} [1 - \beta(t_i - x|t)]dtdx;
\end{aligned}
$$

$$
\begin{aligned}
&P(\text{Case } 2, H_{K_1}|T = t_{K_1+K}) \\
&= \sum_{j=K_1+1}^{K_1+K} \left\{ \sum_{i=0}^{j-1} \int_{t_{i-1}}^{t_i} w(x) \int_{t_{j-1}-x}^{t_j-x} q(t) \prod_{r=i}^{j-1} [1 - \beta(t_r - x|t)]dtdx \right. \\
&\quad \left. + \int_{t_{j-1}}^{t_j} w(x)[1 - Q(t_j - x)]dx \right\}; \qquad (5.42)
\end{aligned}
$$

$$P(\text{Case } 3, H_{K_1}|T = t_{K_1+K})$$
$$= \sum_{j=K_1}^{K_1+K-1} \left\{ \sum_{i=0}^{j-1} \int_{t_{i-1}}^{t_i} w(x) \int_{t_j - x}^{t_{K_1+K}-x} q(t)\beta(t_j - x|t) \right.$$
$$\times \prod_{r=i}^{j-1} [1 - \beta(t_r - x|t)] dt dx$$
$$\left. + \int_{t_{j-1}}^{t_j} w(x) \int_{t_j - x}^{t_{K_1+K}-x} q(t)\beta(t_j - x|t) dt dx \right\}; \tag{5.43}$$

$$P(\text{Case } 4, H_{K_1}|T = t_{K_1+K})$$
$$= \sum_{j=K_1}^{K_1+K-1} \left\{ \sum_{i=0}^{j-1} \int_{t_{i-1}}^{t_i} w(x) \int_{t_{K_1+K}-x}^{\infty} q(t)\beta(t_j - x|t) \right.$$
$$\times \prod_{r=i}^{j-1} [1 - \beta(t_r - x|t)] dt dx$$
$$\left. + \int_{t_{j-1}}^{t_j} w(x) \int_{t_{K_1+K}-x}^{\infty} q(t)\beta(t_j - x|t) dt dx \right\}. \tag{5.44}$$

For a person at current age t_{K_1}, if she will follow a future screening schedule at ages $t_{K_1} < t_{K_1+1} < \cdots < t_{K_1+K} < \ldots$, then the number of her future exams $K = n$, if her lifetime T falls in the interval (t_{K_1+n-1}, t_{K_1+n}), $n = 1, 2, \ldots$, hence the probability of each case when the lifetime T is *random* can be obtained by the weighted average:

$$P(\text{Case } i, H_{K_1}|T > t_{K_1})$$
$$= \int_{t_{K_1}}^{\infty} P(\text{Case } i, H_{K_1}|K = K(T), T = t) f_T(t|T > t_{K_1}) dt, \quad i = 1, 2, 3, 4,$$

where the lifetime distribution $f_T(t|T > t_{K_1}) = \frac{f_T(t)}{1 - F_T(t_{K_1})}$ (for $t > t_{K_1}$) was derived from the US Social Security Administration (SSA) actuarial life table.

Exercise 5.10. Prove that for any $K_1 \geq 0, K \geq 1$,

$$\sum_{i=1}^{4} P(\text{Case } i|H_{K_1}, T > t_{K_1}) = \sum_{i=1}^{4} \frac{P(\text{Case } i, H_{K_1}|T > t_{K_1})}{P(H_{K_1}|T > t_{K_1})} = 1.$$

Therefore, the derived probabilities are correct.

And when $K_1 = 0$, it is the case of no screening history. Using estimated posterior samples $\theta_j^* = (b_0, b_1, \mu, \sigma^2, \kappa, \rho)_j^*$, The Bayesian inference will be used to estimate the probability of each outcome:

$$P(\text{Case } i|T > t_{K_1}, H_{K_1}, DATA) \approx \frac{1}{n} \sum_{j=1}^{n} P(\text{Case } i|T > t_{K_1}, H_{K_1}, \theta_j^*).$$

The probability of *overdiagnosis* among the *screen-detected* is

$$\frac{P(\text{Case } 4|T > t_{K_1}, H_{K_1}, DATA)}{P(\text{Case } 3|T > t_{K_1}, H_{K_1}, DATA) + P(\text{Case } 4|T > t_{K_1}, H_{K_1}, DATA).}$$

We haven't done any simulations using this method. The reader can explore this further.

5.5 Bibliographic notes

I started to work on the problem of overdiagnosis in 2009 when it causes a hot debate in the medical and public health community. And have decided to solve the problem from a different approach: look at all possible outcomes for the whole cohort, and include overdiagnosis as one outcome. This provides a systematic approach to evaluating the long-term outcomes of regular screening for asymptomatic individuals with or without a screening history. All asymptomatic participants in a screening program can be separated into four mutually exclusive groups: symptom-free-life, no-early-detection, true-early-detection, and overdiagnosis. The probability of each group shows that it depends on the current age, the three key parameters, the past and future screening frequency, and the lifetime distribution.

The first result was presented in the ENAR 2009[1] and then in the 2010 JSM, and it was published in the Joint Statistical Meeting (JSM) 2010 Conference Proceedings (Wu and Rosner 2010 [78]). The methodology paper for asymptomatic people without a screening history (section 5.2) was published in Wu et al 2014 [71]. The methodology paper for asymptomatic people with a screening history (section 5.3) was published in Wu et al 2018 [70]. Methods in section 5.4 are just developed and are not published yet.

There are other papers that applied the two methods in sections 5.2 and 5.3 to some specific screening data: Wu et al 2011 applied the probability method to the Mayo Lung Project data to evaluate long-term outcomes and overdiagnosis for male heavy smokers without a screening history [64]. Luo et al 2012 applied the method (without a screening history) to the Minnesota Colon Cancer Control Study (MCCCS) data with annual FOBT screenings for colorectal cancer [35]. Chen et al 2014 applied the method (without a screening history) to the data collected at the Memorial Sloan Kettering Cancer Center lung cancer screening program (MSKC-LCSP) [8], with annual chest X-ray screening for male heavy smokers. Wu et al 2016 applied the method (with and without a screening history) to the NLST-CT data for male and female heavy smokers as a combined group [73]. There are other publications, Wu and Perez 2011 presented a good review article in this area [74], Wu 2012 presented

[1] International Biometric Society Eastern North American Region (ENAR) Spring Meeting, March 2009. San Antonio, TX.

an editorial article regarding overdiagnosis [56]. Our simulation suggests that the probability of overdiagnosis increases as people age, so it seems wise to reduce the number of screening exams for older age groups.

This is the first approach to handling the whole cohort regarding long-term outcomes, and not deal with overdiagnosis alone. The methods are predictive: we use existing data to obtain information on the three key parameters, then use these parameters and the probability model to predict the probability of true-early-detection, no-early-detection, overdiagnosis and symptom-free-life, for different age groups with different screening histories, and different future screening frequencies. This may help policymakers evaluate a screening program's long-term outcomes more appropriately.

5.6 Solution for some exercises

Exercise 5.2:
Proof: We combine the probability of cases 3 and 4, denoted as $\mathbf{A_1}$:

$$\begin{aligned}
&P(\text{Case } 3, A|T = t_K) + P(\text{Case } 4, A|T = t_K) \\
&= \sum_{j=1}^{K-1} \beta_j \left\{ \sum_{i=0}^{j-1} (1-\beta_i)\cdots(1-\beta_{j-1}) \int_{t_{i-1}}^{t_i} w(x)Q(t_j - x)dx \right. \\
&\quad \left. + \int_{t_{j-1}}^{t_j} w(x)Q(t_j - x)dx \right\} + \beta_0 \int_0^{t_0} w(x)Q(t_0 - x)dx \equiv \mathbf{A_1}.
\end{aligned}$$

We simplify the probability of case 2 into four parts of $\mathbf{B}, \mathbf{C}, \mathbf{D}, \mathbf{E}$.

$$\begin{aligned}
&P(\text{Case } 2, A|T = t_K) = I_{K,1} + I_{K,2} + \cdots + I_{K,K} \\
&= \sum_{j=1}^{K} \left\{ \sum_{i=0}^{j-1} (1-\beta_i)\cdots(1-\beta_{j-1}) \int_{t_{i-1}}^{t_i} w(x)[Q(t_{j-1} - x) - Q(t_j - x)]dx \right. \\
&\quad \left. + \int_{t_{j-1}}^{t_j} w(x)[1 - Q(t_j - x)]dx \right\} \\
&= \sum_{j=1}^{K} \sum_{i=0}^{j-1} (1-\beta_i)\cdots(1-\beta_{j-1}) \int_{t_{i-1}}^{t_i} w(x)Q(t_{j-1} - x)dx \\
&\quad - \sum_{j=1}^{K} \sum_{i=0}^{j-1} (1-\beta_i)\cdots(1-\beta_{j-1}) \int_{t_{i-1}}^{t_i} w(x)Q(t_j - x)dx \\
&\quad + \sum_{j=1}^{K} \int_{t_{j-1}}^{t_j} w(x)dx - \sum_{j=1}^{K} \int_{t_{j-1}}^{t_j} w(x)Q(t_j - x)dx \\
&\equiv \mathbf{B} - \mathbf{C} + \mathbf{D} - \mathbf{E}.
\end{aligned}$$

Rewrite the part $\mathbf{B}$, let $l = j - 1$, then change the index l back to j:

$$\begin{aligned}
\mathbf{B} &= \sum_{j=2}^{K}\sum_{i=0}^{j-1}(1-\beta_i)\cdots(1-\beta_{j-1})\int_{t_{i-1}}^{t_i} w(x)Q(t_{j-1}-x)dx \\
&\quad +(1-\beta_0)\int_0^{t_0} w(x)Q(t_0-x)dx. \quad (\text{let } l = j-1) \\
&= \sum_{l=1}^{K-1}\sum_{i=0}^{l}(1-\beta_i)\cdots(1-\beta_l)\int_{t_{i-1}}^{t_i} w(x)Q(t_l-x)dx \\
&\quad +(1-\beta_0)\int_0^{t_0} w(x)Q(t_0-x)dx. \quad (\text{let } j = l) \\
&= \sum_{j=1}^{K-1}\sum_{i=0}^{j}(1-\beta_i)\cdots(1-\beta_j)\int_{t_{i-1}}^{t_i} w(x)Q(t_j-x)dx \\
&\quad +(1-\beta_0)\int_0^{t_0} w(x)Q(t_0-x)dx \\
&= \sum_{j=1}^{K-1}(1-\beta_j)\left\{\sum_{i=0}^{j-1}(1-\beta_i)\cdots(1-\beta_{j-1})\int_{t_{i-1}}^{t_i} w(x)Q(t_j-x)dx\right. \\
&\quad \left.+\int_{t_{j-1}}^{t_j} w(x)Q(t_j-x)dx\right\} + (1-\beta_0)\int_0^{t_0} w(x)Q(t_0-x)dx.
\end{aligned}$$

Now add $\mathbf{A_1}$ and $\mathbf{B}$:

$$\begin{aligned}
\mathbf{A_1}+\mathbf{B} &= \sum_{j=1}^{K-1}\left\{\sum_{i=0}^{j-1}(1-\beta_i)\cdots(1-\beta_{j-1})\int_{t_{i-1}}^{t_i} w(x)Q(t_j-x)dx\right. \\
&\quad \left.+\int_{t_{j-1}}^{t_j} w(x)Q(t_j-x)dx\right\} + \int_0^{t_0} w(x)Q(t_0-x)dx \\
&= \sum_{j=1}^{K-1}\sum_{i=0}^{j-1}(1-\beta_i)\cdots(1-\beta_{j-1})\int_{t_{i-1}}^{t_i} w(x)Q(t_j-x)dx \\
&\quad +\sum_{j=1}^{K-1}\int_{t_{j-1}}^{t_j} w(x)Q(t_j-x)dx + \int_0^{t_0} w(x)Q(t_0-x)dx.
\end{aligned}$$

Some terms will be canceled if we minus part $\mathbf{C}$:

$$\begin{aligned}
\mathbf{A_1}+\mathbf{B}-\mathbf{C} &= \sum_{j=1}^{K-1}\int_{t_{j-1}}^{t_j} w(x)Q(t_j-x)dx + \int_0^{t_0} w(x)Q(t_0-x)dx \\
&\quad -\sum_{i=0}^{K-1}(1-\beta_i)\cdots(1-\beta_{K-1})\int_{t_{i-1}}^{t_i} w(x)Q(t_K-x)dx.
\end{aligned}$$

Since $\mathbf{D} = \int_{t_0}^{t_K} w(x)dx$,

$$\begin{aligned}
&P(\text{Case } 2, A|T = t_K) + P(\text{Case } 3, A|T = t_K) + P(\text{Case } 4, A|T = t_K) \\
&= \mathbf{A_1} + \mathbf{B} - \mathbf{C} + \mathbf{D} - \mathbf{E} \\
&= \int_0^{t_0} w(x)Q(t_0 - x)dx - \sum_{i=0}^{K-1}(1-\beta_i)\cdots(1-\beta_{K-1})\int_{t_{i-1}}^{t_i} w(x)Q(t_K - x)dx \\
&\quad + \int_{t_0}^{t_K} w(x)dx - \int_{t_{K-1}}^{t_K} w(x)Q(t_K - x)dx.
\end{aligned}$$

Compare with

$$\begin{aligned}
P(\text{Case } 1, A|T = t_K) &= 1 - \int_0^{t_K} w(x)dx + \int_{t_{K-1}}^{t_K} w(x)Q(t_K - x)dx \\
&\quad + \sum_{j=0}^{K-1}(1-\beta_j)\cdots(1-\beta_{K-1})\int_{t_{j-1}}^{t_j} w(x)Q(t_K - x)dx.
\end{aligned}$$

We have

$$\begin{aligned}
&\sum_{i=1}^{4} P(\text{Case } i, A|T = t_K) \\
&= P(\text{Case } 1, A|T = t_K) + \mathbf{A_1} + \mathbf{B} - \mathbf{C} + \mathbf{D} - \mathbf{E} \\
&= 1 - \int_0^{t_K} w(x)dx + \int_0^{t_0} w(x)Q(t_0 - x)dx + \int_{t_0}^{t_K} w(x)dx \\
&= 1 - \int_0^{t_0} w(x)dx + \int_0^{t_0} w(x)Q(t_0 - x)dx \\
&= P(A|T > t_0).
\end{aligned}$$

This finishes the proof.

Exercise 5.6:

Proof: First, we combine the last two probabilities:

$$\begin{aligned}
\mathbf{I} &= P(\text{Case } 3, H_{K_1}|T = t_{K_1+K}) + P(\text{Case } 4, H_{K_1}|T = t_{K_1+K}) \\
&= \sum_{j=K_1}^{K_1+K-1} \beta_j \left\{ \sum_{i=0}^{j-1}(1-\beta_i)\cdots(1-\beta_{j-1})\int_{t_{i-1}}^{t_i} w(x)Q(t_j - x)dx \right. \\
&\quad \left. + \int_{t_{j-1}}^{t_j} w(x)Q(t_j - x)dx \right\}.
\end{aligned}$$

Next, we split the $P(\text{Case } 2, H_{K_1}|T = t_{K_1+K})$ into four terms and call them **II**, **III**, **IV**, **V** as follows:

$$\begin{aligned}
& P(\text{Case } 2, H_{K_1}|T = t_{K_1+K}) \\
= \; & I_{K_1+K,K_1+1} + I_{K_1+K,K_1+2} + \cdots + I_{K_1+K,K_1+K} \\
= \; & \sum_{j=K_1+1}^{K_1+K} \left\{ \sum_{i=0}^{j-1} (1-\beta_i)\cdots(1-\beta_{j-1}) \int_{t_{i-1}}^{t_i} w(x)[Q(t_{j-1}-x) \right. \\
& \left. -Q(t_j - x)]dx + \int_{t_{j-1}}^{t_j} w(x)[1 - Q(t_j - x)]dx \right\} \\
= \; & \sum_{j=K_1+1}^{K_1+K} \sum_{i=0}^{j-1} (1-\beta_i)\cdots(1-\beta_{j-1}) \int_{t_{i-1}}^{t_i} w(x)Q(t_{j-1}-x)dx \\
& - \sum_{j=K_1+1}^{K_1+K} \sum_{i=0}^{j-1} (1-\beta_i)\cdots(1-\beta_{j-1}) \int_{t_{i-1}}^{t_i} w(x)Q(t_j - x)dx \\
& + \sum_{j=K_1+1}^{K_1+K} \int_{t_{j-1}}^{t_j} w(x)dx - \sum_{j=K_1+1}^{K_1+K} \int_{t_{j-1}}^{t_j} w(x)Q(t_j - x)dx \\
= \; & \mathbf{II} - \mathbf{III} + \mathbf{IV} - \mathbf{V}.
\end{aligned}$$

Now we combine **I** and **II**, and cancel redundant items. To achieve that, change index $l = j - 1$ in **II**, then change index l back to j to make cancelation:

$$\begin{aligned}
\mathbf{II} \; = \; & \sum_{l=K_1}^{K_1+K-1} \sum_{i=0}^{l} (1-\beta_i)\cdots(1-\beta_l) \int_{t_{i-1}}^{t_i} w(x)Q(t_l - x)dx \\
= \; & \sum_{j=K_1}^{K_1+K-1} \sum_{i=0}^{j} (1-\beta_i)\cdots(1-\beta_j) \int_{t_{i-1}}^{t_i} w(x)Q(t_j - x)dx \\
= \; & \sum_{j=K_1}^{K_1+K-1} (1-\beta_j) \left\{ \sum_{i=0}^{j-1} (1-\beta_i)\cdots(1-\beta_{j-1}) \int_{t_{i-1}}^{t_i} w(x)Q(t_j - x)dx \right. \\
& \left. + \int_{t_{j-1}}^{t_j} w(x)Q(t_j - x)dx \right\}
\end{aligned}$$

Hence,

$$\begin{aligned}
\mathbf{I} + \mathbf{II} \; = \; & \sum_{j=K_1}^{K_1+K-1} \sum_{i=0}^{j-1} (1-\beta_i)\cdots(1-\beta_{j-1}) \int_{t_{i-1}}^{t_i} w(x)Q(t_j - x)dx \\
& + \sum_{j=K_1}^{K_1+K-1} \int_{t_{j-1}}^{t_j} w(x)Q(t_j - x)dx
\end{aligned}$$

Notice that the first term in **I+II** is similar to that of **III**, and the second term in **I + II** is similar to that of **V**, and notice that **IV** $= \int_{t_{K_1}}^{t_{K_1+K}} w(x)dx$. This implies that

$$\sum_{i=2}^{4} P(\text{Case } i, H_{K_1}|T = t_{K_1+K}) = \mathbf{I} + \mathbf{II} - \mathbf{III} + \mathbf{IV} - \mathbf{V}$$

$$\begin{aligned}
&= \sum_{i=0}^{K_1-1} (1-\beta_i)\cdots(1-\beta_{K_1-1}) \int_{t_{i-1}}^{t_i} w(x)Q(t_{K_1}-x)dx \\
&\quad - \sum_{i=0}^{K_1+K-1} (1-\beta_i)\cdots(1-\beta_{K_1+K-1}) \int_{t_{i-1}}^{t_i} w(x)Q(t_{K_1+K}-x)dx \\
&\quad + \int_{t_{K_1-1}}^{t_{K_1}} w(x)Q(t_{K_1}-x)dx - \int_{t_{K_1+K-1}}^{t_{K_1+K}} w(x)Q(t_{K_1+K}-x)dx \\
&\quad + \int_{t_{K_1}}^{t_{K_1+K}} w(x)dx
\end{aligned}$$

Compare with

$$\begin{aligned}
&P(\text{Case } 1, H_{K_1}|T = t_{K_1+K}) \\
&= 1 - \int_0^{t_{K_1+K}} w(x)dx + \int_{t_{K_1+K-1}}^{t_{K_1+K}} w(x)Q(t_{K_1+K}-x)dx \\
&\quad + \sum_{j=0}^{K_1+K-1} (1-\beta_j)\cdots(1-\beta_{K_1+K-1}) \int_{t_{j-1}}^{t_j} w(x)Q(t_{K_1+K}-x)dx.
\end{aligned}$$

Many terms will be canceled, and we have

$$\begin{aligned}
&\sum_{i=1}^{4} P(\text{Case } i, H_{K_1}|T = t_{K_1+K}) \\
&= 1 - \int_0^{t_{K_1}} w(x)dx + \sum_{i=0}^{K_1-1} (1-\beta_i)\cdots(1-\beta_{K_1-1}) \int_{t_{i-1}}^{t_i} w(x)Q(t_{K_1}-x)dx \\
&\quad + \int_{t_{K_1-1}}^{t_{K_1}} w(x)Q(t_{K_1}-x)dx \\
&= P(H_{K_1}|T > t_{K_1}).
\end{aligned}$$

This finishes the proof.

6

Scheduling the First Exam for Asymptomatic Individuals

CONTENTS

Early detection and effective treatments are critical to increasing the cure rate and prolonging the survival of cancer patients. The primary technique for early detection is a screening exam, with the goal that the disease may be found before the symptoms are present. Although screening programs for different kinds of cancer have been carried out in the past six decades in North America, there are still many unanswered questions in the design of screening. One major concern is: at what age should a screening program be initiated [1]? Suppose a superficially healthy person goes to a physician for a regular health checkup, should the physician give any advice on when to initiate screening for a certain type of cancer, based on the person's current age and other factors? We will address two problems in this and the next chapter: (i) for an asymptomatic individual currently at age a_0 and without any screening history, when should s/he start the first screening exam? and (ii) for an asymptomatic individual currently at age a_0 who has taken some screening exams with negative results (including false positives), when to schedule

DOI: 10.1201/9781003404125-6

the next screening exam? We believe clinical physicians face these questions almost daily, and the method here can help them to provide informed and satisfying advice to individuals in such a situation. This chapter is dedicated to addressing the first problem.

6.1 Introduction

There is almost no research in this area. There was some research regarding optimal schedules of screening; however, these existing methods usually deal with how to schedule $(n+1)$ exams in a fixed age interval using some utility function [30, 88]. There were some other approaches to solving the scheduling of exams [39, 40], but all of them involved a utility function requiring specified costs or weights, and none of them focus on scheduling the first exam.

We will develop an approach to handle the problem. We will not use any utility function, costs, or weights, which are subjective. Instead, we will study the probability (or risk) of incidence from one's current age, assuming one is asymptomatic and hasn't taken any screening exam so far. The first screening time (or age) is chosen, such that the *probability of incidence* is limited by some preselected small value, such as 10% or less. Therefore, with 90% or more chance, individuals at risk would not become a clinical incidence case before the first screening exam if they follow this screening schedule. And for those who would be diagnosed with cancer at the first exam, we derive the lead time distribution and the probability of overdiagnosis. This provides predictive information regarding the initial screening age on a personal level. Policymakers or individuals can use this information to make informed decisions. We start with the probability method when the sensitivity is a function of age, then we extend the method to the situation with the sensitivity as a function of the ratio of time in the preclinical state and the sojourn time. We use lung cancer screening as an example in this research since it is the leading cause of cancer death in the United States and counts for about 22.4% of all cancer deaths [38]. The developed method can be applied to other kinds of screening as well.

6.2 Scheduling the first screening exam

Suppose a woman at her current age a_0 is asymptomatic and has not taken any screening so far, should she start her first exam immediately, or wait for some time? And how long should she wait? This is the first problem that we want to address. We will use female lung cancer as an example in the

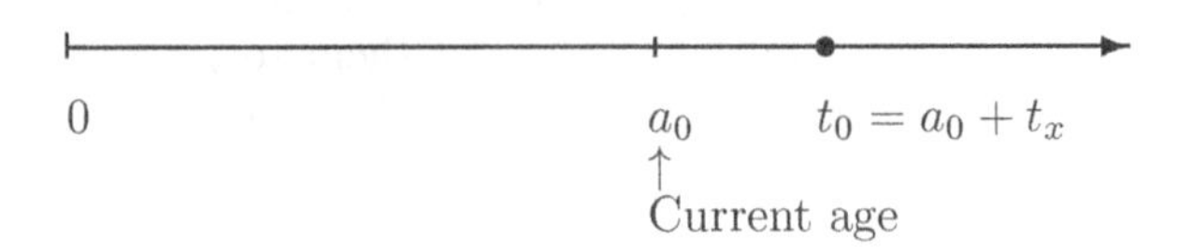

FIGURE 6.1
An individual's current age and the first exam.

modeling description, and the method developed is applicable to other kinds of screening. We start with a simple protocol to help with this decision-making. The goal is to make sure that the probability of clinical incidence from now until her first exam is limited to a small value, such as 0.1 or 0.2.

6.2.1 Probability of incidence and first exam age

We use the same disease progressive model as before where the disease develops through three states $S_0 \to S_p \to S_c$ [87]. S_0 refers to the disease-free state or the state in which the disease cannot be detected; S_p refers to the preclinical disease state, in which an asymptomatic individual unknowingly has a disease that a screening exam can detect; and S_c refers to the disease state at which the disease manifests itself in clinical symptoms.

Suppose that her first screening time will happen at her age $t_0 = a_0 + t_x$, with $t_x > 0$; see Figure 6.1. We want to find the value t_x, such that the probability of incidence is limited to some pre-selected value p. We define a few events:

$$\begin{aligned}
H_0 &= \{\text{One has no screening exam and is asymptomatic in } [0, a_0]\}; \\
A_0 &= \left\{\begin{array}{l}\text{One is asymptomatic in } (a_0, t_0), \\ \text{and has a negative screening result at } t_0\end{array}\right\} \cap H_0; \\
I_0 &= \{\text{One is a clinical incident case in } (a_0, t_0)\} \cap H_0; \\
D_0 &= \{\text{One is diagosed with cancer at age } t_0\} \cap H_0.
\end{aligned}$$

The last three events are mutually exclusive, and they form a partition of the historic sample space H_0:

$$I_0 \cup D_0 \cup A_0 = H_0.$$

We let β be the sensitivity of the exam at age t_0, i.e., the probability that the screening result is positive given that an individual is in the preclinical state S_p. We let X be the time duration in the disease-free state S_0, with a PDF $w(x)$, and we let Y be the sojourn time, with a PDF $q(y)$; and $Q(y) = P(Y > y) = \int_y^\infty q(x)dx$ be the survival function of the sojourn time Y. We assume that the sojourn time Y and the time duration in the disease-free state X are independent.

People at risk are those who belong to events I_0 or D_0, and the probability of incidence among the people at risk can be calculated by

$$P(I_0|I_0 \cup D_0) = \frac{P(I_0)}{P(I_0 \cup D_0)} = \frac{P(I_0)}{P(I_0) + P(D_0)} \,. \tag{6.1}$$

The numerator is the probability of incidence in (a_0, t_0), which could happen in two cases: (i) she enters the preclinical state at age $x \in (0, a_0)$ and her sojourn time is between $(a_0 - x)$ and $(t_0 - x)$; or (ii) she enters the preclinical state at age $x \in (a_0, t_0)$ and her sojourn time is less than $(t_0 - x)$. Hence,

$$P(I_0) = \int_0^{a_0} w(x)[Q(a_0 - x) - Q(t_0 - x)]dx + \int_{a_0}^{t_0} w(x)[1 - Q(t_0 - x)]dx. \tag{6.2}$$

And $P(D_0)$ is the probability of detection at the first exam:

$$P(D_0) = \beta \int_0^{t_0} w(x)Q(t_0 - x)dx. \tag{6.3}$$

Since $P(I_0|I_0 \cup D_0)$ is monotonically increasing with the time interval t_x, and remember $t_0 = a_0 + t_x$, this probability is increasing with t_0. For any given p between 0 and 1, there is a unique solution t_0, such that

$$P(I_0|I_0 \cup D_0) = p.$$

We can use the binary search method to find the t_0 for any given $p \in (0, 1)$.

Exercise 6.1.

(a) Find the $P(H_0)$.

(b) Find the $P(A_0)$.

(c) Prove that: $P(H_0) = P(A_0) + P(I_0) + P(D_0)$.

(d) Prove that under the regularity condition:

$$w(t_0)\left\{\int_0^{a_0} w(x)[Q(a_0 - x) - Q(t_0 - x)]dx + \int_{a_0}^{t_0} w(x)[1 - Q(t_0 - x)]dx\right\}$$
$$< I(t_0)\left\{\int_0^{a_0} w(x)Q(a_0 - x)dx + \int_{a_0}^{t_0} w(x)dx\right\},$$

the incidence probability $P(I_0|I_0 \cup D_0)$ is monotonically increasing with t_x, where $I(t) = \int_0^t w(x)q(t - x)dx$ is the probability of incidence at age t without screening. See Chapter 2, equation (2.1).

In fact, it is easy to verify that $\int_0^\infty I(t)dt = \int_0^\infty w(t)dt < 1$. Hence, for most functions of $w(t)$ and the survival function $Q(x)$, the above inequality is easy to satisfy, although it is hard to mathematically prove this inequality for all forms of $w(\cdot)$ and $Q(\cdot)$.

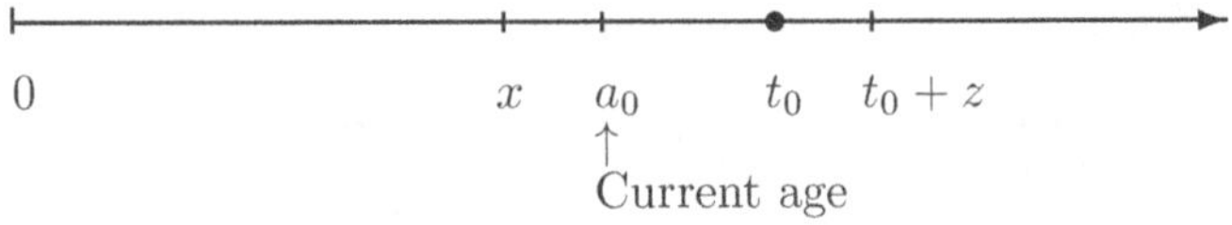

FIGURE 6.2
Lead time at the first exam. x is the onset age of S_p; it must be less than t_0.

6.2.2 Lead time distribution at the first exam

After we find the numerical solution $t_0 = t_0(p)$, we can derive the distribution of the lead time at age t_0 if one would be diagnosed with cancer at the first exam. The lead time is defined as the diagnosis time advanced by screening; in other words, the lead time is the time interval between the diagnosis and the presence of clinical symptoms.

Suppose one would be diagnosed with cancer at the first exam at her (future) age t_0, the probability density function (PDF) of the lead time should be

$$f_L(z|D_0) = \frac{f_L(z, D_0)}{P(D_0)}, \quad \text{for } z \in (0, \infty), \tag{6.4}$$

where the numerator

$$f_L(z, D_0) = \beta \int_0^{t_0} w(x) q(t_0 + z - x) dx. \tag{6.5}$$

That is because she must have entered the preclinical state at age $x \in (0, t_0)$, and her lead time is z means that her sojourn time should be $(t_0 + z - x)$; i.e., if she were not screened, she would be a clinical incident case at age $(t_0 + z)$. See Figure 6.2. The denominator $P(D_0)$ was given in equation (6.3).

Exercise 6.2.

(a) Prove that

$$\int_0^{\infty} f_L(z, D_0) dz = \beta \int_0^{t_0} w(x) Q(t_0 - x) dx = P(D_0).$$

(b) Prove that

$$\int_0^{\infty} f_L(z|D_0) dz = 1.$$

Thus the derived formula is a valid PDF.

6.2.3 Probability of overdiagnosis at the first exam

We can find the probability of overdiagnosis and true-early-detection if one were diagnosed with cancer at the future age t_0 of the first exam. Given a fixed lifetime $T = t(> t_0)$, the probability of overdiagnosis and true-early-detection at t_0 would be

$$\begin{aligned} P(\text{OverD}|D_0, T = t) &= \frac{P(\text{OverD}, D_0|T = t)}{P(D_0|T = t)}, \\ P(\text{TrueED}|D_0, T = t) &= \frac{P(\text{TrueED}, D_0|T = t)}{P(D_0|T = t)}. \end{aligned} \tag{6.6}$$

Since $P(D_0|T = t) = P(D_0)$, we only need to find out the two numerators. To calculate $P(\text{OverD}, D_0|T = t)$, that is, one would be diagnosed with cancer at the first exam at her age t_0, but the symptom would not appear until after her lifetime t; therefore, she must have entered the preclinical state at age $x \in (0, t_0)$, and her sojourn time is longer than $(t - x)$.

$$P(\text{OverD}, D_0|T = t) = \beta \int_0^{t_0} w(x)Q(t - x)dx. \tag{6.7}$$

For true-early-detection, her symptom would have appeared before her lifetime t; therefore, her sojourn time is between $(t_0 - x)$ and $(t - x)$:

$$P(\text{TrueED}, D_0|T = t) = \beta \int_0^{t_0} w(x)[Q(t_0 - x) - Q(t - x)]dx. \tag{6.8}$$

Exercise 6.3. Prove that

$$P(\text{OverD}, D_0|T = t) + P(\text{TrueED}, D_0|T = t) = P(D_0).$$

Therefore,

$$P(\text{OverD}|D_0, T = t) + P(\text{TrueED}|D_0, T = t) = 1.$$

Now if we allow the human lifetime T to be random, then

$$\begin{aligned} P(\text{OverD}|D_0, T > t_0) &= \int_{t_0}^{\infty} P(\text{OverD}|D_0, T = t) f_T(t|T > t_0)dt, \\ P(\text{TrueED}|D_0, T > t_0) &= \int_{t_0}^{\infty} P(\text{TrueED}|D_0, T = t) f_T(t|T > t_0)dt. \end{aligned} \tag{6.9}$$

The conditional PDF of human lifetime $f_T(t|T > t_0) = \frac{f_T(t)}{1-F_T(t_0)}$, if $t > t_0$. And it is obtained by transforming the actuarial life table from the US Social Security Administration[1]; for details, see Wu et al 2012 [72].

Exercise 6.4. Prove that

$$P(\text{OverD}|D_0, T > t_0) + P(\text{TrueED}|D_0, T > t_0) = 1.$$

[1] http://www.ssa.gov/OACT/STATS/table4c6.html, last access 11/19/2020.

6.2.4 Simulation study

The probability of incidence $P(I_0|I_0 \cup D_0)$ is a function of one's current age a_0, the three key parameters (sensitivity β, sojourn time distribution $q(x)$ or $Q(x)$, transition density $w(t)$). It is monotonically increasing with the first screening age t_0. We can find the optimal initial screening age t_0 based on the other given factors. We use the female lifetime distribution in the simulation, simulations using the male lifetime distribution are similar. Specifically, we selected the following parameters for the simulation:

1. Four values of the probability of incidence: $p = 0.05, 0.10, 0.15, 0.20$;
2. Three different screening sensitivities: $\beta = 0.8, 0.9$, and 0.95;
3. Four different mean sojourn time (MST): 1.5, 2.5, 5, and 10 years;
4. Three different current age a_0: 45, 50, 55.

We want to point out that the probability formula that we derived in the section is very general. It is applicable to any estimation of the three key parameters, including the case of semi-parametric or non-parametric estimates of the three key parameters. However, based on our previous research in cancer screening, we use the parametric model of the transition density and the sojourn time in this simulation:

$$\begin{aligned} w(t|\mu, \sigma^2) &= \frac{0.3}{\sqrt{2\pi}\sigma t} \exp\{-(\log t - \mu)^2/(2\sigma^2)\}, \\ Q(x|\lambda, \alpha) &= \exp(-\lambda x^\alpha), \quad \lambda > 0, \alpha > 0, \\ q(x|\lambda, \alpha) &= \alpha\lambda x^{\alpha-1} \exp(-\lambda x^\alpha). \end{aligned} \tag{6.10}$$

For $w(t)$, the input parameters of μ and σ^2 were chosen, so that the mean/median/mode of the lung cancer transition age into the preclinical state was around 70 years old [32], that will give $\mu = 4.25$. Based on our previous lung cancer screening estimates, the σ^2 has a mean value of 0.021 for males, 0.026 for females, and 0.022 for both genders [32], so we picked $\sigma^2 = 0.02$ in the simulation.

For $q(x)$, the parameters (λ, α) were chosen for four different mean sojourn times of 1.5, 2.5, 5, and 10 years (correspondingly represents fast, moderate, and slow-growing tumors) with: $\alpha = 3.0$, and $\lambda = 0.21098, 0.04557, 0.00570, 0.00071$.

Exercise 6.5. Numerically reproduce Table 6.1 using the parameters in the simulation in this section, rounding to two decimal places.

Table 6.1 provides the optimal initial screening age t_0^* using the method and the binary search. This is how to read the table: under the block "MST = 2.5 years", the numbers under $a_0 = 45$ and $\beta = 0.95$ are 45.24, 45.53, 45.91 and 46.40. That is, if someone wants to have a 95% probability of no incidence before the first exam, then she should take the screening at the age of 45.24 (or after 3 months since her current age is 45); or if someone wants to have

TABLE 6.1
Optimal initial screening age t_0^* (in years) found by binary search.

p	MST = 1.5 years								
	$a_0 = 45$			$a_0 = 50$			$a_0 = 55$		
	$\beta = 0.8$	$\beta = 0.9$	$\beta = 0.95$	$\beta = 0.8$	$\beta = 0.9$	$\beta = 0.95$	$\beta = 0.8$	$\beta = 0.9$	$\beta = 0.95$
0.05	45.09	45.10	45.11	50.08	50.09	50.10	55.07	55.08	55.09
0.10	45.19	45.22	45.23	50.17	50.19	50.21	55.16	55.18	55.19
0.15	45.32	45.36	45.38	50.28	50.31	50.33	55.25	55.28	55.30
0.20	45.46	45.53	45.56	50.40	50.45	50.48	55.36	55.41	55.43
p	MST = 2.5 years								
	$a_0 = 45$			$a_0 = 50$			$a_0 = 55$		
	$\beta = 0.8$	$\beta = 0.9$	$\beta = 0.95$	$\beta = 0.8$	$\beta = 0.9$	$\beta = 0.95$	$\beta = 0.8$	$\beta = 0.9$	$\beta = 0.95$
0.05	45.20	45.22	45.24	50.16	50.18	50.19	55.14	55.16	55.17
0.10	45.44	45.50	45.53	50.35	50.40	50.42	55.30	55.34	55.36
0.15	45.74	45.85	45.91	50.57	50.65	50.69	55.48	55.54	55.58
0.20	46.13	46.31	46.40	50.84	50.96	51.03	55.69	55.79	55.84
p	MST = 5.0 years								
	$a_0 = 45$			$a_0 = 50$			$a_0 = 55$		
	$\beta = 0.8$	$\beta = 0.9$	$\beta = 0.95$	$\beta = 0.8$	$\beta = 0.9$	$\beta = 0.95$	$\beta = 0.8$	$\beta = 0.9$	$\beta = 0.95$
0.05	45.84	45.96	46.03	50.54	50.62	50.65	55.40	55.45	55.47
0.10	47.17	47.55	47.76	51.25	51.44	51.54	55.87	55.99	56.05
0.15	49.16	49.88	50.24	52.19	52.55	52.73	56.45	56.65	56.76
0.20	51.52	52.44	52.88	53.42	53.98	54.26	57.15	57.46	57.62
p	MST = 10.0 years								
	$a_0 = 45$			$a_0 = 50$			$a_0 = 55$		
	$\beta = 0.8$	$\beta = 0.9$	$\beta = 0.95$	$\beta = 0.8$	$\beta = 0.9$	$\beta = 0.95$	$\beta = 0.8$	$\beta = 0.9$	$\beta = 0.95$
0.05	52.13	52.92	53.28	53.46	53.98	54.23	56.84	57.10	57.23
0.10	57.37	58.24	58.64	57.63	58.44	58.82	59.20	59.76	60.03
0.15	60.84	61.75	62.17	60.94	61.82	62.24	61.69	62.44	62.80
0.20	63.56	64.49	64.92	63.60	64.53	64.96	64.02	64.87	65.27

Adapted from Table 1 in Wu 2022[59].

TABLE 6.2
Estimated mean, median, mode, and standard deviation of the lead time at the optimal age t_0^* when $a_0 = 50$.

		MST = 1.5 years	
p	$\beta = 0.8$	$\beta = 0.9$	$\beta = 0.95$
0.05	0.91, 0.85, 0.63, 0.58	0.91, 0.85, 0.63, 0.58	0.91, 0.85, 0.63, 0.58
0.10	0.91, 0.85, 0.63, 0.58	0.91, 0.85, 0.63, 0.58	0.91, 0.85, 0.63, 0.58
0.15	0.91, 0.85, 0.63, 0.58	0.91, 0.85, 0.63, 0.58	0.91, 0.85, 0.63, 0.58
0.20	0.91, 0.85, 0.63, 0.58	0.91, 0.85, 0.62, 0.58	0.91, 0.85, 0.62, 0.58
		MST = 2.5 years	
p	$\beta = 0.8$	$\beta = 0.9$	$\beta = 0.95$
0.05	1.59, 1.51, 1.28, 0.98	1.59, 1.51, 1.28, 0.98	1.59, 1.51, 1.28, 0.98
0.10	1.59, 1.50, 1.28, 0.98	1.59, 1.50, 1.28, 0.98	1.59, 1.50, 1.28, 0.98
0.15	1.59, 1.50, 1.27, 0.98	1.59, 1.50, 1.27, 0.98	1.59, 1.50, 1.27, 0.98
0.20	1.58, 1.49, 1.26, 0.98	1.58, 1.49, 1.26, 0.98	1.58, 1.49, 1.25, 0.98
		MST = 5.0 years	
p	$\beta = 0.8$	$\beta = 0.9$	$\beta = 0.95$
0.05	3.51, 3.39, 3.23, 1.96	3.51, 3.39, 3.22, 1.96	3.50, 3.39, 3.22, 1.96
0.10	3.48, 3.36, 3.18, 1.96	3.47, 3.35, 3.17, 1.96	3.47, 3.35, 3.16, 1.96
0.15	3.44, 3.32, 3.11, 1.96	3.43, 3.30, 3.09, 1.96	3.42, 3.29, 3.08, 1.96
0.20	3.39, 3.26, 3.03, 1.96	3.37, 3.23, 2.99, 1.96	3.36, 3.22, 2.97, 1.96
		MST = 10.0 years	
p	$\beta = 0.8$	$\beta = 0.9$	$\beta = 0.95$
0.05	7.74, 7.59, 7.42, 3.87	7.69, 7.54, 7.36, 3.87	7.66, 7.51, 7.33, 3.88
0.10	7.33, 7.14, 6.89, 3.90	7.25, 7.05, 6.78, 3.90	7.21, 7.01, 6.72, 3.90
0.15	7.00, 6.76, 6.39, 3.90	6.91, 6.66, 6.25, 3.90	6.87, 6.61, 6.18, 3.90
0.20	6.74, 6.45, 5.93, 3.90	6.64, 6.34, 5.75, 3.90	6.60, 6.29, 5.67, 3.90

Adapted from Table 3 in Wu 2022 [59].

an 80% chance of not being a clinical case before her first exam, she can come back for screening at the age of 46.40 (or after 1 year and 5 months). As the sensitivity increases from 0.8 to 0.95, the first exam age is slightly increased if other factors were the same. However, the first screening age is dramatically increasing as the incidence probability p increases, or as the MST increases. The optimal first screening age t_0^* also changes with one's current age a_0: the time interval $(t_0^* - a_0)$ is decreasing as a_0 increases if other factors are the same.

Table 6.2 presents the estimated mean, median, mode, and the standard deviation of the lead time at the optimal first screening time t_0^*, when the current age a_0 is 50 years. We omitted the cases when a_0 is 45 or 55 since the patterns are the same. The result shows: As the current age a_0 increases, the mean, median, and mode of the lead time becomes smaller. As the mean

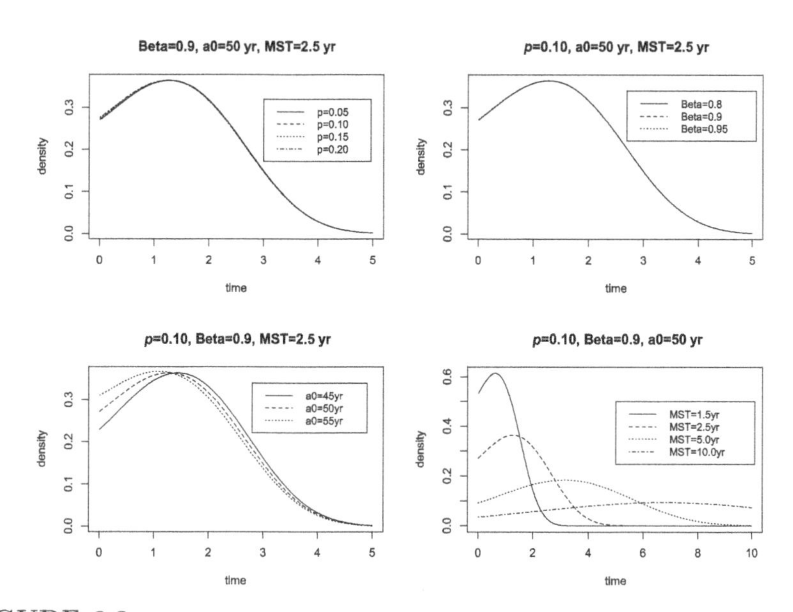

FIGURE 6.3
The lead time PDF under the four factors: Fix three factors and allow one to change. Adapted from Figure 2 in Wu 2022 [59].

sojourn time increases, the mean, median, and mode of the lead time increase as well. The lead time distribution depends very little on the incidence probability p and the sensitivity β using the optimal scheduling time t_0^*. We want to point out that once the t_0^* is found, the lead time distribution $f_L(z|D_0)$ and the probability of overdiagnosis $P(\text{OverD}|D_0, T > t_0^*)$ don't directly depend on β, p and a_0, but they depend on $t_0^*, w(t)$ and $Q(x)$. This is clearly shown by the formulas in subsections 6.2.2, 6.2.3, and is verified by the simulations.

The lead time density curves under different factors: p, β, a_0, and MST were plotted in Figure 6.3. The four panels in Figure 6.3 showed the estimated lead time density when the optimal first screening age t_0^* was used, with three factors fixed and only the fourth factor was allowed to change. It shows that given t_0^*, the lead time distribution barely changes with the incidence probability p and the sensitivity β. However, it changes quite a bit with one's current age a_0 and the mean sojourn time (MST): as the a_0 increases, the mean, median, and mode of the lead time slightly decrease; and as the MST increases, the mean, median, and mode of the lead time increase.

Table 6.3 provides the estimated probability of overdiagnosis (in percentage) if one takes the first exam at the age t_0^* and would be diagnosed with cancer. The probability of overdiagnosis is increasing as the MST increases;

TABLE 6.3
Estimated probability of overdiagnosis (in percentage) at the initial screening age t_0^*

p	MST = 1.5 years								
	$a_0 = 45$			$a_0 = 50$			$a_0 = 55$		
	$\beta = 0.8$	$\beta = 0.9$	$\beta = 0.95$	$\beta = 0.8$	$\beta = 0.9$	$\beta = 0.95$	$\beta = 0.8$	$\beta = 0.9$	$\beta = 0.95$
0.05	0.19	0.19	0.19	0.30	0.30	0.30	0.43	0.43	0.43
0.10	0.19	0.20	0.20	0.30	0.30	0.30	0.43	0.43	0.43
0.15	0.20	0.20	0.20	0.30	0.30	0.30	0.43	0.43	0.43
0.20	0.20	0.20	0.20	0.30	0.30	0.30	0.43	0.43	0.43
p	MST = 2.5 years								
	$a_0 = 45$			$a_0 = 50$			$a_0 = 55$		
	$\beta = 0.8$	$\beta = 0.9$	$\beta = 0.95$	$\beta = 0.8$	$\beta = 0.9$	$\beta = 0.95$	$\beta = 0.8$	$\beta = 0.9$	$\beta = 0.95$
0.05	0.36	0.36	0.36	0.54	0.54	0.54	0.76	0.76	0.76
0.10	0.37	0.37	0.37	0.55	0.55	0.55	0.76	0.76	0.76
0.15	0.38	0.38	0.38	0.56	0.56	0.56	0.77	0.77	0.77
0.20	0.39	0.39	0.40	0.57	0.57	0.58	0.78	0.78	0.79
p	MST = 5.0 years								
	$a_0 = 45$			$a_0 = 50$			$a_0 = 55$		
	$\beta = 0.8$	$\beta = 0.9$	$\beta = 0.95$	$\beta = 0.8$	$\beta = 0.9$	$\beta = 0.95$	$\beta = 0.8$	$\beta = 0.9$	$\beta = 0.95$
0.05	0.96	0.97	0.98	1.35	1.35	1.36	1.79	1.80	1.80
0.10	1.07	1.09	1.11	1.41	1.43	1.43	1.84	1.85	1.86
0.15	1.23	1.29	1.32	1.49	1.52	1.54	1.90	1.92	1.93
0.20	1.43	1.51	1.55	1.60	1.65	1.68	1.98	2.00	2.02
p	MST = 10.0 years								
	$a_0 = 45$			$a_0 = 50$			$a_0 = 55$		
	$\beta = 0.8$	$\beta = 0.9$	$\beta = 0.95$	$\beta = 0.8$	$\beta = 0.9$	$\beta = 0.95$	$\beta = 0.8$	$\beta = 0.9$	$\beta = 0.95$
0.05	4.15	4.33	4.43	4.44	4.57	4.64	5.39	5.50	5.54
0.10	5.62	5.94	6.08	5.66	5.96	6.09	6.26	6.47	6.62
0.15	7.01	7.46	7.71	7.00	7.43	7.68	7.37	7.78	7.96
0.20	8.47	9.04	9.29	8.42	8.99	9.24	8.72	9.19	9.50

Adapted from Table 5 in Wu 2022[59].

it is increasing as p increases, and it is increasing as one's current age a_0 increases, but it barely changes with the sensitivity β. In general, when the MST is less than or equal to 5 years, the probability of overdiagnosis usually is less than 2%, which is negligible. The probability of overdiagnosis is very small in all cases, and the largest value of the probability of overdiagnosis is less than 10% when the MST is 10 years. We did more simulation when the current age $a_0 = 0$, and the result was in the supplementary material of Wu 2022 [59].

In summary, the time interval between one's current age and the first screening time slightly increases with the sensitivity if other factors were the same; it also increases as the incidence probability increases. If one were diagnosed with cancer at the first exam, the lead time barely changes with the incidence probability and the sensitivity; however, the mean, median, and mode of lead time slightly decrease as one's current age increases; and the lead time is positively correlated to the mean sojourn time: longer mean sojourn time means longer mean lead time. Using the calculated first screening age, the probability of overdiagnosis is positively correlated with the mean sojourn time, the incidence probability, and one's current age, and it barely changes with the sensitivity, especially when the MST is less than 2 years.

6.2.5 Application: The NLST-CT study of lung cancer

We now apply the method of scheduling to the NLST low-dose CT data for male and female heavy smokers separately. Section 1.10 provides some background information on the NLST-CT data, and we have estimated the three key parameters $\beta(t), w(t)$ and $q(x)$ for male and female heavy smokers using the NLST-CT data. See section 2.4.6.

Liu et al 2015 estimated the three key parameters for the cohorts of male and female heavy smokers using the NLST-CT data: the sensitivity $\beta(t)$, the PDF of sojourn time $q(x)$, and the transition density $w(t)$ [32]. The sensitivity was modeled as a function of age $\beta(t|b_0, b_1) = \{1 + \exp(-b_0 - b_1(t - m))\}^{-1}$, and $w(t), q(x)$ and $Q(x)$ were the same as in the equations (6.10). The unknown parameters were $\theta = (b_0, b_1, \mu, \sigma^2, \lambda, \alpha)$. Using Markov Chain Monte Carlo (MCMC) with Gibbs sampler and the likelihood function, 1000 Bayesian posterior samples (θ_j^*) for each gender were obtained. For each gender, there were three hypothetic age cohorts in the simulation with different current ages $a_0 = 45, 50, 55$. And we used the 1000 posterior samples $\theta_j^*, j = 1, 2, \ldots, 1000$ to make Bayesian inference on the optimal scheduling time/age.

Given the probability of incidence p, for each θ_j^*, using $P(I_0|I_0 \cup D_0, \theta_j^*) = p$, a scheduling age t_j^* $(j = 1, 2, \ldots, 1000)$ can be found. We calculated the mean, the standard error, and the 95% highest posterior density (HPD) interval of the future screening age t_j^* (in years) and summarized the results for male and female heavy smokers using the NLST-CT data in Table 6.4. The results show that the optimal first screening times are very close for male and female heavy smokers under similar situations, such as the same current age a_0 and same incidence probability p.

TABLE 6.4
Estimated first screening age t_0^* and its 95% HPD interval using the NLST low-dose CT data.

	MALE								
	$a_0 = 45$			$a_0 = 50$			$a_0 = 55$		
p	mean	s.e.	95% CI	mean	s.e.	95% CI	mean	s.e.	95% CI
0.05	45.10	0.013	(45.08, 45.12)	50.09	0.011	(50.07, 50.11)	55.09	0.014	(55.07, 55.12)
0.10	45.21	0.029	(45.16, 45.27)	50.19	0.025	(50.15, 50.24)	55.18	0.022	(55.14, 55.22)
0.15	45.35	0.050	(45.26, 45.44)	50.31	0.041	(50.24, 50.39)	55.28	0.036	(55.22, 55.35)
0.20	45.51	0.076	(45.38, 45.65)	50.45	0.061	(50.34, 50.57)	55.40	0.053	(55.31, 55.51)
	FEMALE								
	$a_0 = 45$			$a_0 = 50$			$a_0 = 55$		
p	mean	s.e.	95% CI	mean	s.e.	95% CI	mean	s.e.	95% CI
0.05	45.11	0.018	(45.08, 45.14)	50.10	0.015	(50.07, 50.13)	55.09	0.014	(55.07, 55.12)
0.10	45.24	0.039	(45.17, 45.31)	50.22	0.033	(50.16, 50.28)	55.20	0.029	(55.15, 55.26)
0.15	45.39	0.066	(45.27, 45.51)	50.35	0.054	(50.24, 50.45)	55.32	0.048	(55.24, 55.42)
0.20	45.57	0.102	(45.39, 45.76)	50.50	0.081	(50.35, 50.65)	55.46	0.069	(55.34, 55.60)

Adapted from Table 6 in Wu 2022 [59].

After the optimal first screening time was determined, we can further evaluate the lead time distribution and the probability of overdiagnosis. One lead time distribution can be obtained by using each pair of (θ_j^*, t_j^*), with $j = 1, 2, \ldots, 1000$. The posterior distribution of the lead time is the average:

$$f_L(z|NLST) \approx \frac{1}{1000} \sum_{j=1}^{1000} f_L(z|\theta_j^*).$$

We then calculate the mean, median, mode, and standard deviation of the lead time using the $f_L(z|NLST)$. The result is presented in Table 6.5. The estimated lead time density curves under different current ages a_0 and different incidence probability p are plotted using the NLST low-dose CT male and female heavy smokers data in Figure 6.4. It shows that the lead time curve didn't change much with the incidence probability p if the optimal scheduling time t_0^* were used. The density curves do change with the current age a_0: larger a_0 corresponds to a higher spike in the density curve, which translates to a slightly smaller mode value.

Finally, we use each pair $(\theta_j^*, t_j^*), j = 1, 2, \ldots, 1000$, to estimate the probability of overdiagnosis. And we can calculate the posterior mean, standard error, and the 95% HPD interval of the probability (or percentage) of overdiagnosis. Correspondingly, the probability of true-early-detection is just 1 minus the probability of overdiagnosis. The posterior mean, the standard error, and the 95% HPD interval are listed in Table 6.6. The probability of overdiagnosis is very low at the first screening for heavy smokers using the parameters derived from the NLST-CT data ($< 0.5\%$). This risk of overdiagnosis slightly increases with one's current age for both genders. And it is slightly higher for male heavy smokers than their female counterparts. The probability of overdiagnosis slightly increases when p increases. However, the maximum probability of overdiagnosis was less than 1% for both genders in our simulation. Therefore, overdiagnosis is not an issue at the first screening exam using low-dose CT for lung cancer.

The result is compatible with the simulation. The probability of overdiagnosis is negligible at the first screening. Based on our research, overdiagnosis is more related to a person's lifetime. Since the first screening time happens at a comparatively younger age, the possibility of overdiagnosis is very small.

We want to point out that the estimated optimal first screening time is a function of the three key parameters: sensitivity, sojourn time in the preclinical state, and transition density into the preclinical state. Therefore, the accuracy of the proposed method depends on the accurate estimation of the three key parameters. And these three key parameters uniquely determine the process of periodic screening. In summary, this is the first study to work on the optimal screening time for an asymptomatic person for a certain type of cancer based on their current age.

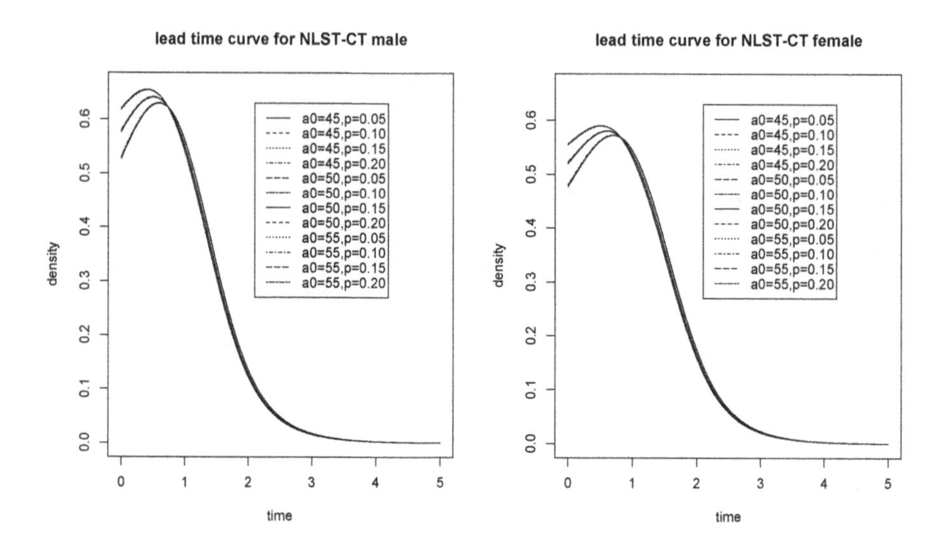

FIGURE 6.4
Estimated lead time density curve for heavy smokers in the NLCT-CT study. Adapted from Figure 3 in Wu 2022 [59].

TABLE 6.5
Estimated mean, median, mode, and standard deviation of lead time using NLST-CT data.

		MALE	
p	$a_0 = 45$	$a_0 = 50$	$a_0 = 55$
0.05	0.93, 0.83, 0.59, 0.65	0.91, 0.80, 0.50, 0.65	0.89, 0.78, 0.41, 0.64
0.10	0.93, 0.83, 0.59, 0.65	0.91, 0.80, 0.50, 0.65	0.89, 0.78, 0.41, 0.64
0.15	0.93, 0.83, 0.59, 0.65	0.91, 0.80, 0.50, 0.65	0.89, 0.78, 0.41, 0.64
0.20	0.93, 0.83, 0.59, 0.65	0.91, 0.80, 0.50, 0.65	0.89, 0.78, 0.40, 0.64
		FEMALE	
p	$a_0 = 45$	$a_0 = 50$	$a_0 = 55$
0.05	1.02, 0.92, 0.70, 0.69	0.99, 0.89, 0.61, 0.69	0.97, 0.87, 0.51, 0.68
0.10	1.02, 0.92, 0.70, 0.69	0.99, 0.89, 0.60, 0.69	0.97, 0.86, 0.51, 0.68
0.15	1.01, 0.92, 0.69, 0.69	0.99, 0.89, 0.60, 0.69	0.97, 0.86, 0.50, 0.68
0.20	1.01, 0.92, 0.69, 0.69	0.99, 0.89, 0.60, 0.69	0.97, 0.86, 0.50, 0.68

Adapted from Table 7 in Wu 2022 [59].

TABLE 6.6
Probability of overdiagnosis (in %) at the t_0^* using the NLST-CT data.

p	MALE								
	$a_0 = 45$			$a_0 = 50$			$a_0 = 55$		
	mean	s.e.	95% CI	mean	s.e.	95% CI	mean	s.e.	95% CI
0.05	0.304	0.059	(0.214, 0.423)	0.472	0.091	(0.336, 0.657)	0.712	0.135	(0.490, 0.967)
0.10	0.306	0.059	(0.214, 0.426)	0.475	0.092	(0.324, 0.650)	0.715	0.136	(0.492, 0.973)
0.15	0.308	0.061	(0.215, 0.432)	0.479	0.094	(0.326, 0.658)	0.720	0.138	(0.493, 0.980)
0.20	0.313	0.063	(0.217, 0.440)	0.484	0.096	(0.328, 0.668)	0.725	0.140	(0.496, 0.991)
	FEMALE								
	$a_0 = 45$			$a_0 = 50$			$a_0 = 55$		
	mean	s.e.	95% CI	mean	s.e.	95% CI	mean	s.e.	95% CI
0.05	0.212	0.042	(0.139, 0.291)	0.326	0.064	(0.216, 0.448)	0.467	0.089	(0.322, 0.649)
0.10	0.214	0.043	(0.141, 0.296)	0.329	0.065	(0.217, 0.452)	0.470	0.091	(0.323, 0.653)
0.15	0.216	0.044	(0.142, 0.300)	0.331	0.066	(0.218, 0.458)	0.473	0.092	(0.324, 0.659)
0.20	0.219	0.046	(0.147, 0.311)	0.335	0.068	(0.221, 0.467)	0.477	0.094	(0.325, 0.667)

Adapted from Table 8 in Wu 2022 [59].

6.3 Improved method: Scheduling the first exam when sensitivity is a function of sojourn time

In this section, we will provide an improved method for the same problem. The major improvement is that the screening sensitivity is a function of the sojourn time and time spent in the preclinical state. In the previous method, we assumed that the screening sensitivity and the sojourn time are uncorrelated. But in reality, the screening sensitivity may depend on how long one has entered and stayed in the preclinical state with respect to the sojourn time: the longer one has stayed in the preclinical state (relative to the sojourn time), the easier for the tumor to be detected. Based on this fact, we make an extension to derive the corresponding probability formula when the sensitivity and the sojourn time are correlated for asymptomatic individuals based on their current age. And after the first screening time is decided, we further evaluate the lead time and probability of overdiagnosis at the future screening time. This approach provides individuals with more accurate predictive information regarding the expected time of early diagnosis and the expected probability of overdiagnosis.

We use the same disease progressive model where the disease develops through three states $S_0 \rightarrow S_p \rightarrow S_c$ [87]. We let X be the time duration in the disease-free state S_0, with a pdf $w(x)$; We let Y be the sojourn time in the preclinical state S_p, with a pdf $q(y)$; and $Q(z) = \int_z^\infty q(y)dy$ is the survival function of the sojourn time Y. The sojourn time Y and the time duration in the disease-free state X are assumed to be independent. We let $\beta(s|Y)$ be the screening sensitivity, i.e., the probability that the screening is positive given that an individual is in the preclinical state S_p. Here s is the length of time that one has stayed in the preclinical state S_p, and Y represents one's sojourn time in the S_p, a random variable. And the sensitivity β will increase as s increases, and it will decrease as Y increases. We will use female smokers for lung cancer in the setup of the modeling, the result is applicable to other kinds of screening as well.

6.3.1 Probability of incidence and first screening time

Assume a woman has never taken any screening exams so far, and she is asymptomatic at her current age a_0. Should she start her first exam immediately, or wait for some time? We will adopt the same protocol to help with this decision-making as in Wu 2022 [59]; however, since sensitivity is a function of the sojourn time and time spent in the preclinical state, the formulas are dramatically different. The goal is to ensure that the probability of clinical incidence from her current age until her first screening time is limited to a small value, such as 0.1 or 0.2. Let t_x represent the screening time interval from her current a_0; that is, her first exam will happen at her age $t_0 = a_0 + t_x$, with

$t_x > 0$. We want to find the value t_x such that the probability of incidence is limited to a pre-selected value p.

We use the same events H_0, A_0, I_0, and D_0 defined in section 6.2.1. The last three events are mutually exclusive and $I_0 \cup D_0 \cup A_0 = H_0$. Since most people will have no cancer symptoms during their lifetime, we are more concerned with those who would develop cancer before the first exam. So we need to calculate the conditional probability of an interval case in (a_0, t_0) among those who would develop cancer in that interval, and this probability is

$$P(I_0|I_0 \cup D_0) = \frac{P(I_0)}{P(I_0 \cup D_0)} = \frac{P(I_0)}{P(I_0) + P(D_0)}. \tag{6.11}$$

The numerator is the probability of incidence in (a_0, t_0), which is the same as in equation (6.2):

$$P(I_0) = \int_0^{a_0} w(x)[Q(a_0 - x) - Q(t_0 - x)]dx + \int_{a_0}^{t_0} w(x)[1 - Q(t_0 - x)]dx.$$

The probability of D_0 is the probability of a screen-detected case at the first exam at her age t_0. That is, she must have entered the preclinical state S_p at some age $x \in (0, t_0)$, and her sojourn time is larger than $(t_0 - x)$. Let $t > (t_0 - x)$ be her sojourn time in the S_p. Since her time in the S_p would be $(t_0 - x)$ at the first exam t_0, her sensitivity would be $\beta(t_0 - x|t)$. Hence,

$$P(D_0) = \int_0^{t_0} w(x) \int_{t_0 - x}^{\infty} q(t)\beta(t_0 - x|t)dtdx. \tag{6.12}$$

Since $P(I_0|I_0 \cup D_0)$ is monotonically increasing with the time interval t_x, and remember $t_0 = a_0 + t_x$, this probability is increasing with t_0. For any given value p between 0 and 1, there is a unique solution t_0, such that

$$P(I_0|I_0 \cup D_0) = p. \tag{6.13}$$

We can use the binary search method to find the age t_0 for any given $p \in (0, 1)$.

6.3.2 Lead time distribution at the first exam

After the numerical solution $t_0 = t_0(p)$ is found, the distribution of the lead time at the first screening can be derived if one would be diagnosed with cancer. Let L be the lead time, the conditional probability density function of the lead time given one would be diagnosed at t_0 is

$$f_L(z|D_0) = \frac{f_L(z, D_0)}{P(D_0)}, \qquad \text{for } z > 0,$$

where the denominator $P(D_0)$ is the same as in equation (6.12), and the numerator,

$$f_L(z, D_0) = \int_0^{t_0} w(x)q(t_0 + z - x)\beta(t_0 - x|t_0 + z - x)dx. \qquad (6.14)$$

That is, she must have entered the preclinical state at some age x in the interval $(0, t_0)$, and her lead time is z, so her sojourn time would be (t_0+z-x), and the time she has stayed in the preclinical state would be $(t_0 - x)$ at t_0; i.e., her screening sensitivity would be $\beta(t_0 - x|t_0 + z - x)$. And we simply "add" all these possible cases using the integration.

Exercise 6.6. Prove that

$$\int_0^{\infty} f_L(z|D_0)dz = 1.$$

So the derived probability density function is valid.

6.3.3 Probability of overdiagnosis and true-early-detection

The probabilities of overdiagnosis and that of true-early-detection, given that one would be diagnosed at t_0 with a fixed lifetime $T = t(> t_0)$, are

$$P(\text{OverD}|D_0, T = t) = \frac{P(\text{OverD}, D_0|T = t)}{P(D_0|T = t)},$$

$$P(\text{TrueED}|D_0, T = t) = \frac{P(\text{TrueED}, D_0|T = t)}{P(D_0|T = t)}.$$

Since $P(D_0|T = t) = P(D_0)$ is the same as in equation (6.12), we only need to find out the two numerators. To calculate $P(\text{OverD}, D_0|T = t)$, the probability of overdiagnosis at the first exam at age t_0; but no symptom would present until after her lifetime $T = t$; she must have entered the preclinical state at age $x \in (0, t_0)$, her time in the preclinical state would be $(t_0 - x)$ at the age t_0, and her sojourn time would be longer than $(t - x)$ so that no clinical symptom would appear in her lifetime. Therefore,

$$P(\text{OverD}, D_0|T = t) = \int_0^{t_0} w(x) \int_{t-x}^{\infty} q(y)\beta(t_0 - x|y)dydx. \qquad (6.15)$$

For the case of true-early-detection, her symptom would have appeared before her lifetime t; therefore, her sojourn time would be between $(t_0 - x)$ and $(t - x)$:

$$P(\text{TrueED}, D_0|T = t) = \int_0^{t_0} w(x) \int_{t_0-x}^{t-x} q(y)\beta(t_0 - x|y)dydx. \qquad (6.16)$$

And it is easy to verify that

$$P(\text{OverD}, D_0|T = t) + P(\text{TrueED}, D_0|T = t) = P(D_0).$$

Hence the conditional probabilities given D_0 would add up to 1:

$$P(\text{OverD}|D_0, T = t) + P(\text{TrueED}|D_0, T = t) = 1.$$

Now we allow the human lifetime T to be random and let $f_T(t|T > t_0)$ be the conditional PDF of the lifetime T, then

$$\begin{aligned} &P(\text{OverD}|D_0, T > t_0) \\ &= \int_{t_0}^{\infty} P(\text{OverD}|D_0, T = t) f_T(t|T > t_0) dt, \qquad (6.17) \\ &P(\text{TrueED}|D_0, T > t_0) \\ &= \int_{t_0}^{\infty} P(\text{TrueED}|D_0, T = t) f_T(t|T > t_0) dt. \qquad (6.18) \end{aligned}$$

The conditional PDF of human lifetime $f_T(t|T > t_0) = \frac{f_T(t)}{1-F_T(t_0)}$, if $t > t_0$. And it is obtained by transforming the actuarial life table from the US Social Security Administration; for details, see Wu et al (2012).

Exercise 6.7. Prove that

$$P(\text{OverD}|D_0, T > t_0) + P(\text{TrueED}|D_0, T > t_0) = 1.$$

6.3.4 Simulation

Simulations were carried out using the above methods. The incidence probability $P(I_0|I_0 \cup D_0)$ is a function of one's current age and the three key parameters. Therefore, when this probability is limited to a small value, the next screening time interval is a function of the above-mentioned variables. We explore the effects of these factors on the first screening age; specifically, we select the following scenarios for simulation:

(a) Four different probability of incidence: $p = 0.05, 0.10, 0.15, 0.20$;

(b) Three different screening sensitivities: $\beta_i(s|Y), i = 1, 2, 3$;

(c) Three different mean sojourn time (MST): 2, 5, and 10 years;

(d) Two different transition mode for $w(t)$: 65 and 69 years;

(e) Three different current ages a_0: 55, 60, and 65 years.

The conditional probability of incidence $P(I_0|I_0 \cup D_0)$ is controlled by four pre-selected values $p = 0.05, 0.1, 0.15, 0.2$. We let the sensitivity be

$$\beta(s|Y) = [1 + \exp(-b_0 - b_1 \cdot \frac{s}{Y})]^{-1}, \quad 0 \le s \le Y, \qquad (6.19)$$

where s is the time one has stayed in the preclinical state S_p and Y is the (total) sojourn time in S_p [76]. We choose three different pairs of $(b_0, b_1) =$

(0.85, 2.65), (1.40, 2.10), and (2.20, 1.30), so that the corresponding sensitivity at the onset of S_p would be $[1+\exp(-b_0)]^{-1} = 0.7, 0.8$, and 0.9, and at the end of S_p (or the onset of S_c), the sensitivity would be $[1+\exp(-b_0-b_1)]^{-1} = 0.97$ for all three cases.

We use the same parametric model of the transition density and the sojourn time defined in (6.10) in section 6.2.4. The transition probability density $w(t)$ was a lognormal (μ, σ^2) with an upper limit of 30%, which is applicable to people with a high risk for cancer (i.e., heavy smokers of lung cancer, or people with BRCA1 or BRCA2 genes for breast cancer). The input parameters of μ and σ^2 were chosen, so that the mode of the transition age into the preclinical state was around 65 (for breast cancer [83]) or 69 (for lung cancer [76]) years old. The mode of a lognormal PDF is $\exp(\mu - \sigma^2)$, and based on our previous research, we pick $(\mu, \sigma^2) = (4.25, 0.02)$, which would have a mode around 69, to mimic lung cancer, and $(\mu, \sigma^2) = (4.35, 0.175)$, which would have a mode around 65, to mimic breast cancer.

The sojourn time distribution was a Weibull (λ, α), with parameters chosen so that the mean sojourn times are 2, 5, and 10 years (corresponding roughly to fast, moderate, and slow-growing tumors). The parameters were chosen: $\alpha = 2.5, \lambda = 0.13109, 0.01326, 0.00234$. Using equation (6.13), the optimal scheduling time t^* was found and summarized in Table 6.7.

In Table 6.7, p in the first column is the preselected probability of incidence in the simulation; it takes on values of 0.05 to 0.20. Columns 2 to 10 present the calculated optimal scheduling time (in years) of the next exam, given values of p, the current age a_0, the sensitivity β, and the mean sojourn time (MST) with different transition modes of $w(t)$ at 69 or 65 years old. The result shows that the $w(t)$ will affect the first screening age, and the density curves of the $w(t)$ are plotted in Figure 6.5 for comparison purposes. Although the modes are very close to each other (69 vs. 65), the shapes of the two $w(t)$s are very different, and the variance of $w(t)$ is mainly controlled by the parameter σ^2: a larger σ^2 will produce a flat and more spreading $w(t)$; and this, in turn, will affect the first screening age/time.

It shows that the mean sojourn time (MST) plays an important role in the timing of the first screening: longer MST (slowly growing tumors or low-risk people) means one can wait a longer time to take the first screening exam. However, it is impossible to predict the MST, even though people could be identified as high or low risk, so this information is somewhat academic. Higher probability of incidence p translates to longer screening intervals in the future (consistent with our intuition). A person's current age a_0 obviously plays a role in the scheduling: older people should come back for their first exam earlier than their younger counterparts. Finally, the sensitivity function β seems not to affect the first screening time much. Under the same risk p, the same current age a_0 and the same MST, the first screening time barely changes with the three different β. We would say that the three different β are all pretty high and reflect today's screening technology.

TABLE 6.7
Optimal initial screening age t_0^* (in years).

when $(\mu, \sigma^2) = (4.25, 0.02)$, or mode of $w(t)$ around 69.

				MST = 2 years					
	$a_0 = 55$			$a_0 = 60$			$a_0 = 65$		
p	$^a\beta_1$	β_2	β_3	β_1	β_2	β_3	β_1	β_2	β_3
0.05	55.11	55.11	55.12	60.10	60.10	60.11	65.10	65.10	65.10
0.10	55.23	55.24	55.25	60.21	60.22	60.23	65.20	65.21	65.22
0.15	55.37	55.39	55.40	60.34	60.36	60.37	65.32	65.33	65.34
0.20	55.54	55.56	55.58	60.49	60.51	60.53	65.45	65.47	65.49
				MST = 5 years					
	$a_0 = 55$			$a_0 = 60$			$a_0 = 65$		
p	β_1	β_2	β_3	β_1	β_2	β_3	β_1	β_2	β_3
0.05	55.39	55.41	55.43	60.32	60.34	60.35	65.28	65.29	65.30
0.10	55.86	55.91	55.96	60.69	60.73	60.76	65.59	65.61	65.63
0.15	56.44	56.52	56.60	61.13	61.18	61.23	65.94	65.97	66.01
0.20	57.15	57.27	57.39	61.63	61.71	61.78	66.34	66.39	66.44
				MST = 10 years					
	$a_0 = 55$			$a_0 = 60$			$a_0 = 65$		
p	β_1	β_2	β_3	β_1	β_2	β_3	β_1	β_2	β_3
0.05	56.52	56.63	56.74	61.05	61.11	61.17	65.78	65.81	65.85
0.10	58.59	58.84	59.09	62.32	62.46	62.59	66.66	66.74	66.82
0.15	61.03	61.38	61.72	63.81	64.02	64.23	67.66	67.79	67.91
0.20	63.50	63.89	64.26	65.47	65.74	65.99	68.77	68.94	69.10

when $(\mu, \sigma^2) = (4.35, 0.175)$, or mode of $w(t)$ around 65.

				MST = 2 years					
	$a_0 = 55$			$a_0 = 60$			$a_0 = 65$		
p	$^a\beta_1$	β_2	β_3	β_1	β_2	β_3	β_1	β_2	β_3
0.05	55.09	55.10	55.10	60.09	60.09	60.10	65.09	65.09	65.10
0.10	55.19	55.20	55.21	60.19	60.20	60.21	65.19	65.20	65.20
0.15	55.31	55.32	55.33	60.31	60.32	60.33	65.30	65.31	65.33
0.20	55.44	55.45	55.47	60.43	60.45	60.46	65.43	65.45	65.46
				MST = 5 years					
	$a_0 = 55$			$a_0 = 60$			$a_0 = 65$		
p	β_1	β_2	β_3	β_1	β_2	β_3	β_1	β_2	β_3
0.05	55.24	55.25	55.26	60.24	60.24	60.25	65.23	65.24	65.25
0.10	55.51	55.53	55.55	60.50	60.52	60.54	65.49	65.51	65.52
0.15	55.81	55.84	55.88	60.79	60.82	60.85	65.78	65.81	65.83
0.20	56.16	56.20	56.24	61.12	61.17	61.21	66.10	66.14	66.18
				MST = 10 years					
	$a_0 = 55$			$a_0 = 60$			$a_0 = 65$		
p	β_1	β_2	β_3	β_1	β_2	β_3	β_1	β_2	β_3
0.05	55.54	55.56	55.58	60.51	60.53	60.55	65.49	65.50	65.52
0.10	56.14	56.19	56.23	61.07	61.11	61.16	66.02	66.06	66.10
0.15	56.82	56.89	56.97	61.71	61.77	61.84	66.63	66.69	66.75
0.20	57.59	57.69	57.80	62.43	62.52	62.61	67.31	67.39	67.48

$^a\beta_i = \beta_i(s|Y) = [1 + \exp(-b_0 - b_1 \cdot \frac{s}{Y})]^{-1}, 0 \leq s \leq Y$, where the values of (b_0, b_1) equal to (0.85, 2.65), (1.40, 2.10), (2.20, 1.30) for $\beta_1, \beta_2, \beta_3$ respectively.

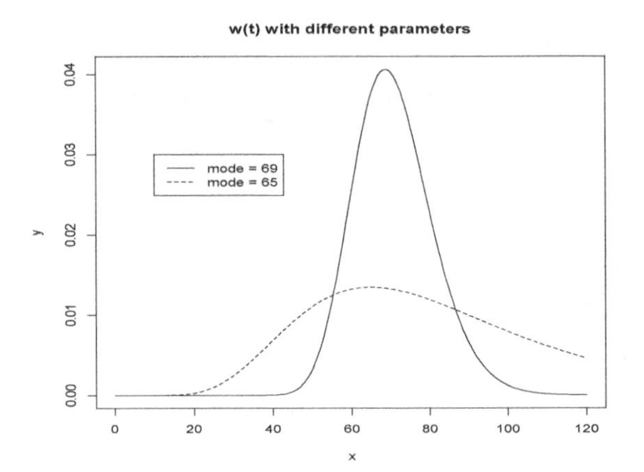

FIGURE 6.5
$w(t)$ under two sets of parameters $(\mu, \sigma^2) = (4.25, 0.02)$ with a mode around 69, and $(\mu, \sigma^2) = (4.35, 0.175)$ with a mode around 65.

Figures 6.6 and 6.7 illustrate how the lead time density curves are changing with the four factors of p, β, age, and the MST, with the two different $w(t)$ at the first exam t_0^*. The only difference between Figures 6.6 and 6.7 are the different choices of the $w(t)$. In the four panels in these two figures, we fix three factors and allow only one factor to change. For example, the panel in the upper left corner shows how the density curve of the lead time changes with p when $\beta = \beta_2(s|Y)$, MST $= 2$ years, and current age $a_0 = 60$ years. It shows that the density curve of the lead time barely changes with p, but it changes with the screening sensitivity β and the MST. It changes slightly with the one's current age a_0 when the mode of $w(t)$ is 69 (Figure 6.6 lower left panel), and barely changes with a_0 when the mode of $w(t)$ is 65 (Figure 6.7 lower left panel).

We evaluated the probability of overdiagnosis at the first exam t_0, and the results are summarized in Table 6.8. Longer MST may cause a larger probability of overdiagnosis. However, the possibility is less than 4% when the MST is 5 years or less, showing that overdiagnosis won't be a big problem at the first screening exam. The risk of overdiagnosis will slightly increase as the sensitivity increases; It increases faster as one's current age increases. Since overdiagnosis is closely related to one's lifetime and age, this is compatible with our intuition. When the probability of incidence p increases from 0.05 to 0.2, the probability of overdiagnosis slightly increases, when the other three factors are the same. Finally, the possibility of overdiagnosis changes with

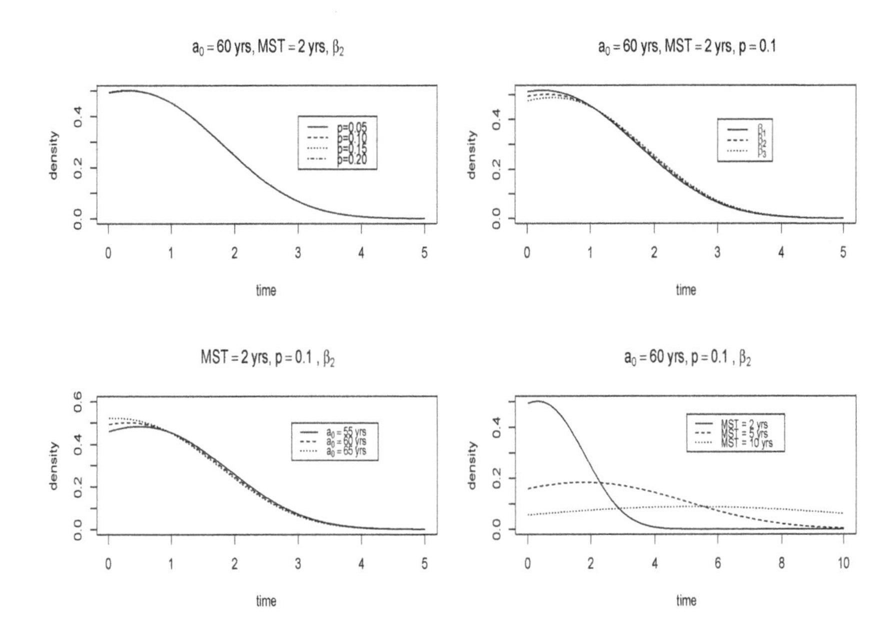

FIGURE 6.6
Lead time density under the four factors when the mode is 69: Fix three and allow one to change.

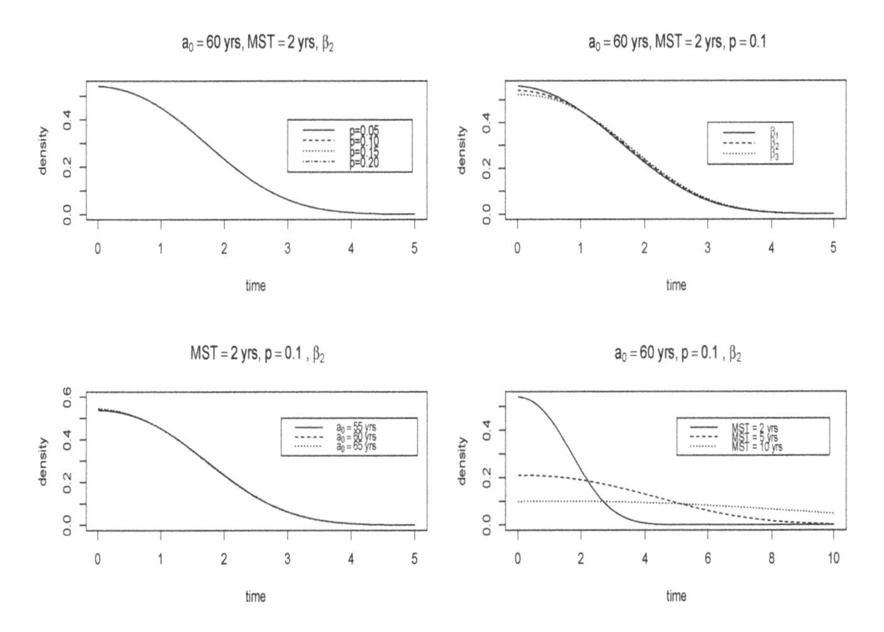

FIGURE 6.7
Lead time density when the mode is 65: Only allow one factor to change.

TABLE 6.8

Estimated probability of overdiagnosis (in percentage) at the t_0^* .

when $(\mu, \sigma^2) = (4.25, 0.02)$, or mode of $w(t)$ around 69.

	$a_0 = 55$			$a_0 = 60$			$a_0 = 65$		
MST = 2 years									
p	β_1	β_2	β_3	β_1	β_2	β_3	β_1	β_2	β_3
0.05	0.595	0.610	0.623	0.820	0.840	0.858	1.148	1.176	1.208
0.10	0.598	0.613	0.627	0.824	0.845	0.863	1.161	1.190	1.216
0.15	0.602	0.617	0.635	0.829	0.850	0.868	1.169	1.198	1.224
0.20	0.611	0.626	0.640	0.834	0.860	0.879	1.178	1.208	1.234
MST = 5 years									
p	β_1	β_2	β_3	β_1	β_2	β_3	β_1	β_2	β_3
0.05	1.864	1.919	1.956	2.481	2.539	2.590	3.431	3.514	3.587
0.10	1.924	1.981	2.019	2.527	2.603	2.655	3.508	3.619	3.695
0.15	1.988	2.046	2.098	2.606	2.667	2.737	3.624	3.711	3.813
0.20	2.070	2.128	2.181	2.687	2.769	2.825	3.727	3.818	3.926
MST = 10 years									
p	β_1	β_2	β_3	β_1	β_2	β_3	β_1	β_2	β_3
0.05	5.535	5.686	5.819	7.186	7.398	7.541	9.769	10.080	10.291
0.10	6.192	6.444	6.640	7.790	8.026	8.238	10.399	10.732	11.037
0.15	7.186	7.488	7.830	8.590	8.915	9.216	11.160	11.521	11.938
0.20	8.362	8.797	9.217	9.566	10.009	10.366	12.076	12.562	12.921

when $(\mu, \sigma^2) = (4.35, 0.175)$, or mode of $w(t)$ around 65.

	$a_0 = 55$			$a_0 = 60$			$a_0 = 65$		
MST = 2 years									
p	β_1	β_2	β_3	β_1	β_2	β_3	β_1	β_2	β_3
0.05	0.553	0.567	0.579	0.784	0.803	0.820	1.126	1.154	1.179
0.10	0.557	0.573	0.586	0.788	0.807	0.829	1.133	1.161	1.193
0.15	0.564	0.578	0.590	0.794	0.816	0.834	1.148	1.176	1.202
0.20	0.568	0.582	0.595	0.802	0.822	0.8840	1.157	1.186	1.212
MST = 5 years									
p	β_1	β_2	β_3	β_1	β_2	β_3	β_1	β_2	β_3
0.05	1.582	1.619	1.653	2.213	2.266	2.314	3.224	3.302	3.372
0.10	1.615	1.653	1.688	2.245	2.313	2.362	3.279	3.383	3.456
0.15	1.652	1.692	1.727	2.294	2.366	2.416	3.365	3.475	3.550
0.20	1.686	1.736	1.772	2.359	2.416	2.482	3.478	3.564	3.642
MST = 10 years									
p	β_1	β_2	β_3	β_1	β_2	β_3	β_1	β_2	β_3
0.05	3.960	4.061	4.150	5.571	5.716	5.845	8.168	8.443	8.638
0.10	4.123	4.229	4.347	5.786	5.974	6.112	8.586	8.816	9.083
0.15	4.320	4.431	4.560	6.089	6.252	6.441	9.028	9.274	9.562
0.20	4.525	4.672	4.808	6.420	6.638	6.841	9.577	9.843	10.151

$w(t)$ as well: a larger mode of $w(t)$ may not mean waiting longer for the first exam, but it surely means a larger probability of overdiagnosis.

6.3.5 Application: The NLST-CT data

The NLST study enrolled approximately 54,000 male and female heavy smokers aged 55 to 74 between August 2002 and April 2004 [53]. Participants were randomized into two intervention arms in equal proportions: low-dose CT or traditional chest X-ray; and they were offered three annual screening exams. We applied our method to the low-dose CT data separated by gender. The methods can be applied to data from other screening trials as well. We know that the probability of incidence is a function of the next screening time interval, the three key parameters ($\beta(t)$, $w(t)$, and $Q(x)$ or $q(x)$), and a person's current age a_0.

TABLE 6.9
Initial screening t_0^* and 95% HPD interval using the NLST-CT data.

	MALE					
	$a_0 = 50$		$a_0 = 60$		$a_0 = 70$	
p	mean (s.e.)	95% CI	mean (s.e.)	95% CI	mean (s.e.)	95% CI
0.05	50.09 (0.012)	(50.06, 50.11)	60.08 (0.011)	(60.06, 60.10)	70.07 (0.010)	(70.05, 70.09)
0.10	50.19 (0.027)	(50.13, 50.24)	60.16 (0.023)	(60.12, 60.20)	70.14 (0.021)	(70.11, 70.19)
0.15	50.31 (0.045)	(50.22, 50.39)	60.26 (0.037)	(60.19, 60.33)	70.23 (0.033)	(70.17, 70.30)
0.20	50.44 (0.067)	(50.32, 50.58)	60.36 (0.053)	(60.27, 60.47)	70.33 (0.047)	(70.25, 70.42)
	FEMALE					
	$a_0 = 50$		$a_0 = 60$		$a_0 = 70$	
p	mean (s.e.)	95% CI	mean (s.e.)	95% CI	mean (s.e.)	95% CI
0.05	50.09 (0.016)	(50.06, 50.12)	60.08 (0.014)	(60.05, 60.10)	70.07 (0.012)	(70.05, 70.10)
0.10	50.20 (0.036)	(50.13, 50.26)	60.17 (0.029)	(60.12, 60.22)	70.15 (0.026)	(70.11, 70.20)
0.15	50.32 (0.059)	(50.21, 50.43)	60.27 (0.047)	(60.18, 60.36)	70.24 (0.041)	(70.17, 70.32)
0.20	50.46 (0.088)	(50.30, 50.62)	60.38 (0.067)	(60.26, 60.51)	70.34 (0.058)	(70.25, 70.46)

Wu et al 2022 [76] estimated the three key parameters using the NLST-CT data and the $w(t), Q(x), q(x)$ defined in (6.10) . The sensitivity was a function of the time spent in the S_p and the sojourn time.

$$\beta(s|Y) = \{1 + \exp[-b_0 - b_1 \frac{s}{Y}]\}^{-1}, \ 0 < s < Y,$$

where Y is the sojourn time and s is the time spent in the S_p at the time of the exam. The unknown parameters in this model were $\theta = (b_0, b_1, \mu, \sigma^2, \lambda, \alpha)$. For each gender, using Markov Chain Monte Carlo (MCMC) with Gibbs sampler and a likelihood function, 6000 samples were generated; after 1000 burn-in and thinning every 50 iterations, a posterior sample of 100 from each chain was obtained. Running eight parallel chains with over-dispersed initial values provided 800 Bayesian posterior samples $\theta_j^*, j = 1, 2, \ldots, 800$ for each gender. For more details, see Wu et al 2022. We will use these 800 posterior samples from each gender to make Bayesian inference on optimal scheduling time/age.

We assume that for each gender, there are three hypothetic cohorts with the different current age: $a_0 = 50, 60, 70$. Given the probability of incidence p, for each θ_j^*, using $P(I_0|I_0 \cup D_0, \theta_j^*) = p$, a scheduling age t_{0j}^* $(j = 1, 2, \ldots, 800)$ could be found. We calculated the mean, the standard error, and the 95% highest posterior density (HPD) interval of the future screening age using t_{0j}^* (in years) and summarized the results for male and female heavy smokers using the NLST CT data in Table 6.9. The results show that the optimal first screening times are very close for male and female heavy smokers in similar situations, such as the same current age a_0 and same incidence probability p.

After the optimal first screening time was determined, we can further evaluate the lead time distribution and the probability of overdiagnosis. One lead time distribution can be obtained by using each pair of (θ_j^*, t_j^*), with $j = 1, 2, \ldots, 800$. The posterior distribution of the lead time is the average:

$$f_L(z|NLST) \approx \frac{1}{800} \sum_{j=1}^{800} f_L(z|\theta_j^*).$$

We then calculate the mean, median, mode, and standard deviation of the lead time using $f_L(z|NLST)$. The result is presented in Table 6.10. The estimated

TABLE 6.10
Estimated mean, median, mode, and standard deviation of lead time using NLST-CT data.

	MALE		
p	$a_0 = 50$	$a_0 = 60$	$a_0 = 70$
0.05	0.94, 0.75, 0.53, 0.63	0.89, 0.71, 0.28, 0.64	0.86, 0.68, 0.01, 0.63
0.10	0.94, 0.75, 0.53, 0.63	0.89, 0.71, 0.28, 0.64	0.86, 0.68, 0.01, 0.63
0.15	0.94, 0.75, 0.53, 0.63	0.89, 0.71, 0.28, 0.64	0.86, 0.68, 0.01, 0.63
0.20	0.94, 0.75, 0.52, 0.63	0.89, 0.71, 0.28, 0.64	0.86, 0.68, 0.01, 0.63
[a]95% C.I.	(0, 1.78)	(0, 1.78)	(0, 1.77)
	FEMALE		
p	$a_0 = 50$	$a_0 = 60$	$a_0 = 70$
0.05	0.92, 0.76, 0.68, 0.59	0.88, 0.72, 0.45, 0.59	0.85, 0.70, 0.01, 0.59
0.10	0.92, 0.76, 0.68, 0.59	0.88, 0.72, 0.44, 0.59	0.85, 0.70, 0.01, 0.59
0.15	0.92, 0.76, 0.67, 0.59	0.87, 0.72, 0.44, 0.59	0.85, 0.70, 0.01, 0.59
0.20	0.92, 0.76, 0.67, 0.59	0.87, 0.72, 0.44, 0.59	0.85, 0.70, 0.01, 0.59
95% C.I.	(0, 1.72)	(0, 1.71)	(0, 1.70)

[a]The 95% CI is the 95% highest probability density (HPD) interval using the Bayesian empirical method. Since the lead time curve for different p are almost the same, we list the largest interval for different p if there is a small discrepancy.

lead time density curves under different current age a_0 and different incidence probability p were plotted using the NLST low-dose CT male and female heavy smokers data in Figure 6.8. Since the lead time density curve doesn't change much with the incidence probability p if the optimal scheduling time t_0^* was used, we only plot the cases when $p = 0.05$ for each current age a_0. The density curves did change with the current age a_0: larger a_0 corresponds to a higher spike in the density curve, which translates to a slightly smaller mode value.

Finally, we use each pair $(\theta_j^*, t_j^*), j = 1, 2, \ldots, 800$, to estimate the probability of overdiagnosis. And we can calculate the posterior mean, standard error, and 95% HPD interval of the probability (or percentage) of overdiagnosis. Correspondingly, the probability of true-early-detection is just one minus the probability of overdiagnosis. The posterior mean, the standard error, and the 95% HPD interval are listed in Table 6.11. The probability of overdiagnosis is very low at the first screening for male and female heavy smokers using the parameters derived from the NLST-CT data ($< 0.5\%$). This risk of overdiagnosis slightly increases with one's current age for both genders. And it is slightly higher for male heavy smokers than their female counterparts. The probability of overdiagnosis slightly increases when p increases. However, the maximum probability of overdiagnosis was less than 1% for both genders in

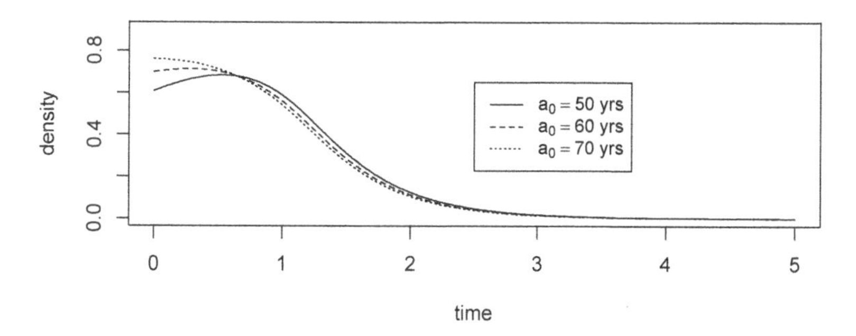

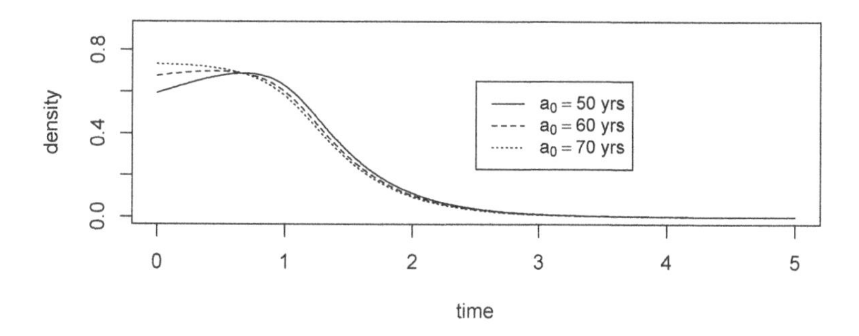

FIGURE 6.8
Lead time density when $p = 0.05$ using the NLST-CT data.

our simulation. Therefore, overdiagnosis is not an issue at the first screening exam using low-dose CT for lung cancer.

TABLE 6.11
Probability of overdiagnosis at the initial screening age t_0^* for the NLST-CT data (in percentage).

	MALE					
	$a_0 = 50$		$a_0 = 60$		$a_0 = 70$	
p	mean (s.e.)	95% CI	mean (s.e.)	95% CI	mean (s.e.)	95% CI
0.05	0.464 (0.107)	(0.270, 0.659)	0.990 (0.224)	(0.578, 1.391)	1.892 (0.428)	(1.176, 2.737)
0.10	0.467 (0.108)	(0.276, 0.669)	0.995 (0.226)	(0.579, 1.405)	1.902 (0.432)	(1.179, 2.754)
0.15	0.470 (0.110)	(0.265, 0.665)	1.000 (0.228)	(0.580, 1.413)	1.912 (0.438)	(1.181, 2.773)
0.20	0.476 (0.112)	(0.273, 0.678)	1.007 (0.232)	(0.582, 1.423)	1.925 (0.444)	(1.186, 2.794)
	FEMALE					
	$a_0 = 50$		$a_0 = 60$		$a_0 = 70$	
p	mean (s.e.)	95% CI	mean (s.e.)	95% CI	mean (s.e.)	95% CI
0.05	0.284 (0.069)	(0.169, 0.414)	0.579 (0.137)	(0.349, 0.836)	1.248 (0.297)	(0.751, 1.803)
0.10	0.286 (0.070)	(0.169, 0.417)	0.582 (0.138)	(0.350, 0.841)	1.256 (0.300)	(0.753, 1.821)
0.15	0.288 (0.071)	(0.170, 0.423)	0.585 (0.140)	(0.350, 0.846)	1.265 (0.305)	(0.754, 1.844)
0.20	0.291 (0.073)	(0.171, 0.430)	0.589 (0.142)	(0.348, 0.854)	1.276 (0.311)	(0.757, 1.861)

6.4 Bibliographic notes

There is limited research on the theory of optimal scheduling, and there is almost no research on the first scheduling time before. The method in this chapter is the first one in this area, and it avoids using utility functions (which are subjective) such as cost or weight, but using the risk of incidence directly. This is a method that could be directly used by physicians or diagnostic radiologists to schedule a person's future screening exam.

The method in section 6.2 was in fact developed after the method in section 7.2, because this could be considered a special case of section 7.2. The first result was presented at the 2021 Conference on Statistical Practice (CSP) and at the 2021 International Biometric Society Eastern North American Region (ENAR) spring meeting. Later, it was published in *Statistics and Its Interface* [59]. The method in section 6.3 was presented at the 2022 Symposium on Data Science and Statistics (SDSS) and at the 2022 Joint Statistical Meeting (JSM). It was not published yet, and the materials came from the draft of Wu 2023 [62].

The model can be improved to accommodate more variables, such as one's perceived cancer risk: if the risk is high, such as a family history of cancer or close relatives have cancer, then the distribution of the disease-free time $w(t)$ and the survival function of the sojourn time $Q(x)$ could be modified to reflect the changes. I want to emphasize that all tables in the simulations are reproducible using the provided parameters. The tables in the applications are also reproducible if the posterior samples are available. The modeling approach is just one way of thinking about the problem. Other models and approaches are possible. The important point is to recognize that screening has outcomes and consequences that one should consider, especially for policy purposes. We hope that this research would provide a theoretical and practical basis to guide individuals or physicians towards an informed decision.

6.5 Solution for some exercises

Exercise 6.1

(a) $P(H_0) = 1 - \int_0^{a_0} w(x)dx + \int_0^{a_0} w(x)Q(a_0 - x)dx$.

(b) $P(A_0) = 1 - \int_0^{t_0} w(x)dx + (1-\beta)\int_0^{t_0} w(x)Q(t_0 - x)dx$.

(d) **Proof:** Since

$$P(I_0|I_0 \cup D_0) = \frac{P(I_0)}{P(I_0) + P(D_0)} = \frac{1}{1 + \frac{P(D_0)}{P(I_0)}}.$$

We only need to prove that $\frac{P(D_0)}{P(I_0)}$ is monotone decreasing with t_x, or it is monotone decreasing with $t_0 = a_0 + t_x$. We let $t = t_0$ and define

$$H(t) = \frac{P(D_0)}{P(I_0)}.$$

We only need to check the first derivative $H'(t) < 0$ or not. Since

$$H'(t) = \frac{P'_t(D_0)P(I_0) - P(D_0)P'_t(I_0)}{P^2(I_0)}$$

Now we only need to check whether the numerator $P'_t(D_0)P(I_0) - P(D_0)P'_t(I_0)$ is less than 0 or not. Since $t = t_0$, and

$$P(D_0) = \beta \int_0^t w(x)Q(t-x)dx.$$

Using the Leibnitz's rule[2], recall $Q(0) = 1, Q'(t) = -q(t), I(t) = \int_0^t w(x)q(t-x)dx$:

$$\begin{aligned}
P'_t(D_0) &= \beta\left\{w(t)Q(t-t) + \int_0^t w(x)\cdot[-q(t-x)]dx\right\} \\
&= \beta\left\{w(t) - \int_0^t w(x)q(t-x)dx\right\} \\
&= \beta[w(t) - I(t)].
\end{aligned}$$

Similarly, since

$$P(I_0) = \int_0^{a_0} w(x)[Q(a_0-x) - Q(t-x)]dx + \int_{a_0}^t w(x)[1-Q(t-x)]dx.$$

Using the Leibnitz's rule, and remember that $0 < a_0 < t$,

$$\begin{aligned}
P'_t(I_0) &= \int_0^{a_0} w(x)q(t-x)dx + w(t)[1-Q(t-t)] + \int_{a_0}^t w(x)q(t-x)dx \\
&= \int_0^{a_0} w(x)q(t-x)dx + \int_{a_0}^t w(x)q(t-x)dx \\
&= \int_0^t w(x)q(t-x)dx = I(t).
\end{aligned}$$

---

[2]Leibnitz's rule: if $f(x,\theta), a(\theta), b(\theta)$ are differentiable with respect to θ, then

$$\frac{d}{d\theta}\int_{a(\theta)}^{b(\theta)} f(x,\theta)dx = f(b(\theta),\theta)\frac{d}{d\theta}b(\theta) - f(a(\theta),\theta)\frac{d}{d\theta}a(\theta) + \int_{a(\theta)}^{b(\theta)} \frac{\partial}{\partial\theta}f(x,\theta)dx.$$

Now check the numerator

$$
\begin{aligned}
&[P_t'(D_0)P(I_0) - P(D_0)P_t'(I_0)]/\beta \\
&= [w(t) - I(t)] \\
&\quad \times \left\{ \int_0^{a_0} w(x)[Q(a_0 - x) - Q(t-x)]dx + \int_{a_0}^{t} w(x)[1 - Q(t-x)]dx \right\} \\
&\quad -I(t) \int_0^t w(x)Q(t-x)dx \\
&= w(t) \left\{ \int_0^{a_0} w(x)[Q(a_0 - x) - Q(t-x)]dx + \int_{a_0}^{t} w(x)[1 - Q(t-x)]dx \right\} \\
&\quad -I(t) \left\{ \int_0^{a_0} w(x)[Q(a_0 - x) - Q(t-x)]dx + \int_{a_0}^{t} w(x)[1 - Q(t-x)]dx \right\} \\
&\quad -I(t) \left\{ \int_0^{a_0} w(x)Q(t-x)dx + \int_{a_0}^{t} w(x)Q(t-x)dx \right\} \\
&= w(t) \left\{ \int_0^{a_0} w(x)[Q(a_0 - x) - Q(t-x)]dx + \int_{a_0}^{t} w(x)[1 - Q(t-x)]dx \right\} \\
&\quad -I(t) \left\{ \int_0^{a_0} w(x)Q(a_0 - x)dx + \int_{a_0}^{t} w(x)dx \right\} \\
&< 0.
\end{aligned}
$$

This finishes the proof.

Exercise 6.6

The proof is straightforward, by switching the order of dx and dz, we can show that

$$
\begin{aligned}
\int_0^\infty f_L(z, D_0)dz &= \int_0^\infty \int_0^{t_0} w(x)q(t_0 + z - x)\beta(t_0 - x|t_0 + z - x)dxdz \\
&= \int_0^{t_0} \int_0^\infty w(x)q(t_0 + z - x)\beta(t_0 - x|t_0 + z - x)dzdx \\
&= \int_0^{t_0} w(x) \int_0^\infty q(t_0 + z - x)\beta(t_0 - x|t_0 + z - x)dzdx \\
&= \int_0^{t_0} w(x) \int_{t_0 - x}^\infty q(t)\beta(t_0 - x|t)dtdx.
\end{aligned}
$$

The last step is achieved by replacing the variable z with $t = t_0 + z - x$. Therefore,

$$\int_0^\infty f_L(z, D_0)dz = P(D_0).$$

And dividing $P(D_0)$ on both sides to obtain

$$\int_0^\infty f_L(z|D_0)dz = 1.$$

7

Scheduling the Upcoming Exam for Individuals with a Screening History

CONTENTS

In Chapter 6, we addressed the problem of scheduling the first exam for asymptomatic people who has no screening history, a more realistic question is: for those who have taken screening exams in the past with negative results and who look healthy right now, when to schedule their next exam? We will provide a solution to this question using probability of incidence, and also derive the lead time distribution and probability of overdiagnosis if one would be diagnosed with cancer at the future scheduling time. This could be helpful for physicians and individuals at risk to make informed decisions.

DOI: 10.1201/9781003404125-7

7.1 Introduction

Some research has been done on optimal scheduling. Zelen 1993 developed a utility function to find the optimal scheduling for $(n+1)$ exams [88]. "This is equivalent to a fixed budget which allows only $(n+1)$ examinations" (quote from Zelen 1993). The utility function assigns different weights to cases diagnosed by the first exam, cases diagnosed at subsequent exams, and interval cases. The optimal spacing of the exams is to find a sequence of time $(t_0, t_1, \cdots, t_n)$ to maximize the utility function. Zelen found that for the optimal intervals to be equal, the sensitivity must be 1, which cannot be achieved in reality. Another concern is the choice of weights in the utility function, which is subjective in nature.

Lee and Zelen 1998 developed a threshold method [30]. Their threshold method calculates the probability of being in the preclinical state S_p, and exams are scheduled whenever this probability reaches the same value as that at the initial age (which is 0.0018 in their simulation when the initial age is 50 years old and the mean sojourn time is 4 years). They found that the screening interval is getting smaller as people become older. They also introduced a concept of schedule sensitivity to measure the effectiveness of a screening program. The schedule sensitivity calculates the ratio of the expected number of cases diagnosed on scheduled exams to the expected number of the total cancer cases (the screen-detected and the interval cases). They tried to use predetermined schedule sensitivity to plan future screening programs. However, "prespecifying the screening horizon schedule sensitivity does not necessarily result in unique schedules" (quote from Lee and Zelen 1998). As their example shows, to maintain the same schedule sensitivity $(R = \sum D_i/(\sum D_i + \sum I_i))$, one can either choose a later age to start and a higher threshold probability of being in the preclinical state S_p, or an earlier age to start and a slightly lower threshold probability. Hence schedule sensitivity will increase if more screenings would be scheduled in a fixed time interval. Again, costs or weights were involved in their schedule sensitivity. Their main contributions are to the scheduling for $(n+1)$ exams in a fixed age interval and with a fixed budget. There are other papers on optimal scheduling [39, 40]. They all use some utility functions that involve cost.

We will not use any concept of weight or cost, or utility function. Instead, we will use incidence probability as in Chapter 6 to handle the scheduling of screening. We will derive the probability of incidence before the next exam, given one's current age and personal screening history. The next screening interval will be chosen, such that this probability of incidence will be limited to some preselected small values, such as 10% or less. Hence, with a 90% or more chance, an individual will not become a clinical incident case before the next exam if one would follow this schedule. After this scheduling time is found, we can derive the lead time distribution and the probability of overdiagnosis at this future time point if one would be diagnosed with cancer at the exam. This provides important predictive information regarding how early the diagnosis of cancer could be if one would develop cancer and the risk of overdiagnosis, should one follows this schedule. This research provides a theoretical and practical basis to guide individuals or physicians to make an informed decision in the screening exam. Specifically, the research may solve the problem of when screening should be performed for individuals with different risks of disease in the near future.

7.2 Scheduling upcoming exam for asymptomatic people with negative screening results

Suppose a woman has taken a few exams with negative screening results (including false positive), and she is asymptomatic and without any history of cancer so far, what kind of suggestion should a physician provide to her regarding her next screening time? Should she come back after 6, 12, 18 months, or longer? What kind of criteria should be used to back up the suggestion or decision? We will provide a probability method in this area.

When we think about optimal scheduling in cancer screening, intuition tells us that more screening seems to guarantee that one would be detected early if one would develop clinical disease. However, too many screening exams may lead to false-positive results and also incur a huge cost to individuals and insurance companies. Since the possibility of disease incidence before the next screening exam will be monotonic increasing as the time interval increases, we will use the conditional probability of incidence as the main criterion: given a woman has a screening history with negative results and is asymptomatic so far, we will derive the conditional probability of incidence before her next screening exam. This conditional probability will be a function of the time interval before her next exam, so that we can choose a future time interval such that this conditional probability is less than some preselected small values, such as 10% or 5%. In other words, with a 90% or 95% chance she would not end up being a clinical incident case (i.e., poor prognosis) before her next scheduled exam.

We let $\beta(t)$ be the screening sensitivity, where t is the individual's age at the exam. We define $w(t)$ as the probability density function (PDF) of time duration in the disease-free state S_0; let $q(x)$ be the PDF of the sojourn time in the S_p, and let $Q(z) = \int_z^\infty q(x)dx$ be the survival function of the sojourn time in the preclinical state S_p. Throughout this chapter, the time variable t represents the participating individual's age.

To derive the conditional probability of incidence, we will illustrate the key idea using as an example, an asymptomatic woman with a history of two screening exams. We will provide the general results for an asymptomatic woman with any number of examinations in her screening history at the end of this section.

7.2.1 Probability of incidence with $K = 2$ exams in the past

Suppose a woman has gone through two screening exams at her ages t_0 and $t_1(> t_0)$ with negative results at both exams and her current age is $a_0(\geq t_1)$. We let $t_{-1} = 0$, and let t_x represent her next screening time interval; that is, her future screening will be at her age $t_2 = a_0 + t_x$. See Figure 7.1.

We define four events:

$$
\begin{aligned}
H_2 &= \{\text{One is asymptomatic in } [0, a_0] \text{ after taking two exams at } t_0 < t_1\}; \\
A_2 &= \left\{ \begin{array}{l} \text{One is asymptomatic in } (a_0, t_2), \\ \text{and has a negative test result at } t_2 \end{array} \right\} \cap H_2; \\
I_2 &= \{\text{One is a clinical incident case in } (a_0, t_2)\} \cap H_2; \\
D_2 &= \{\text{One is diagnosed with cancer at } t_2 = a_0 + t_x\} \cap H_2.
\end{aligned}
$$

Three possible events could happen in the time interval $(a_0, a_0 + t_x]$: (i) event A_2: she has no symptoms of breast cancer until age $t_2 = a_0 + t_x$, and her exam result at t_2 is negative; or (ii) event I_2: she is a clinical incident case in $(a_0, a_0 + t_x)$; or (iii) event D_2: she is diagnosed with cancer at $a_0 + t_x$. The three events (A_2, I_2, D_2) are mutually exclusive and form a partition of the sample space H_2. That is,

$$A_2 \cup I_2 \cup D_2 = H_2.$$

Since most people will be symptom-free, we are more concerned about those who would develop cancer before the next exam. So we need to calculate the conditional probability of interval incidence case in $(t_1, t_1 + t_x)$ among those who would develop cancer in that time interval. Hence the probability of incidence is

$$P(I_2 | I_2 \cup D_2) = \frac{P(I_2)}{P(I_2 \cup D_2)} = \frac{P(I_2)}{P(I_2) + P(D_2)}. \tag{7.1}$$

We need to calculate two probabilities: $P(I_2)$ and $P(D_2)$.

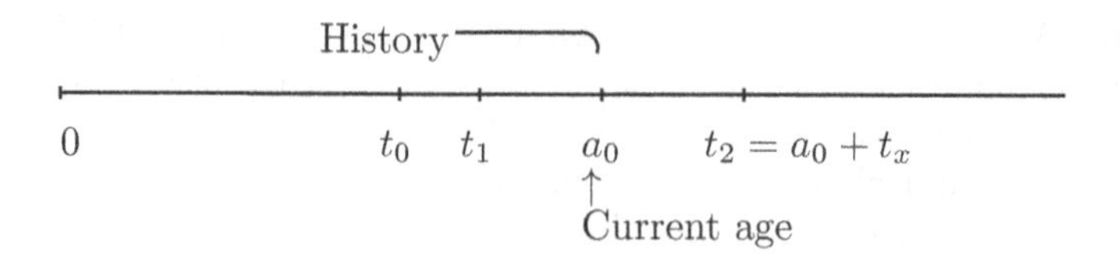

FIGURE 7.1
Illustration of screening examinations.

For the event I_2, she will be an incident case in (a_0, t_2) with her screening history. There are four possible events: (i) she enters the preclinical state at x in $(0, t_0)$ and gets false-negative screening results at t_0 and t_1; (ii) she enters the preclinical state at $x \in (t_0, t_1)$ and gets a false-negative result at t_1; (iii) she enters the preclinical state at $x \in (t_1, a_0)$; or (iv) she enters the preclinical state at $x \in (a_0, t_2)$. Here x is her onset age of the preclinical state S_p. In the first three cases, her sojourn time is between $(a_0 - x)$ and $(t_2 - x)$, while in case (iv), her sojourn time is less than $(t_2 - x)$. Therefore,

$$\begin{aligned} P(I_2) &= (1-\beta_0)(1-\beta_1)\int_0^{t_0} w(x)[Q(a_0-x)-Q(t_2-x)]dx \\ &\quad +(1-\beta_1)\int_{t_0}^{t_1} w(x)[Q(a_0-x)-Q(t_2-x)]dx \\ &\quad +\int_{t_1}^{a_0} w(x)[Q(a_0-x)-Q(t_2-x)]dx \\ &\quad +\int_{a_0}^{t_2} w(x)[1-Q(t_2-x)]dx. \end{aligned}$$

To obtain $P(D_2)$, she will be diagnosed with cancer at $t_2 = a_0 + t_x$, there are three possible events: (i) she enters the preclinical state at $x \in (0, t_0)$ and gets false-negative screening results at t_0 and t_1; (ii) she enters the preclinical state in (t_0, t_1), and gets a false-negative result at t_1; or (iii) she enters the preclinical state after t_1. In all three cases, her sojourn time is longer than $(t_2 - x)$, let $\beta_2 = \beta(t_2)$, therefore

$$\begin{aligned} P(D_2) &= \beta_2(1-\beta_0)(1-\beta_1)\int_0^{t_0} w(x)Q(t_2-x)dx \\ &\quad +\beta_2(1-\beta_1)\int_{t_0}^{t_1} w(x)Q(t_2-x)dx \\ &\quad +\beta_2\int_{t_1}^{t_2} w(x)Q(t_2-x)dx. \end{aligned}$$

This incidence probability $P(I_2|I_2 \cup D_2)$ is monotone increasing as the next screening interval t_x increases; therefore, for any preselected small value $p \in (0, 1)$, there exists a unique solution t^*, satisfying

$$P(I_2|I_2 \cup D_2) = p$$

which means, with probability $(1-p)$, an individual would not be an incident case before her next screening if she chooses to take her next exam at her age $a_0 + t^*$ (or at time t^* from now on). People may choose p =5%, 10% or 20% based on their perception of risk tolerance. Notice that, to guarantee a 100% probability of no clinical incidence/symptoms before the next exam, then one must take the screening exam every day, which is impractical and harmful.

Exercise 7.1.

(a) Find $P(H_2)$.

(b) Find $P(A_2)$.

(c) Prove that $P(H_2) = P(A_2) + P(I_2) + P(D_2)$.

7.2.2 Probability of incidence with any K exams in the past

Now we generalize this approach to the case of an asymptomatic woman with any screening history. Assume a woman has taken $K(\geq 1)$ screening exams with negative screening results at her ages $t_0 < t_1 < \cdots < t_{K-1}$, and she is asymptomatic at her current age $a_0(\geq t_{K-1})$. We let $t_{-1} = 0$. See Figure 7.2. Let K = number of screening in the past, and t_x represents her next screening time interval, and let $t_K = a_0 + t_x$. We define four events as follows:

$$\begin{aligned}
H_K &= \left\{ \begin{array}{l} \text{One is asymptomatic in } [0, a_0] \text{ after} \\ \text{taking } K \text{ exams at } t_0 < t_1 < \cdots < t_{K-1} \end{array} \right\}; \\
A_K &= \left\{ \begin{array}{l} \text{One is asymptomatic in } (a_0, t_K), \\ \text{and has a negative test result at } t_K \end{array} \right\} \cap H_K; \\
I_K &= \{\text{One is an incident case in } (a_0, t_K)\} \cap H_K; \\
D_K &= \{\text{One is diagnosed at } t_K\} \cap H_K.
\end{aligned} \tag{7.2}$$

The three mutually exclusive events (I_K, D_K, A_K) is a partition of the sample space:

$$I_K \cup D_K \cup A_K = H_K.$$

The probability of incidence among those at risk before the next exam at $t_K = a_0 + t_x$ is

$$P(I_K | I_K \cup D_K) = \frac{P(I_K)}{P(I_K \cup D_K)} = \frac{P(I_K)}{P(I_K) + P(D_K)}. \tag{7.3}$$

We need to calculate $P(I_K)$ and $P(D_K)$. The probability $P(I_K)$ is the probability of incidence in $(a_0, t_K = a_0 + t_x)$, and it could happen in $(K+2)$ mutually exclusive events, depending on when she enters the preclinical state:

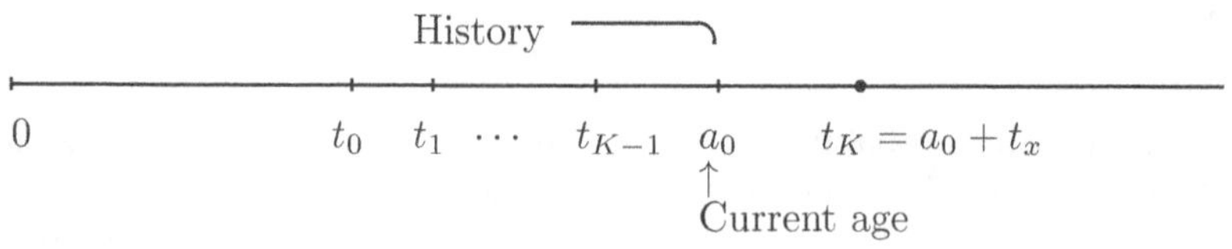

History

0 t_0 t_1 $\cdots$ t_{K-1} a_0 $t_K = a_0 + t_x$

↑ Current age

FIGURE 7.2
Illustration of K screening exams.

(i) she enters the preclinical state at $x \in (t_{i-1}, t_i)$ with $i = 0, 1, \ldots, K-1$, her cancer was undetected, and her sojourn time is in $(a_0 - x, t_K - x)$, these are K disjoint events; (ii) she enters the preclinical state at $x \in (t_{K-1}, a_0)$ and her sojourn time is between $(a_0 - x, t_K - x)$; or (iii) she enters the preclinical state at $x \in (a_0, t_K)$ and her sojourn time is less than $(t_K - x)$. We simply add all these probabilities and obtain

$$\begin{aligned} P(I_K) &= \sum_{i=0}^{K-1} (1-\beta_i)\cdots(1-\beta_{K-1}) \int_{a_0}^{t_K} \int_{t_{i-1}}^{t_i} w(x)q(t-x)dxdt \\ &\quad + \int_{a_0}^{t_K} \int_{t_{K-1}}^{a_0} w(x)q(t-x)dxdt + \int_{a_0}^{t_K} \int_{a_0}^{t} w(x)q(t-x)dxdt \\ &= \sum_{i=0}^{K-1} (1-\beta_i)\cdots(1-\beta_{K-1}) \int_{t_{i-1}}^{t_i} w(x)[Q(a_0-x) - Q(t_K-x)]dx \\ &\quad + \int_{t_{K-1}}^{a_0} w(x)[Q(a_0-x) - Q(t_K-x)]dx \\ &\quad + \int_{a_0}^{t_K} w(x)[1 - Q(t_K-x)]dx. \end{aligned} \tag{7.4}$$

And the probability $P(D_K)$ is getting diagnosed with cancer for the first time at t_K:

$$\begin{aligned} P(D_K) &= \beta_K \left\{ \sum_{i=0}^{K-1} (1-\beta_i)\cdots(1-\beta_{K-1}) \int_{t_{i-1}}^{t_i} w(x)Q(t_K-x)dx \right. \\ &\quad \left. + \int_{t_{K-1}}^{t_K} w(x)Q(t_K-x)dx \right\}. \end{aligned} \tag{7.5}$$

This conditional probability is monotone increasing as t_x increases. Hence for any given value $p \in (0,1)$, there exists a unique numerical solution t^*, such that

$$P(I_K | I_K \cup D_K) = \frac{P(I_K)}{P(I_K) + P(D_K)} = p. \tag{7.6}$$

This means, with probability $(1-p)$ she would not be a clinical incident case before her next screening if she would take her next exam at her age $t_K = a_0 + t^*$ (or at time t^* from now on). People may choose p to be 5% or 10%, or any other preferred small value to meet their needs.

A special case is when $a_0 = t_{K-1}$, and in this case, the formula of $P(D_K)$ does not change at all, except that $t_K = a_0 + t_x = t_{K-1} + t_x$, but the $P(I_K)$

will be slightly changed to

$$P(I_K) = \sum_{i=0}^{K-1}(1-\beta_i)\cdots(1-\beta_{K-1})\int_{t_{i-1}}^{t_i} w(x)[Q(a_0-x)-Q(t_K-x)]dx + \int_{t_{K-1}}^{t_K} w(x)[1-Q(t_K-x)]dx. \tag{7.7}$$

Exercise 7.2.

(a) Find the probability $P(H_K)$.

(b) Find the probability $P(A_K)$.

(c) Prove that $P(H_K) = P(A_K) + P(I_K) + P(D_K)$.

7.2.3 Lead time distribution at $t_K = a_0 + t^*$

Once the upcoming exam time t^* is found, we can evaluate the conditional distribution of the lead time on an individual basis. If a woman plans to take her next screening at the scheduled time $(a_0 + t^*)$ and is diagnosed with cancer, then how early could it be for her diagnosis due to screening? Or what is the most possible lead time (the mode of the lead time) for her case due to screening?

We let L be the lead time, and let $t_K = a_0 + t^*$, the lead time distribution given that one is first diagnosed with cancer at t_K (i.e., the event D_K happens) is

$$f_L(z|D_K) = \frac{f_L(z, D_K)}{P(D_K)}, \qquad \text{for } z \in (0, \infty), \tag{7.8}$$

where the numerator

$$\begin{aligned} f_L(z, D_K) &= \sum_{i=0}^{K} f_L(z, D_K, \text{she enters the } S_p \text{ state in } (t_{i-1}, t_i)) \\ &= \beta_K \left\{ \sum_{i=0}^{K-1}(1-\beta_i)\cdots(1-\beta_{K-1})\int_{t_{i-1}}^{t_i} w(x)q(t_K+z-x)dx \right. \\ &\quad \left. + \int_{t_{K-1}}^{t_K} w(x)q(t_K+z-x)dx \right\} \qquad \text{for } z > 0. \end{aligned} \tag{7.9}$$

And the denominator $P(D_K)$ is the same as in equation (7.5).

Exercise 7.3. Prove that

$$\int_0^\infty f_L(z|D_K)dz = 1. \tag{7.10}$$

Hence, the lead time distribution is a valid PDF.

7.2.4 Probability of overdiagnosis and true-early-detection

Given one would be diagnosed at $t_K = a_0 + t^*$ and one's lifetime $T = t(> t_K)$, the probability of true-early-detection and overdiagnosis can be derived as

$$\begin{aligned} P(\text{TrueED}|D_K, T = t) &= \frac{P(\text{TrueED}, D_K|T = t)}{P(D_K|T = t)}, \\ P(\text{OverD}|D_K, T = t) &= \frac{P(\text{OverD}, D_K|T = t)}{P(D_K|T = t)}. \end{aligned}$$

Notice that $P(D_K|T = t) = P(D_K)$ which is given in equation (7.5), we only need to figure out $P(\text{TrueED}, D_K|T = t)$ and $P(\text{OverD}, D_K|T = t)$.

To calculate $P(\text{TrueED}, D_K|T = t)$, she must have entered the preclinical state S_p before t_K. Let x represent the onset of the preclinical state, then $x \in (t_{i-1}, t_i), i = 0, \ldots, K$, and we let $t_{-1} = 0$ (see Figure 7.2). She was not detected by the previous exams before t_K, and her sojourn time must be in the interval $(t_K - x, t - x)$. Hence,

$$\begin{aligned} & P(\text{TrueED}, D_K|T = t) \\ = \; & \beta_K \left\{ \sum_{i=0}^{K-1} (1 - \beta_i) \cdots (1 - \beta_{K-1}) \int_{t_{i-1}}^{t_i} w(x)[Q(t_K - x) - Q(t - x)]dx \right. \\ & \left. + \int_{t_{K-1}}^{t_K} w(x)[Q(t_K - x) - Q(t - x)]dx \right\}. \end{aligned} \tag{7.11}$$

Similarly, overdiagnosis means that her sojourn time must be longer than $(t - x)$:

$$\begin{aligned} & P(\text{OverD}, D_K|T = t) \\ = \; & \beta_K \left\{ \sum_{i=0}^{K-1} (1 - \beta_i) \cdots (1 - \beta_{K-1}) \int_{t_{i-1}}^{t_i} w(x)Q(t - x)dx \right. \\ & \left. + \int_{t_{K-1}}^{t_K} w(x)Q(t - x)dx \right\}. \end{aligned} \tag{7.12}$$

Exercise 7.4. Prove that

$$P(\text{TrueED}, D_K|T = t) + P(\text{OverD}, D_K|T = t) = P(D_K).$$

Therefore

$$P(\text{TrueED}|D_K, T = t) + P(\text{OverD}|D_K, T = t) = 1.$$

Now we allow lifetime T to be a random variable, and let $f_T(t|T > t_k)$ be the conditional PDF of the lifetime T, then

$$\begin{aligned} P(\text{TrueED}|D_K, T > t_K) &= \int_{t_K}^{\infty} P(\text{TrueED}|D_K, T = t) f_T(t|T > t_K)dt, \\ P(\text{OverD}|D_K, T > t_K) &= \int_{t_K}^{\infty} P(\text{OverD}|D_K, T = t) f_T(t|T > t_K)dt. \end{aligned}$$

And the probability formulas are valid since

$$P(\text{TrueED}|D_K, T > t_K) + P(\text{OverD}|D_K, T > t_K) = 1.$$

7.2.5 Simulations

We conducted simulations using the above methods. The conditional probability $P(I_K|I_K \cup D_K)$ is a function of the next screening interval, the past screening history, and the three model parameters (sensitivity, sojourn time, transition density from S_0 to S_p); To explore the effects of these factors on the probability of incidence before the next exam, we selected the following scenarios for simulation:

1. The probability of incidence: $p = 0.05, 0.10, 0.15$, or 0.20;
2. The initial screening age $t_0 = 50$, the last screening age $t_{K-1} = 62$;
3. The current age $a_0 = t_{K-1} = 62$;
4. The past screening interval $\Delta = 1.0, 1.5, 2.0$ years;
5. Three different screening sensitivities: $\beta = 0.7, 0.8$, and 0.9;
6. Three different mean sojourn time (MST): 2, 5, 10, and 15 years.

Notice that we choose the current age $a_0 = t_{K-1}$ because when a_0 is larger than t_{K-1}, the result depends less on the past screening interval. We will present some simulation results when $a_0 > t_{K-1}$ in the NLST-CT applications in section 7.2.7. Since the past screening intervals $\Delta = 1.0, 1.5, 2.0$ years from age 50 to age 62, the corresponding past screening number would be $K = 13, 9, 7$. The sojourn time distribution was chosen to be a log-logistic PDF (see section 2.4.3), with parameters chosen so that the mean sojourn times are 2, 5, 10, and 15 years (corresponding roughly to fast-growing, moderate-growing, slow-growing, and extremely slow-growing tumors). The parameters chosen for the log-logistic PDF were $\kappa = 2.5, \rho = 0.661, 0.264, 0.132, 0.088$. The transition probability density $w(t)$ was chosen to be a lognormal PDF, with a single mode around 60 years old, and with an upper limit of 20%, which is applicable to different kinds of cancer, including breast cancer; and the parameters for $w(t)$ are chosen as $(\mu, \sigma^2) = (4.2, 0.1)$. The simulation results are summarized in Table 7.1.

In Table 7.1, the first column p is the probability of incidence (from 0.05 to 0.20) before the next exam in the simulation. Columns 2 to 10 present the future screening time interval (in years) found by using equation (7.6) under the probability of incidence, with different values of the test sensitivity β and different screening histories. It shows that sensitivity plays an important role in the optimal time for the next screening: under the same control probability of incidence, higher sensitivity leads to lower screening frequencies (longer screening intervals). For example, in row 5 where the mean sojourn time (MST) is 2 years and $p = 0.20$ (probability of incidence before the next

TABLE 7.1
Estimated scheduling time interval t^* (in years) when initial exam age $t_0 = 50$, current age $a_0 = t_{K-1} = 62$ years old.

	$^a MST = 2$ **yrs**								
		$\beta = 0.7$			$\beta = 0.8$			$\beta = 0.9$	
$^b p\backslash\Delta$	1.0	1.5	2.0	1.0	1.5	2.0	1.0	1.5	2.0
0.05	0.13	0.10	0.09	0.21	0.14	0.11	0.47	0.31	0.23
0.10	0.33	0.24	0.21	0.56	0.40	0.33	0.84	0.75	0.69
0.15	0.58	0.45	0.39	0.86	0.72	0.64	1.12	1.05	1.01
0.20	0.83	0.69	0.62	1.11	1.01	0.94	1.36	1.31	1.28
	$MST = 5$ **yrs**								
		$\beta = 0.7$			$\beta = 0.8$			$\beta = 0.9$	
$p\backslash\Delta$	1.0	1.5	2.0	1.0	1.5	2.0	1.0	1.5	2.0
0.05	0.87	0.53	0.38	1.31	0.98	0.69	1.67	1.52	1.35
0.10	1.65	1.28	1.00	2.07	1.84	1.61	2.42	2.31	2.21
0.15	2.25	1.94	1.67	2.67	2.48	2.30	3.03	2.95	2.86
0.20	2.78	2.52	2.28	3.22	3.06	2.91	3.60	3.53	3.46
	$MST = 10$ **yrs**								
		$\beta = 0.7$			$\beta = 0.8$			$\beta = 0.9$	
$p\backslash\Delta$	1.0	1.5	2.0	1.0	1.5	2.0	1.0	1.5	2.0
0.05	2.69	2.22	1.74	3.19	2.92	2.61	3.59	3.47	3.34
0.10	4.03	3.66	3.29	4.56	4.35	4.13	5.00	4.91	4.82
0.15	5.11	4.79	4.47	5.69	5.51	5.32	6.18	6.10	6.02
0.20	6.09	5.81	5.53	6.73	6.57	6.40	7.29	7.21	7.14
	$MST = 15$ **yrs**								
		$\beta = 0.7$			$\beta = 0.8$			$\beta = 0.9$	
$p\backslash\Delta$	1.0	1.5	2.0	1.0	1.5	2.0	1.0	1.5	2.0
0.05	4.43	4.02	3.56	5.00	4.77	4.50	5.46	5.36	5.25
0.10	6.35	6.02	5.66	6.99	6.81	6.61	7.54	7.47	7.38
0.15	7.91	7.61	7.30	8.63	8.46	8.29	9.27	9.20	9.12
0.20	9.33	9.06	8.78	10.14	9.99	9.83	10.87	10.81	10.74

[a]MST is the mean sojourn time.
[b]$p\backslash\Delta$: p is the probability in the first column, while Δ is the past screening interval in years in the corresponding row.

exam is no more than 0.20), a woman should return in 0.83 years (or at her age 62.83) if the sensitivity is 0.7, or in 1.36 years (or at her age 63.36) if the sensitivity is 0.9. Table 7.1 also shows that the past screening history (or the number of previous negative screens) plays an important role in future screening: when one's past screening interval is longer, to maintain the same probability of incidence, she should come back more frequently, and vice versa. Thus, for example, in row 3, where MST = 5 years, an individual who had annual (negative) prior screens and who wishes to keep the incidence probability p below 0.1 can return 7.8, 5.5, and 2.5 months later than those who underwent biannual screening when sensitivity changed from 0.7 to 0.9.

TABLE 7.2
Estimated mean, median, mode, standard deviation, and 95% CI of the lead time under the optimal scheduling: $t_0 = 50$, current age $t_{K-1} = 62$, MST = 2 or 5 years.

		$^a MST = 2$ **yrs,** $\beta = 0.7$	
$^b p\backslash\Delta$	1.0	1.5	2.0
0.05	1.69,1.18,0.68,2.10(0,4.75)	1.67,1.13,0.56,2.19(0,4.84)	1.68,1.11,0.47,2.27(0,4.95)
0.10	1.70,1.19,0.72,2.10(0,4.75)	1.70,1.16,0.65,2.17(0,4.84)	1.70,1.15,0.59,2.25(0,4.94)
0.15	1.68,1.17,0.67,2.10(0,4.73)	1.69,1.17,0.66,2.16(0,4.82)	1.71,1.16,0.64,2.22(0,4.92)
0.20	1.65,1.13,0.61,2.11(0,4.72)	1.67,1.14,0.62,2.15(0,4.80)	1.69,1.15,0.62,2.21(0,4.88)
		$^a MST = 2$ **yrs,** $\beta = 0.8$	
$p\backslash\Delta$	1.0	1.5	2.0
0.05	1.73,1.24,0.79,2.06(0,4.75)	1.70,1.19,0.70,2.13(0,4.80)	1.70,1.15,0.61,2.20(0,4.89)
0.10	1.70,1.20,0.73,2.06(0,4.71)	1.72,1.21,0.74,2.10(0,4.78)	1.73,1.20,0.72,2.16(0,4.86)
0.15	1.65,1.14,0.64,2.07(0,4.68)	1.68,1.16,0.66,2.10(0,4.74)	1.69,1.17,0.67,2.14(0,4.80)
0.20	1.63,1.11,0.56,2.09(0,4.68)	1.64,1.12,0.58,2.12(0,4.72)	1.66,1.13,0.59,2.14(0,4.77)
		$^a MST = 2$ **yrs,** $\beta = 0.9$	
$p\backslash\Delta$	1.0	1.5	2.0
0.05	1.74,1.25,0.81,2.03(0,4.71)	1.76,1.27,0.83,2.06(0,4.77)	1.77,1.27,0.83,2.10(0,4.83)
0.10	1.67,1.17,0.68,2.04(0,4.66)	1.68,1.18,0.70,2.06(0,4.69)	1.70,1.19,0.72,2.07(0,4.72)
0.15	1.63,1.12,0.59,2.07(0,4.65)	1.64,1.13,0.60,2.08(0,4.67)	1.65,1.13,0.61,2.09(0,4.69)
0.20	1.61,1.09,0.52,2.09(0,4.67)	1.62,1.09,0.53,2.10(0,4.68)	1.62,1.10,0.53,2.11(0,4.70)
		$^a MST = 5$ **yrs,** $\beta = 0.7$	
$p\backslash\Delta$	1.0	1.5	2.0
0.05	4.28,3.16,2.04,4.39(0,11.77)	4.25,3.11,1.99,4.43(0,11.80)	4.18,3.02,1.85,4.48(0,11.83)
0.10	4.12,2.97,1.79,4.42(0,11.65)	4.16,3.00,1.83,4.44(0,11.72)	4.17,3.00,1.83,4.47(0,11.80)
0.15	4.02,2.85,1.59,4.45(0,11.61)	4.05,2.88,1.63,4.46(0,11.67)	4.08,2.90,1.67,4.48(0,11.75)
0.20	3.97,2.77,1.42,4.48(0,11.63)	3.99,2.79,1.46,4.49(0,11.67)	4.01,2.81,1.49,4.51(0,11.73)
		$^a MST = 5$ **yrs,** $\beta = 0.8$	
$p\backslash\Delta$	1.0	1.5	2.0
0.05	4.24,3.11,1.97,4.39(0,11.70)	4.27,3.14,2.03,4.40(0,11.77)	4.28,3.14,2.03,4.43(0,11.82)
0.10	4.07,2.91,1.70,4.42(0,11.60)	4.10,2.94,1.74,4.42(0,11.65)	4.13,2.97,1.79,4.44(0,11.70)
0.15	3.99,2.80,1.50,4.45(0,11.59)	4.00,2.82,1.53,4.46(0,11.62)	4.02,2.84,1.57,4.47(0,11.66)
0.20	3.94,2.73,1.33,4.49(0,11.63)	3.95,2.74,1.36,4.50(0,11.65)	3.96,2.75,1.38,4.50(0,11.67)
		$^a MST = 5$ **yrs,** $\beta = 0.9$	
$p\backslash\Delta$	1.0	1.5	2.0
0.05	4.19,3.05,1.90,4.38(0,11.65)	4.21,3.07,1.93,4.39(0,11.68)	4.24,3.11,1.98,4.39(0,11.72)
0.10	4.03,2.87,1.63,4.42(0,11.58)	4.05,2.88,1.65,4.42(0,11.59)	4.06,2.90,1.67,4.43(0,11.61)
0.15	3.96,2.77,1.42,4.46(0,11.59)	3.97,2.77,1.44,4.46(0,11.60)	3.97,2.78,1.46,4.47(0,11.61)
0.20	3.92,2.70,1.25,4.51(0,11.65)	3.92,2.70,1.26,4.51(0,11.65)	3.93,2.71,1.28,4.51(0,11.66)

[a]MST is the mean sojourn time.
[b]$p\backslash\Delta$: p is the probability in the first column, while Δ is the past screening interval in years in the corresponding row.

The mean sojourn time (MST) affects the next screening interval in a positive way: longer MST (slow-growing tumor or low-risk people) means she can wait longer to take the next screening exams. Unfortunately, MST is unknown to individuals, so this information is somewhat academic. Finally, a lower probability of incidence translates to shorter screening intervals in the future (consistent with our intuition).

Based on the optimal screening time t^* in Table 7.1, we further evaluated the lead time distribution given that if one would follow this schedule and is diagnosed with cancer at her next exam. The estimated mean, median, mode, standard deviation, and 95% credible interval (C.I.) of each scenario are listed in Tables 7.2 and 7.3. The estimated standard deviation of the lead time

TABLE 7.3
Estimated mean, median, mode, standard deviation, and 95% CI of the lead time under the optimal scheduling: $t_0 = 50$, current age $t_{K-1} = 62$, MST = 10 or 15 years.

	[a]$MST = 10$ **yrs**, $\beta = 0.7$		
[b]$p\backslash\Delta$	1.0	1.5	2.0
0.05	8.10,6.22,3.96,7.32(0,23.38)	8.15,6.27,4.03,7.33(0,23.46)	8.18,6.31,4.08,7.34(0,23.53)
0.10	7.78,5.86,3.45,7.35(0,23.19)	7.82,5.90,3.51,7.36(0,23.24)	7.86,5.94,3.57,7.37(0,23.30)
0.15	7.60,5.64,3.07,7.39(0,23.15)	7.63,5.66,3.12,7.39(0,23.18)	7.66,5.69,3.17,7.40(0,23.22)
0.20	7.49,5.49,2.75,7.43(0,23.20)	7.51,5.51,2.78,7.43(0,23.22)	7.52,5.53,2.82,7.44(0,23.25)
	[a]$MST = 10$ **yrs**, $\beta = 0.8$		
$p\backslash\Delta$	1.0	1.5	2.0
0.05	8.02,6.13,3.84,7.32(0,23.31)	8.05,6.17,3.89,7.33(0,23.35)	8.10,6.21,3.95,7.33(0,23.41)
0.10	7.72,5.78,3.32,7.36(0,23.15)	7.74,5.80,3.36,7.36(0,23.17)	7.76,5.82,3.40,7.37(0,23.20)
0.15	7.55,5.57,2.93,7.40(0,23.15)	7.56,5.58,2.96,7.40(0,23.16)	7.58,5.60,2.99,7.41(0,23.18)
0.20	7.45,5.43,2.60,7.45(0,23.23)	7.45,5.44,2.62,7.45(0,23.24)	7.46,5.45,2.64,7.45(0,23.25)
	[a]$MST = 10$ **yrs**, $\beta = 0.9$		
$p\backslash\Delta$	1.0	1.5	2.0
0.05	7.96,6.06,3.74,7.33(0,23.26)	7.97,6.07,3.76,7.33(0,23.28)	7.99,6.09,3.79,7.33(0,23.30)
0.10	7.66,5.71,3.21,7.37(0,23.13)	7.67,5.72,3.23,7.37(0,23.14)	7.68,5.73,3.24,7.37(0,23.15)
0.15	7.51,5.51,2.81,7.42(0,23.16)	7.51,5.52,2.82,7.42(0,23.16)	7.52,5.52,2.84,7.42(0,23.17)
0.20	7.41,5.38,2.46,7.47(0,23.28)	7.42,5.38,2.47,7.47(0,23.28)	7.42,5.39,2.48,7.47(0,23.28)
	[a]$MST = 15$ **yrs**, $\beta = 0.7$		
$p\backslash\Delta$	1.0	1.5	2.0
0.05	11.42,9.28,5.87,9.44(0,35.02)	11.46,9.33,5.93,9.45(0,35.08)	11.51,9.38,6.01,9.45(0,35.15)
0.10	10.96,8.75,5.12,9.48(0,34.74)	10.99,8.78,5.17,9.48(0,34.78)	11.02,8.82,5.23,9.48(0,34.82)
0.15	10.69,8.42,4.54,9.51(0,34.69)	10.71,8.45,4.59,9.51(0,34.71)	10.73,8.47,4.64,9.51(0,34.74)
0.20	10.51,8.20,4.06,9.55(0,34.76)	10.52,8.21,4.09,9.55(0,34.78)	10.54,8.23,4.13,9.55(0,34.80)
	[a]$MST = 15$ **yrs**, $\beta = 0.8$		
$p\backslash\Delta$	1.0	1.5	2.0
0.05	11.32,9.16,5.72,9.45(0,34.94)	11.34,9.19,5.75,9.45(0,34.97)	11.38,9.23,5.80,9.45(0,35.01)
0.10	10.87,8.64,4.95,9.49(0,34.70)	10.88,8.66,4.97,9.49(0,34.72)	10.90,8.68,5.00,9.49(0,34.74)
0.15	10.61,8.33,4.35,9.52(0,34.70)	10.62,8.34,4.38,9.52(0,34.71)	10.63,8.35,4.40,9.52(0,34.72)
0.20	10.44,8.11,3.83,9.56(0,34.82)	10.45,8.12,3.85,9.57(0,34.82)	10.46,8.13,3.87,9.56(0,34.83)
	[a]$MST = 15$ **yrs**, $\beta = 0.9$		
$p\backslash\Delta$	1.0	1.5	2.0
0.05	11.24,9.07,5.59,9.45(0,34.88)	11.25,9.08,5.61,9.45(0,34.89)	11.26,9.10,5.63,9.45(0,34.90)
0.10	10.80,8.55,4.79,9.49(0,34.68)	10.80,8.56,4.80,9.50(0,34.69)	10.81,8.57,4.82,9.50(0,34.69)
0.15	10.55,8.25,4.18,9.54(0,34.72)	10.55,8.25,4.18,9.54(0,34.72)	10.56,8.26,4.19,9.54(0,34.73)
0.20	10.39,8.04,3.63,9.58(0,34.89)	10.39,8.04,3.64,9.58(0,34.89)	10.39,8.05,3.65,9.58(0,34.89)

[a]MST is the mean sojourn time.
[b]$p\backslash\Delta$: p is the probability in the first column, while Δ is the past screening interval in years in the corresponding row.

is always larger than the corresponding mean value, and the density curves are all skewed to the right, so the median and the mode are more reliable estimations of the lead time than the mean value. It shows that a smaller probability of incidence p may not guarantee a larger mode (the highest value of the PDF curve), and the same with the median. The 95% CI is almost the same for different p under the same mean sojourn time.

Figure 7.3 illustrates how the density of the lead time are changing under different scenarios. There are four factors in our simulation: sensitivity β, mean sojourn time (MST), historic screening interval Δ, and probability of incidence p. In the four plots in Figure 7.3, we fix three factors and allow only one factor change. For example, the plot in the upper left corner shows how

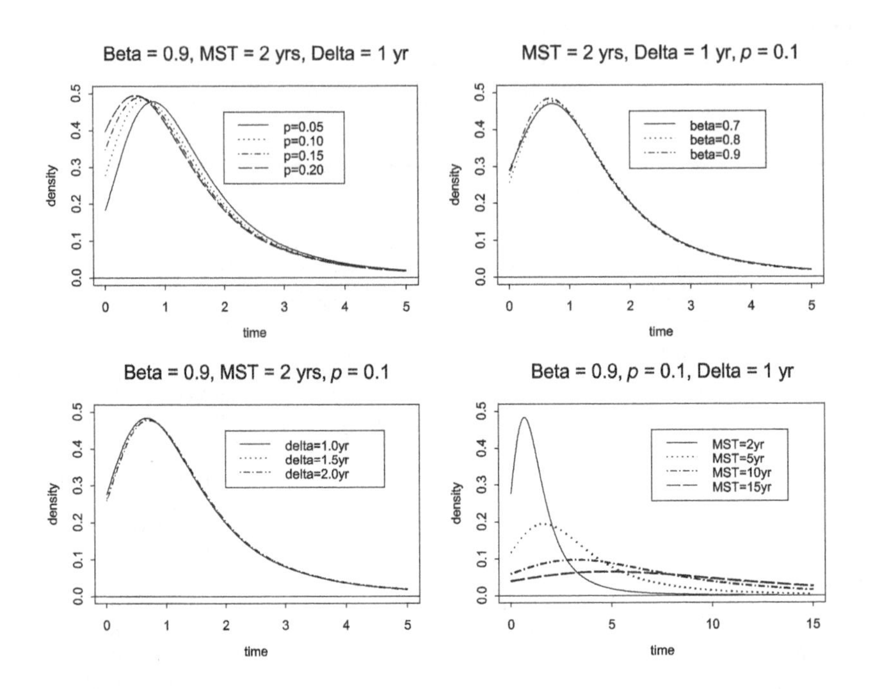

FIGURE 7.3
PDF of the lead time under the four factors: p, β, Δ, and MST.

the PDF of the lead time changes with p when $\beta = 0.9$, MST $= 2$ years, and historic screening interval $\Delta = 1$ year. It shows that the density curve of the lead time changes more with different p and mean sojourn time, and changes less with the sensitivity and historic screening interval Δ if the patient will follow the dynamic scheduling.

We then evaluate the probability of overdiagnosis if the scheduling time was used. The results were summarized in Table 7.4. It seems that the probability of overdiagnosis will slightly increase as the sensitivity increases when other factors are fixed. However, higher sensitivity usually means the future screening time interval will be larger in Table 7.1; hence, the person's age is older, and older age usually causes a larger probability of overdiagnosis. It also showed that for different probabilities of incidence p changing from 0.05 to 0.2, the probability of overdiagnosis won't change very much when the MST is 2 years. In order to investigate how the probability of overdiagnosis would be changing with the future scheduling time, the percentage of overdiagnosis versus the future scheduling time is plotted in Figure 7.4. Four different colors black, red, green, and blue were used to illustrate the corresponding curves under different mean sojourn times of 2, 5, 10, and 15 years. For each mean sojourn time of 2, 5, 10, and 15 years, the percentage of overdiagnosis was

TABLE 7.4
Estimated probability of overdiagnosis (in percentage) under the optimal scheduling when $t_0 = 50$, and current age $t_{K-1} = 62$.

				[a]$MST = 2$ **yrs**					
		$\beta = 0.7$			$\beta = 0.8$			$\beta = 0.9$	
[b]$p\backslash\Delta$	1.0	1.5	2.0	1.0	1.5	2.0	1.0	1.5	2.0
0.05	1.55	1.55	1.57	1.58	1.57	1.57	1.62	1.62	1.63
0.10	1.58	1.58	1.60	1.60	1.60	1.62	1.61	1.61	1.62
0.15	1.59	1.60	1.62	1.61	1.61	1.63	1.62	1.62	1.63
0.20	1.59	1.62	1.64	1.62	1.63	1.64	1.64	1.64	1.64
				$MST = 5$ **yrs**					
		$\beta = 0.7$			$\beta = 0.8$			$\beta = 0.9$	
$p\backslash\Delta$	1.0	1.5	2.0	1.0	1.5	2.0	1.0	1.5	2.0
0.05	5.17	5.01	4.90	5.29	5.21	5.11	5.38	5.34	5.31
0.10	5.31	5.21	5.13	5.43	5.37	5.31	5.53	5.50	5.48
0.15	5.46	5.38	5.31	5.60	5.54	5.49	5.73	5.71	5.68
0.20	5.63	5.55	5.49	5.80	5.75	5.70	5.96	5.93	5.91
				$MST = 10$ **yrs**					
		$\beta = 0.7$			$\beta = 0.8$			$\beta = 0.9$	
$p\backslash\Delta$	1.0	1.5	2.0	1.0	1.5	2.0	1.0	1.5	2.0
0.05	14.27	13.91	13.54	14.61	14.41	14.19	14.88	14.79	14.70
0.10	15.03	14.72	14.44	15.43	15.26	15.08	15.80	15.71	15.63
0.15	15.80	15.52	15.25	16.31	16.14	15.97	16.76	16.69	16.62
0.20	16.64	16.37	16.11	17.27	17.10	16.94	17.86	17.77	17.70
				$MST = 15$ **yrs**					
		$\beta = 0.7$			$\beta = 0.8$			$\beta = 0.9$	
$p\backslash\Delta$	1.0	1.5	2.0	1.0	1.5	2.0	1.0	1.5	2.0
0.05	25.90	25.41	24.86	26.51	26.22	25.90	27.00	26.87	26.74
0.10	27.67	27.24	26.77	28.45	28.19	27.92	29.12	29.02	28.90
0.15	29.45	29.01	28.57	30.42	30.16	29.90	31.32	31.21	31.09
0.20	31.31	30.90	30.47	32.53	32.29	32.03	33.67	33.56	33.44

evaluated for four scenarios: sensitivity β is 0.7 or 0.9, and historic screening interval Δ is 1 or 2 years. It is clear that the mean sojourn time plays the most important role in the estimation of overdiagnosis. And given someone would be diagnosed with cancer at the future scheduled time, the probability of overdiagnosis is not changing much with sensitivity or historic screening interval. The estimation was done for the case of initial screening age at $t_0 = 50$, and current age at $t_{K-1} = 62$. However, if we increase the current age to 84, the probability of overdiagnosis will increase quite a bit, showing that one's current age dramatically affects the probability of overdiagnosis beside the mean sojourn time.

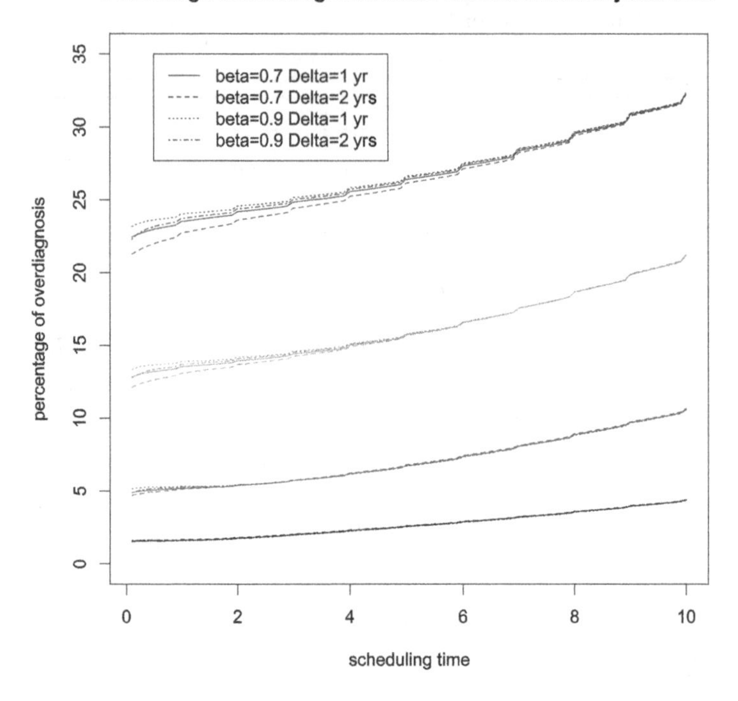

FIGURE 7.4
Percentage of overdiagnosis using different scheduling time t^* and under different mean sojourn time.

7.2.6 Application: Breast cancer using the HIP study

We applied the method to the Health Insurance Plan (HIP) of the Greater New York breast cancer screening data (Shapiro et al 1988 [47]). The conditional probability is a function of the next screening time interval, the three key parameters, a person's current age a_0, and her screening history. For the three key parameters, Wu, Rosner, and Broemeling (2005) estimated them for the HIP data using parametric models as follows [79]:

$$\begin{aligned}
\beta(t) &= \{1+\exp[-b_0-b_1(t-m)]\}^{-1}, \\
w(t) &= \frac{0.2}{\sqrt{2\pi}\sigma t}\exp\left\{-(\log t-\mu)^2/(2\sigma^2)\right\}, \\
Q(x) &= [1+(x\rho)^\kappa]^{-1}, \quad \kappa>0,\, \rho>0,
\end{aligned}$$

where $m = 51.6$ is the average age of women at the time of their entry into the HIP study. The unknown parameters in this model are $\theta = (b_0, b_1, \mu, \sigma^2, \kappa, \rho)$. The 0.2 in the model for $w(t)$ is the upper limit when making a transition from

TABLE 7.5
Optimal time interval (and s.e.) in years using the HIP data.

	$t_0 = 50, t_{K-1} = 62$			$t_0 = 60, t_{K-1} = 72$		
p	$\Delta = 1.0$	$\Delta = 2.0$	$\Delta = 3.0$	$\Delta = 1.0$	$\Delta = 2.0$	$\Delta = 3.0$
0.05	0.30 (0.19)	0.23 (0.15)	0.22 (0.15)	0.42 (0.40)	0.32 (0.25)	0.30 (0.20)
0.10	0.56 (0.31)	0.45 (0.19)	0.43 (0.19)	0.68 (0.55)	0.59 (0.40)	0.55 (0.31)
0.15	0.78 (0.42)	0.67 (0.24)	0.64 (0.21)	0.91 (0.67)	0.82 (0.53)	0.78 (0.43)
0.20	0.99 (0.52)	0.88 (0.32)	0.85 (0.25)	1.11 (0.79)	1.04 (0.65)	1.00 (0.55)

the disease-free state to the preclinical state. Using Markov Chain Monte Carlo (MCMC), 2000 Bayesian posterior samples (θ_j^*) were obtained [79].

We conducted the Bayesian inference in this way: Given a fixed $p \in (0, 1)$, for each posterior sample $\theta_j^*, j = 1, 2, \ldots, 2000$, using

$$P(I_K | I_K \cup D_K, \theta_j^*) = p,$$

we can find a solution of $t_j^*, j = 1, 2, \ldots, 2000$.

We used two hypothetical cohorts of asymptomatic women with $(t_0, t_{K-1}) = (50, 62)$ or (60, 72), the current age $a_0 = t_{K-1}$, with different past screening intervals $\Delta = 1, 2$, and 3 years, which is corresponding to 13, 7, and 5 equally spaced exams in the past. Using $p = 0.05$, 0.1, 0.15, and 0.2 as the incidence probability, the posterior mean of the t_j^* and its standard deviation (in years) based on the 2000 posterior samples are summarized in Table 7.5. It seems that the next screening interval is increasing with a person's current age if other parameters are the same, and it is increasing with the incidence probability p. The next screening interval is changing with the past screening interval Δ: smaller Δ means that they can come back at a later time, while a larger Δ in the past means that they should come back earlier.

We further investigate how the lead time and the probability of overdiagnosis would change in different scenarios for the above cohorts. Using each pair of the 2000 posterior samples θ_j^* and its corresponding t_j^*, one posterior lead time distribution can be obtained:

$$f_L^{HIP}(l) \approx \frac{1}{n} \sum_{i=1}^{n} f_L^{HIP}(l | \theta_j^*, t_j^*),$$

from which we calculate the mean, median, mode, and standard deviation of the lead time using $f_L^{HIP}(l)$. Similarly, the probability of overdiagnosis was calculated using each of the 2000 posterior samples θ_j^* and the corresponding t_j^*. Table 7.6 summarizes the mean, median, mode, and standard deviation of the lead time; Table 7.7 summarizes the mean and percentile of the probability of overdiagnosis based on the 2000 cases. Recall that the probability of true-early-detection equals one minus the probability of overdiagnosis, so they share the same standard deviation.

TABLE 7.6
Estimated mean, median, mode with the standard deviation of the lead time at the optimal scheduling time t^* using the HIP data (in years).

p	$\Delta = 1.0$	$\Delta = 2.0$	$\Delta = 3.0$
		$t_0 = 50, t_{K-1} = 62$	
0.05	1.84,0.97,0.49(3.42)	1.88,0.95,0.47(3.61)	1.92,0.95,0.46(3.77)
0.10	1.80,0.92,0.42(3.42)	1.85,0.93,0.41(3.58)	1.89,0.93,0.41(3.72)
0.15	1.78,0.89,0.35(3.43)	1.83,0.90,0.35(3.58)	1.87,0.91,0.35(3.70)
0.20	1.77,0.87,0.30(3.46)	1.82,0.88,0.30(3.59)	1.85,0.89,0.30(3.70)
		$t_0 = 60, t_{K-1} = 72$	
0.05	1.83,0.96,0.48(3.38)	1.87,0.96,0.47(3.53)	1.90,0.96,0.46(3.67)
0.10	1.78,0.91,0.40(3.39)	1.83,0.92,0.40(3.52)	1.86,0.93,0.40(3.63)
0.15	1.77,0.88,0.34(3.41)	1.81,0.89,0.34(3.52)	1.84,0.90,0.34(3.62)
0.20	1.76,0.86,0.28(3.44)	1.79,0.87,0.29(3.54)	1.82,0.88,0.29(3.63)

From Table 7.6, we can see that the lead time distribution changes slightly with p and one's current age if the other elements are the same: when p increases, the mean, median, and mode of lead time decrease; and when age increases, the mean, median, and mode of lead time decrease. That is, the central location (i.e., mean, median, mode) of the lead time seems to be negatively correlated with the p and one's current age. Also, the mean, median, and mode of lead time increase as the past screening interval Δ increase (positively correlated). However, the changes are small in general using the HIP data; the standard deviation of the lead time is almost double its mean, show-

TABLE 7.7
Estimated mean probability of overdiagnosis with 95% CI (in percentage) under the optimal scheduling using HIP data.

p	$\Delta = 1.0$	$\Delta = 2.0$	$\Delta = 3.0$
		$t_0 = 50, t_{K-1} = 62$	
0.05	2.25(0.57,10.97)	2.38(0.56,12.47)	2.52(0.56,13.80)
0.10	2.26(0.53,11.35)	2.37(0.54,12.61)	2.49(0.54,13.65)
0.15	2.29(0.52,11.37)	2.39(0.52,12.84)	2.50(0.52,13.67)
0.20	2.34(0.51,11.54)	2.43(0.51,12.91)	2.52(0.51,13.80)
		$t_0 = 60, t_{K-1} = 72$	
0.05	4.65(1.40,19.98)	4.76(1.40,20.48)	4.89(1.40,21.45)
0.10	4.68(1.33,20.37)	4.78(1.33,21.39)	4.89(1.33,21.42)
0.15	4.76(1.30,20.76)	4.84(1.31,21.86)	4.94(1.31,21.73)
0.20	4.87(1.30,21.49)	4.93(1.30,22.07)	5.02(1.31,22.57)

ing heavy tails (i.e., skew to the right) of the lead time density curve. The average probability of overdiagnosis is 2.25–2.52% for the 62 years old group, and increases to 4.65–5.02% for the 72 years old group; the corresponding 95% C.I. increases also from Table 7.7. The risk of overdiagnosis is widely recognized to be low in the HIP study, although our model does predict slight increases with one's current age and the past screening interval Δ.

The HIP data suggested that women should have returned at 11.9 months to maintain an 80% early detection probability when the past screening interval was 12 months (as it was in HIP for those that chose to be screened). For a 90% probability of early detection, she would have reduced her screening interval to 6.7 months (possibly because the test sensitivity may have been lower for HIP than it is today). If the optimal time t^* were adopted and one were diagnosed with cancer at that time, the lead time follows similar distribution as shown in Figure 7.3, with the mean lead time slightly changing between 1.76 and 1.92 years, the median lead time changes between 0.86 and 0.97 years, and the mode of lead time (the highest point on the density curve) is between 0.28 and 0.49 years. The probability of overdiagnosis among the screen-detected is comparatively small: with an average of 2.25–2.52%, and a 95% C.I. of (0.51%, 13.80%) for the 62-year-old; and an average of 4.65-5.02%, and a 95% C.I. of (1.30%, 22.57%) for the 72 years old.

7.2.7 Application: Lung cancer using the NLST-CT data

We now apply the scheduling method to the NLST low-dose CT data for male and female heavy smokers. After we found the scheduling time $(a_0 + t^*)$, we will use it to estimate the lead time and probability of overdiagnosis and true-early-detection.

From the two cohorts (male and female heavy smokers) in the NLST CT data, we first estimated the three key parameters: sensitivity $\beta(t)$, PDF of sojourn time $q(x)$, and transition density $w(t)$. These three key parameters are critical since the probability of incidence in equation (1) is a function of these three key parameters. We used a likelihood function and parametric modeling to estimate these three from the NLST CT arm data (Liu et al 2015 [32]), where

$$\begin{aligned}
\beta(t|b_0, b_1) &= \frac{1}{1+\exp(-b_0 - b_1 * (t-m))}, \\
w(t|\mu, \sigma^2) &= \frac{0.3}{\sqrt{2\pi}\sigma t} \exp\left\{-(\log t - \mu)^2/(2\sigma^2)\right\}, \\
Q(x|\lambda, \alpha) &= \exp(-\lambda x^{\alpha}), x > 0, \lambda > 0, \alpha > 0.
\end{aligned}$$

The unknown parameters in the likelihood are $\theta = (b_0, b_1, \mu, \sigma^2, \lambda, \alpha)$. Using Markov Chain Monte Carlo (MCMC) with Gibbs sampler, 130,000 samples were generated; after 30,000 burn-in and thinning every 200 iterations, we obtained a sample of 500 from each chain. Running two initially over-dispersed chains provide 1000 Bayesian posterior samples (θ_j^*) for each gender. For more details, see Liu et al 2015 [32].

We designed hypothetical cohorts in our simulation: For each gender, we have three big cohorts according to the initial screening age t_0 and current age t_{K-1}: $(t_0, t_{K-1}) = (56, 62), (62, 68)$, and $(68, 74)$. Then within each age cohort, we split it into three smaller groups, by assuming that the historical screening time interval Δ from t_0 to t_{K-1} was 1, 2, or 3 years. So, there were 9 cohorts for each gender in the simulation. Then we used the 1000 posterior samples $\theta_j^*, j = 1, 2, \ldots, 1000$ from the MCMC for each gender to make Bayesian inference on optimal scheduling.

For each θ_j^*, using $P(I_K|I_K \cup D_K, \theta_j^*) = p$, a scheduling time $t_j^*(j = 1, 2, \ldots, 1000)$ can be found; We calculated the mean and 95% credible interval (C.I.) of the future screening time interval t_j^* (in years) and summarized the results in Table 7.8. To find the future screening age using Table 7.8, for example, we can look at the big column "Female" and "$t_0 = 56, a_0 = t_{K-1} = 62$", then look at the row when $p = 0.10$. It shows that if $\Delta = 1.0$ years (i.e., one had annual exam from 56 to 62 years old, inclusive), then she should come back at age 63.25 (or after 1.25 years), with a 95% C.I. between 62.96 and 63.59 years, if she wants to have a probability of 90% early detection. Table 7.8 shows that the future scheduling age $t_K^* = a_0 + t^*$ increases as the incidence risk p increases. i.e., heavy smokers can come back at a later time if they want to maintain an 80% early detection rather than a 90% early detection. The mean of t^* slightly decreases as the current age increases; i.e., older smokers should take the next exam earlier than their younger counterparts when other conditions are the same. Under the same conditions, male heavy smokers should take the next exam earlier than their female counterparts. Historic screening interval and the future screening time are negatively correlated: shorter screening interval in the past means larger t^* for the upcoming test, and vice versa. Table 7.9 summarized the simulation results when $a_0 = t_{K-1} + 1$. It shows that one year after the last screening, the historic screening interval Δ almost has no effect on the future screening interval t^*, and in this situation, one's current age seems to have little effect on t^* also. Only the probability of incidence p can affect the future screening time interval t^*. We then estimated the lead time and risk of overdiagnosis if one would be diagnosed with cancer at the future time point $t_K^* = a_0 + t^*$. One lead time density curve can be obtained by using each pair of (θ_j^*, t_j^*), with $j = 1, 2, \ldots, 1000$, and the posterior distribution of the lead time is the average:

$$f_L(x|NLST) = \frac{1}{1000} \sum_{j=1}^{1000} f_L(x|\theta_j^*, t_j^*).$$

We then calculate the mean, median, mode, and standard deviation of the lead time using the $f_L(x|NLST)$. We plot four panels in Figure 7.5 to show the changes in the lead time. In each panel, we only allow one factor to change while the other factors are kept the same. The lead time curves when p changes

TABLE 7.8
Posterior mean scheduling age ($a_0 + t^*$) and the 95% CI when $a_0 = t_{K-1}$.

$t_0 = 56, a_0 = t_{K-1} = 62$

	Female			Male		
$p\backslash\Delta$	1.0	2.0	3.0	1.0	2.0	3.0
0.05	62.89(62.63, 63.14)	62.71(62.21, 63.04)	62.65(62.17, 63.03)	62.64(62.43, 62.85)	62.44(62.11, 62.73)	62.41(62.10, 62.73)
0.10	63.25(62.96, 63.49)	63.16(62.89, 63.47)	63.14(62.82, 63.45)	62.98(62.79, 63.17)	62.87(62.56, 63.11)	62.85(62.49, 63.11)
0.15	63.51(63.25, 63.83)	63.45(63.18, 63.74)	63.44(63.15, 63.71)	63.23(63.05, 63.44)	63.16(62.95, 63.37)	63.15(62.92, 63.37)
0.20	63.74(63.42, 64.09)	63.69(63.40, 64.04)	63.69(63.41, 64.04)	63.45(63.24, 63.67)	63.40(63.21, 63.61)	63.39(63.21, 63.61)

$t_0 = 62, a_0 = t_{K-1} = 68$

	Female			Male		
$p\backslash\Delta$	1.0	2.0	3.0	1.0	2.0	3.0
0.05	68.90(68.64, 69.10)	68.71(68.28, 69.07)	68.65(68.14, 68.97)	68.62(68.39, 68.84)	68.41(68.10, 68.71)	68.38(68.09, 68.71)
0.10	69.24(68.99, 69.49)	69.16(68.91, 69.44)	69.13(68.84, 69.41)	68.96(68.76, 69.17)	68.84(68.47, 69.09)	68.81(68.40, 69.10)
0.15	69.50(69.22, 69.79)	69.44(69.18, 69.71)	69.43(69.16, 69.68)	69.21(69.02, 69.42)	69.13(68.87, 69.36)	69.11(68.83, 69.35)
0.20	69.72(69.39, 70.04)	69.68(69.37, 69.99)	69.67(69.37, 69.97)	69.42(69.21, 69.66)	69.36(69.16, 69.61)	69.35(69.10, 69.56)

$t_0 = 68, a_0 = t_{K-1} = 74$

	Female			Male		
$p\backslash\Delta$	1.0	2.0	3.0	1.0	2.0	3.0
0.05	74.89(74.64, 75.14)	74.69(74.19, 75.04)	74.64(74.13, 75.01)	74.59(74.23, 74.88)	74.40(74.07, 74.74)	74.36(74.06, 74.73)
0.10	75.23(74.99, 75.51)	75.14(74.80, 75.45)	75.11(74.71, 75.45)	74.93(74.60, 75.23)	74.79(74.23, 75.11)	74.76(74.20, 75.08)
0.15	75.48(75.19, 75.77)	75.42(75.14, 75.72)	75.41(75.09, 75.71)	75.17(74.89, 75.48)	75.07(74.55, 75.40)	75.05(74.47, 75.39)
0.20	75.70(75.39, 76.06)	75.66(75.31, 75.97)	75.65(75.34, 75.99)	75.38(75.09, 75.68)	75.31(74.90, 75.66)	75.29(74.85, 75.66)

TABLE 7.9
Posterior mean scheduling age $(a_0 + t^*)$ and the 95% CI when $a_0 = t_{K-1} + 1$.

$t_0 = 56, a_0 = t_{K-1} + 1 = 63$

	Female			Male		
$p\backslash\Delta$	1.0	2.0	3.0	1.0	2.0	3.0
0.05	63.24(63.15, 63.35)	63.23(63.15, 63.33)	63.23(63.15, 63.33)	63.16(63.12, 63.22)	63.16(63.11, 63.21)	63.16(63.11, 63.21)
0.10	63.46(63.29, 63.66)	63.45(63.30, 63.64)	63.45(63.30, 63.64)	63.32(63.23, 63.43)	63.32(63.22, 63.41)	63.32(63.23, 63.42)
0.15	63.66(63.42, 63.92)	63.65(63.42, 63.89)	63.65(63.42, 63.89)	63.48(63.34, 63.64)	63.48(63.34, 63.63)	63.48(63.34, 63.63)
0.20	63.86(63.55, 64.19)	63.85(63.56, 64.18)	63.85(63.56, 64.18)	63.65(63.45, 63.87)	63.64(63.45, 63.85)	63.64(63.45, 63.84)

$t_0 = 62, a_0 = t_{K-1} + 1 = 69$

	Female			Male		
$p\backslash\Delta$	1.0	2.0	3.0	1.0	2.0	3.0
0.05	69.24(69.14, 69.34)	69.23(69.14, 69.32)	69.23(69.15, 69.32)	69.16(69.11, 69.21)	69.15(69.11, 69.20)	69.15(69.11, 69.20)
0.10	69.45(69.27, 69.63)	69.44(69.28, 69.61)	69.44(69.28, 69.61)	69.31(69.22, 69.43)	69.31(69.22, 69.41)	69.31(69.22, 69.41)
0.15	69.65(69.41, 69.90)	69.64(69.40, 69.87)	69.64(69.40, 69.87)	69.47(69.32, 69.63)	69.46(69.32, 69.61)	69.46(69.33, 69.62)
0.20	69.84(69.53, 70.15)	69.83(69.55, 70.16)	69.83(69.53, 70.13)	69.63(69.44, 69.85)	69.62(69.43, 69.81)	69.62(69.42, 69.81)

$t_0 = 68, a_0 = t_{K-1} + 1 = 75$

	Female			Male		
$p\backslash\Delta$	1.0	2.0	3.0	1.0	2.0	3.0
0.05	75.23(75.14, 75.34)	75.23(75.14, 75.32)	75.23(75.14, 75.32)	75.15(75.10, 75.21)	75.15(75.10, 75.21)	75.15(75.10, 75.20)
0.10	75.44(75.27, 75.62)	75.44(75.27, 75.60)	75.43(75.27, 75.60)	75.30(75.21, 75.43)	75.30(75.20, 75.41)	75.30(75.20, 75.40)
0.15	75.64(75.39, 75.87)	75.63(75.40, 75.86)	75.63(75.40, 75.85)	75.45(75.31, 75.62)	75.45(75.30, 75.61)	75.45(75.32, 75.62)
0.20	75.82(75.52, 76.13)	75.81(75.52, 76.10)	75.81(75.52, 76.10)	75.61(75.42, 75.84)	75.60(75.41, 75.81)	75.60(75.41, 75.81)

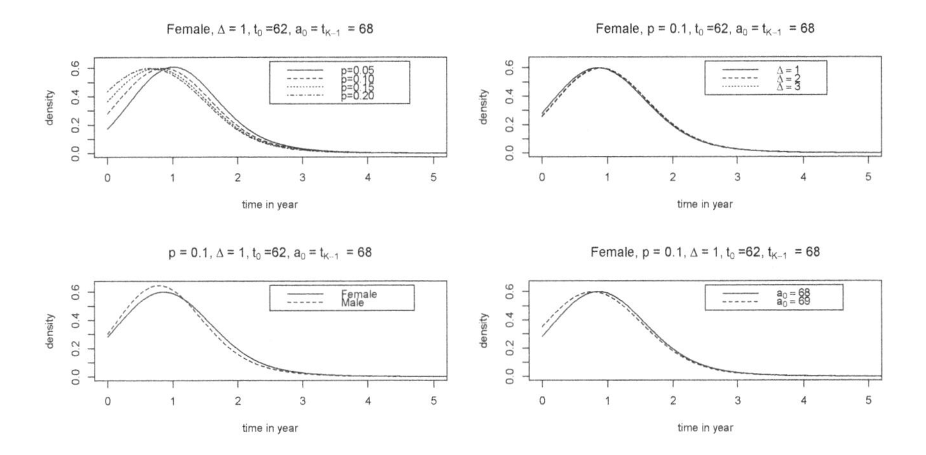

FIGURE 7.5
Lead time density curve when $t_0 = 62$ and $a_0 = t_{K-1} = 68$.

from 0.05 to 0.20 is plotted in the upper left panel: the central location (mean, median, and mode) of the lead time is getting smaller as p increases from 0.05 to 0.20. The upper right panel shows that lead time does not change much as the past screening interval changes from 1 to 3 years. The lower left panel compares the male and female lead time curves under similar conditions: the males seem to have a slightly higher density at the mode than their female counterparts, and the mode of the lead time of male heavy smokers is slightly smaller. The lower right panel compares the lead time differences between $a_0 = t_{K-1}$ and $a_0 = t_{K-1} + 1$. In summary, the incidence probability p has more influence on the lead time distribution than other factors. The distribution of lead time changes slightly with gender: male heavy smokers usually have a relatively shorter central location (mean, median, and mode) of the lead time than their female counterpart at the future screening age $(a_0 + t^*)$. The three age groups (t_0, t_{K-1}) = (56, 62), (62, 68), and (68,74) have almost the same lead time distribution when $a_0 = t_{K-1}$; and the three age groups have almost the same lead time distribution when $a_0 = t_{K-1}+1$, but with a smaller central location compared with that of $a_0 = t_{K-1}$.

Finally, we used each pair (θ_j^*, t_j^*), $j = 1, 2, \ldots, 1000$, to estimate the probability of overdiagnosis at the future screening age. And the probability of true early detection is 1 minus the probability of overdiagnosis. The posterior mean (in percentage) and the standard error are listed in Tables 7.10 and 7.11. The probability of overdiagnosis is very low in the NLST-CT study ($< 4\%$). This probability slightly increases with one's current age for both genders. And it is slightly higher for male heavy smokers than their female counterparts. It slightly decreases when p increases. The maximum probability of overdiagnosis is less than 3.1% for females and less than 3.9% for males in the simulation.

TABLE 7.10
Estimated mean probability of overdiagnosis and s.e. (in percentage) at a_0+t^* when $a_0 = t_{K-1}$.

			$t_0 = 56, a_0 = t_{K-1} = 62$			
		Female			Male	
$p\backslash\Delta$	1.0	2.0	3.0	1.0	2.0	3.0
0.05	1.03(0.20)	1.05(0.20)	1.05(0.20)	1.55(0.28)	1.57(0.26)	1.56(0.25)
0.10	0.97(0.20)	0.98(0.20)	0.98(0.20)	1.45(0.29)	1.47(0.28)	1.47(0.28)
0.15	0.93(0.20)	0.94(0.20)	0.94(0.20)	1.40(0.28)	1.41(0.29)	1.42(0.29)
0.20	0.91(0.20)	0.92(0.20)	0.92(0.20)	1.36(0.28)	1.37(0.28)	1.37(0.28)
			$t_0 = 62, a_0 = t_{K-1} = 68$			
		Female			Male	
$p\backslash\Delta$	1.0	2.0	3.0	1.0	2.0	3.0
0.05	1.68(0.34)	1.71(0.33)	1.71(0.33)	2.31(0.42)	2.32(0.39)	2.30(0.38)
0.10	1.59(0.34)	1.61(0.34)	1.61(0.34)	2.17(0.43)	2.19(0.42)	2.20(0.42)
0.15	1.53(0.34)	1.54(0.34)	1.54(0.34)	2.10(0.43)	2.12(0.43)	2.12(0.43)
0.20	1.51(0.34)	1.51(0.34)	1.51(0.34)	2.04(0.43)	2.05(0.43)	2.05(0.43)
			$t_0 = 68, a_0 = t_{K-1} = 74$			
		Female			Male	
$p\backslash\Delta$	1.0	2.0	3.0	1.0	2.0	3.0
0.05	2.98(0.61)	3.03(0.58)	3.02(0.57)	3.81(0.70)	3.77(0.68)	3.74(0.66)
0.10	2.84(0.61)	2.87(0.61)	2.88(0.61)	3.62(0.72)	3.64(0.69)	3.64(0.68)
0.15	2.74(0.61)	2.76(0.60)	2.76(0.61)	3.53(0.73)	3.55(0.71)	3.56(0.71)
0.20	2.69(0.61)	2.70(0.61)	2.70(0.61)	3.43(0.72)	3.46(0.72)	3.46(0.72)

In summary, overdiagnosis is not a big issue using low-dose CT in lung cancer screening.

We have applied the same method to lung cancer screening using low-dose CT for both males and females heavy smokers. In fact, the method can be applied to any kind of screening for chronic disease, and it can handle any screening history $t_0 < t_1 < ...t_{K-1}$, including those not equally-spaced screening intervals. Theoretically (and verified by simulations) the incidence risk increases as scheduling time for the next exam increases. That is, for those who can tolerate higher incidence risk or consider themselves low risk for specific cancer, they can come back for the next exam at a later date. The scheduling time decreases as one's current age increases if other conditions are the same, which means older smokers should come back earlier than younger ones if other conditions are the same. And male heavy smokers should take their next exam earlier than their female counterparts. The simulation also shows that screening history, especially the length of past screening intervals affects the timing of the next exam. A shorter screening interval in the past means one can come back later for the upcoming test. Robbins et al 2019 analyzed participants who had negative CT results in the NLST study, and using their newly developed Lung Cancer Risk Assessment Tool + CT,

TABLE 7.11
Estimated mean probability of overdiagnosis and s.e. (in percentage) at a_0+t^* when $a_0 = t_{K-1} + 1$.

$t_0 = 56, a_0 = t_{K-1} + 1 = 63$						
	Female			Male		
$p\backslash\Delta$	1.0	2.0	3.0	1.0	2.0	3.0
0.05	0.97(0.20)	0.97(0.20)	0.97(0.20)	1.42(0.29)	1.42(0.28)	1.42(0.28)
0.10	0.94(0.20)	0.94(0.20)	0.94(0.20)	1.38(0.28)	1.38(0.28)	1.38(0.28)
0.15	0.92(0.20)	0.92(0.20)	0.92(0.20)	1.36(0.28)	1.36(0.28)	1.36(0.28)
0.20	0.91(0.20)	0.91(0.20)	0.91(0.20)	1.34(0.28)	1.34(0.28)	1.34(0.28)
$t_0 = 62, a_0 = t_{K-1} + 1 = 69$						
	Female			Male		
$p\backslash\Delta$	1.0	2.0	3.0	1.0	2.0	3.0
0.05	1.59(0.34)	1.59(0.34)	1.59(0.34)	2.12(0.43)	2.12(0.43)	2.12(0.43)
0.10	1.54(0.34)	1.54(0.34)	1.54(0.34)	2.07(0.43)	2.06(0.43)	2.06(0.43)
0.15	1.51(0.34)	1.51(0.34)	1.51(0.34)	2.03(0.43)	2.03(0.43)	2.03(0.43)
0.20	1.50(0.35)	1.50(0.35)	1.50(0.35)	2.00(0.43)	2.00(0.43)	2.00(0.43)
$t_0 = 68, a_0 = t_{K-1} + 1 = 75$						
	Female			Male		
$p\backslash\Delta$	1.0	2.0	3.0	1.0	2.0	3.0
0.05	2.84(0.61)	2.84(0.61)	2.84(0.61)	3.56(0.73)	3.55(0.73)	3.55(0.72)
0.10	2.75(0.61)	2.75(0.61)	2.75(0.61)	3.47(0.73)	3.47(0.72)	3.47(0.72)
0.15	2.70(0.61)	2.70(0.61)	2.70(0.61)	3.40(0.72)	3.40(0.72)	3.40(0.72)
0.20	2.68(0.63)	2.68(0.62)	2.68(0.62)	3.36(0.72)	3.36(0.72)	3.36(0.72)

they predicted short-term lung cancer risk following a negative CT screen. Their results support the idea "that many, but not all, screen-negatives might reasonably lengthen their CT screening interval". Our result seems to be compatible with their findings.

7.3 Scheduling upcoming exam when sensitivity is a function of sojourn time

This is an extension of our previous model for dynamic scheduling of future screening exams based on an asymptomatic individual's current age and screening history. The main improvement is to model the screening sensitivity as a function of the ratio of time spent in the preclinical state and sojourn time. This is based on the reality that screening sensitivity is low when one's cancer just enters the preclinical state, and it would be close to one at the end of the preclinical state. Therefore, sensitivity is a function of the time one has stayed in the preclinical state; relative to the sojourn time. This improvement in the model assumption causes dramatic changes in all probability formulas, and we will use simulations and applications to show this.

7.3.1 Probability of incidence and future screening time

We will use the conditional probability of incidence as before: Given that a woman has been asymptomatic throughout her previous screening exams, we derive the conditional probability of incidence before her next screening exam, which is a function of the time length from now to the next exam, so we can choose a future time interval such that this probability is less than some preselected small values, such as 0.10 or 0.05. In other words, with a probability of 0.90 or 0.95, the case is not likely to become a clinically incident case before her next scheduled exam.

The commonly used disease progressive model is assumed where the disease develops through three states $S_0 \to S_p \to S_c$ [87]. S_0 refers to the disease-free state or the state in which the disease cannot be detected; S_p refers to the preclinical disease state, in which an asymptomatic individual unknowingly has a disease that a screening exam can detect; and S_c refers to the disease state at which the disease manifests itself in clinical symptoms.

We let $\beta(s|Y)$ be the screening sensitivity, where s is the length of time that one has been in the preclinical state S_p, and Y represents the sojourn time in the S_p, a random variable. The sensitivity β will increase as s increases, and it will decrease as Y increases. We let $w(t)$ be the probability density function (PDF) of the time duration in the disease-free state S_0 (a sub-PDF, or a mixture of a point mass at infinity and a continuous PDF, since most people may remain in the S_0 during their lifetime). We let $q(x)$ be the probability density function of the sojourn time in the S_p, and let $Q(z) = \int_z^\infty q(x)dx$ be the survival function of the sojourn time in the preclinical state S_p.

Assume a woman has taken $K(\geq 1)$ screenings at her ages $t_0 < t_1 < \cdots < t_{K-1}$, and she is asymptomatic at her current age $a_0(\geq t_{K-1})$. Let t_x represent the time of her next screening time interval. We let $t_{-1} = 0$, and let $t_K = a_0 + t_x, (t_x > 0)$. See Figure 7.2. We define the four events H_K, A_K, I_K, D_K as in (7.2). The three events (I_K, D_K, A_K) are mutually exclusive, and they form a partition of the whole sample space; i.e., $I_K \cup D_K \cup A_K = H_K$. Since most people will have no symptoms during their lifetime, we are more concerned with those who would develop cancer before the next screening time. So we need to calculate the conditional probability of an interval case in (a_0, t_K) among those who would develop cancer in this interval.

The probability of incidence before the next screening exam, given that someone would have clinical cancer in the time interval (a_0, t_K) is

$$P(I_K|I_K \cup D_K) = \frac{P(I_K)}{P(I_K \cup D_K)} = \frac{P(I_K)}{P(I_K) + P(D_K)}.$$

where the probability $P(I_K)$ is the probability of incidence in (a_0, t_K) for the first time, and it could happen in $(K+2)$ mutually exclusively ways: (i) one enters the preclinical state at age $x \in (t_{i-1}, t_i)$, with $i = 0, 1, \ldots, K-1$, has a sojourn time in $(a_0 - x, t_K - x)$, and cancer were not detected, which are K cases; (ii) one enters the preclinical state at age $x \in (t_{K-1}, a_0)$, and has a sojourn time in $(a_0 - x, t_K - x)$; or (iii) one enters the preclinical state at age $x \in (a_0, t_K)$, and the sojourn time is less than $(t_K - x)$. And we just add these probabilities to get:

$$\begin{aligned} P(I_K) &= \sum_{i=0}^{K-1} \int_{t_{i-1}}^{t_i} w(x) \int_{t_{K-1}-x}^{t_K - x} q(t) \left\{ \prod_{j=i}^{K-1} [1 - \beta(t_j - x|t)] \right\} dtdx \\ &+ \int_{t_{K-1}}^{a_0} w(x)[Q(a_0 - x) - Q(t_K - x)]dx \\ &+ \int_{a_0}^{t_K} w(x)[1 - Q(t_K - x)]dx. \end{aligned} \tag{7.13}$$

When $a_0 = t_{K-1}$, we have

$$\begin{aligned} P(I_K) &= \sum_{i=0}^{K-1} \int_{t_{i-1}}^{t_i} w(x) \int_{t_{K-1}-x}^{t_K - x} q(t) \left\{ \prod_{j=i}^{K-1} [1 - \beta(t_j - x|t)] \right\} dtdx \\ &+ \int_{t_{K-1}}^{t_K} w(x)[1 - Q(t_K - x)]dx. \end{aligned} \tag{7.14}$$

The probability $P(D_K)$ is the probability of screen-detected case at t_K, and it could happen in $(K+1)$ mutually exclusively ways: (i) one enters the preclinical state at age $x \in (t_{i-1}, t_i)$, has a sojourn time longer than $(t_K - x)$, and cancer was undetected by the previous exams at $t_i, \ldots, t_{K-1}$, but was only detected at t_K; with $i = 0, 1, \ldots, K-1$, which are K cases; or (ii) one enters the preclinical state at age $x \in (t_{K-1}, t_K)$, and has a sojourn time longer than $(t_K - x)$. And we add these possibilities to obtain

$$\begin{aligned} P(D_K) &= \sum_{i=0}^{K-1} \int_{t_{i-1}}^{t_i} w(x) \int_{t_K - x}^{\infty} q(t) \left\{ \prod_{j=i}^{K-1} [1 - \beta(t_j - x|t)] \right\} \beta(t_K - x|t)dtdx \\ &+ \int_{t_{K-1}}^{t_K} w(x) \int_{t_K - x}^{\infty} q(t)\beta(t_K - x|t)dtdx. \end{aligned} \tag{7.15}$$

Exercise 7.5.

(a) Find the probability $P(H_K)$.

(b) Find the probability $P(A_K)$.

(c) Prove that

$$P(I_K) + P(D_K) + P(A_K) = P(H_K), \text{ and } P(A_K) = P(H_{K+1}).$$

Since $\frac{P(I_K)}{P(D_K)}$ is monotonically increasing as t_x increases or $\frac{P(D_K)}{P(I_K)}$ is monotonically decreasing as t_x increases, therefore, $1 + \frac{P(D_K)}{P(I_K)}$ is monotonically decreasing as t_x increases. Hence the inverse of that $1/(1 + \frac{P(D_K)}{P(I_K)}) = \frac{P(I_K)}{P(I_K)+P(D_K)}$ is monotonically increasing as t_x increases. For any preselected small value of p, a unique solution t_x can be found by

$$P(I_K|I_K \cup D_K) = p \tag{7.16}$$

Let t^* be the solution, then with probability $(1-p)$, one will not be a clinical incident case before the next screening if one would take the next exam at the age $t_K = a_0 + t^*$. People may choose $p = 5\%, 10\%, 15\%, 20\%$, or any small value to meet their needs of risk tolerance.

7.3.2 Lead time distribution

After t^* is found, the distribution of the lead time (i.e., diagnosis time advanced by screening) can be estimated. Let L be the lead time, and $t_K = a_0 + t^*$. The conditional probability density function of the lead time given someone who is diagnosed at t_K is

$$f_L(z|D_K) = \frac{f_L(z, D_K)}{P(D_K)}, \qquad \text{for } z > 0, \tag{7.17}$$

where $P(D_k)$ is the same as in equation (7.15). To calculate the numerator $f_L(z, D_K)$, since the lead time is z, that is, one will have clinical symptoms appear at age $t_K + z$ if no screening were carried out, there are $(K+1)$ mutually exclusive cases: (i) one enters the preclinical state at age $x \in (t_{i-1}, t_i)$, has a sojourn time equals to $(t_K + z - x)$, and cancer was not detected by the previous exams at $t_i, \ldots, t_{K-1}$, but it was only detected at t_K; with $i = 0, 1, \ldots, K-1$, which are K cases; or (ii) one enters the preclinical state at age $x \in (t_{K-1}, t_K)$, has a sojourn time of $(t_K + z - x)$, and cancer was diagnosed at t_K. And we add these possibilities:

$$\begin{aligned} f_L(z, D_K) &= \sum_{i=0}^{K-1} \int_{t_{i-1}}^{t_i} w(x) q(t_K + z - x) \beta(t_K - x | t_K + z - x) \\ &\quad \times \left\{ \prod_{j=i}^{K-1} [1 - \beta(t_j - x | t_K + z - x)] \right\} dx \\ &\quad + \int_{t_{K-1}}^{t_K} w(x) q(t_K + z - x) \beta(t_K - x | t_K + z - x) dx. \end{aligned} \tag{7.18}$$

Exercise 7.6. Prove that

$$\int_0^\infty f_L(z|D_K) dz = 1.$$

Hence, this probability density function is a valid PDF.

7.3.3 Probability of overdiagnosis and true early detection

Probability of overdiagnosis, and that of true-early-detection, given one would be diagnosed at $t_K = t_{K-1} + t^*$ with a fixed lifetime $T = t(> t_K)$, are

$$
\begin{aligned}
P(\text{OverD}|D_K, T = t) &= \frac{P(\text{OverD}, D_K|T = t)}{P(D_K|T = t)}, \\
P(\text{TrueED}|D_K, T = t) &= \frac{P(\text{TrueED}, D_K|T = t)}{P(D_K|T = t)},
\end{aligned}
$$

where $P(D_K|T = t) = P(D_K)$ is the same as in equation (7.15). To obtain $P(\text{OverD}, D_K|T = t)$, no clinical symptom would have appeared before one's lifetime, so the sojourn time must be longer than $(t - x)$, where x is the onset age of the preclinical state, and $x \in (t_{i-1}, t_i), i = 0, 1, \ldots, K$; however, one was diagnosed at t_K. Therefore,

$$
\begin{aligned}
&P(\text{OverD}, D_K|T = t) \\
&= \sum_{i=0}^{K-1} \int_{t_{i-1}}^{t_i} w(x) \int_{t-x}^{\infty} q(y)\beta(t_K - x|y) \prod_{j=i}^{K-1} [1 - \beta(t_j - x|y)]dydx \\
&\quad + \int_{t_{K-1}}^{t_K} w(x) \int_{t-x}^{\infty} q(y)\beta(t_K - x|y)dydx. \qquad (7.19)
\end{aligned}
$$

And for $P(\text{TrueED}, D_K|T = t)$, the case of true-early-detection, one was diagnosed at t_K and her symptoms would have appeared before death; i.e., the sojourn time is within the interval $(t_K - x, t - x)$. Therefore,

$$
\begin{aligned}
&P(\text{TrueED}, D_K|T = t) \\
&= \sum_{i=0}^{K-1} \int_{t_{i-1}}^{t_i} w(x) \int_{t_K-x}^{t-x} q(y)\beta(t_K - x|y) \prod_{j=i}^{K-1} [1 - \beta(t_j - x|y)]dydx \\
&\quad + \int_{t_{K-1}}^{t_K} w(x) \int_{t_K-x}^{t-x} q(y)\beta(t_K - x|y)dydx. \qquad (7.20)
\end{aligned}
$$

Exercise 7.7. Prove that

$$P(\text{OverD}, D_K|T = t) + P(\text{TrueED}, D_K|T = t) = P(D_K).$$

Therefore,

$$P(\text{OverD}|D_K, T = t) + P(\text{TrueED}|D_K, T = t) = 1.$$

Now we allow human lifetime T to be random, and let $f_T(t|T > t_K)$ be the conditional PDF of the lifetime T, then

$$
\begin{aligned}
P(\text{OverD}|D_K, T > t_K) &= \int_{t_K}^{\infty} P(\text{OverD}|D_K, T = t)f_T(t|T > t_K)dt, \\
P(\text{TrueED}|D_K, T > t_K) &= \int_{t_K}^{\infty} P(\text{TrueED}|D_K, T = t)f_T(t|T > t_K)dt.
\end{aligned}
$$

The probability formulas are correct since we can prove that

$$P(\text{TrueED}|D_K, T > t_K) + P(\text{OverD}|D_K, T > t_K) = 1.$$

7.3.4 Simulation

The conditional probability $P(I_K|I_K \cup D_K)$ is a function of one's screening history (including current age), the three model parameters (sensitivity, sojourn time, transition density from S_0 to S_p); and it is monotonically increasing with the future screening interval. Therefore, when this probability is limited to a small value, the next screening time interval is a function of the above-mentioned factors. We explore the effects of these factors on the next screening time t_x, or age $t_K = t_{K-1} + t_x$. We assumed that the current age $a_0 = t_{K-1}$ and selected the following scenarios for simulation:

(a) Four different probability of incidence: $p = 0.05, 0.10, 0.15, 0.20$;

(b) Three different screening sensitivity functions: $\beta_i(s|Y), i = 1, 2, 3$;

(c) Three different mean sojourn time (MST): 2, 5, and 10 years;

(d) Two sets of initial screening age and current age:

$$(t_0, t_{K-1}) = (55, 61) \text{ and } (60, 66);$$

(e) Three different screening interval in the past Δ: 1, 2, and 3 years.

We let the sensitivity

$$\beta(s|Y) = [1 + \exp(-b_0 - b_1 \cdot \frac{s}{Y})]^{-1}, \quad 0 \leq s \leq Y, \tag{7.21}$$

where s is the time one has stayed in the preclinical state S_p and Y is the sojourn time. We choose three pairs of (b_0, b_1) = (0.85, 2.65), (1.40, 2.10), and (2.20, 1.30), so the corresponding sensitivity at the onset of S_p would be $\beta(s = 0|Y) = [1 + \exp(-b_0)]^{-1} = 0.7$, 0.8, and 0.9, and the sensitivity at the end of S_p (or onset of S_c) would be $\beta(s = Y|Y) = [1+\exp(-b_0-b_1)]^{-1} = 0.97$ for all three cases [76].

We use the parametric model of the transition density and the sojourn time [76]:

$$\begin{aligned} w(t|\mu, \sigma^2) &= \frac{0.3}{\sqrt{2\pi}\sigma t} \exp\{-(\log t - \mu)^2/(2\sigma^2)\}, \\ Q(x|\lambda, \alpha) &= \exp(-\lambda x^\alpha), \quad \lambda > 0, \alpha > 0, \\ q(x|\lambda, \alpha) &= \alpha\lambda x^{\alpha-1} Q(x|\lambda, \alpha). \end{aligned} \tag{7.22}$$

The transition probability density $w(t)$ was a lognormal density with an upper limit of 30%, which is applicable to most kinds of cancer; the input parameters of μ and σ^2 were chosen, so that the mean/median/mode of the lung cancer transition age into the preclinical state was around 70 years old [76], that will give $\mu = 4.25$. Based on our previous research, the σ^2 has a posterior mean of 0.021 for female heavy smokers, 0.017 for their male counterparts, so we picked $\sigma^2 = 0.02$ in the simulation.

The sojourn time distribution was a Weibull (λ, α), with parameters chosen so that the mean sojourn times are 2, 5, and 10 years (corresponding to fast-growing, moderate-growing, and slow-growing tumors). The parameters chosen for the simulation were $\alpha = 3.0, \lambda = 0.08901, 0.00570, 0.00071$. Using equation (7.16), the optimal scheduling time t^* was found and summarized in Table 7.12.

In Table 7.12, p in the first column is the preselected probability of incidence before the next exam in the simulation, taking values from 0.05 to 0.20. Columns 2 to 10 present the calculated optimal scheduling time (in years) of the next exam, given values of p, the test sensitivity β_i, the mean sojourn time (MST), and past screening interval Δ.

Table 7.12 shows that the sensitivity function β_i plays an important role in the optimal time for the next screening: under the same risk p, higher sensitivity leads to lower frequencies (or longer future screening intervals). In another word, sensitivity is positively correlated with the next screening interval. For example, for the age group $(t_0, t_{K-1}) = (55, 61)$, when the mean sojourn time (MST) is 2 years, $\Delta = 2$ years, and $p = 0.20$ (i.e., incidence probability before the next exam is no more than 0.20), a woman should return in 1.91 years (or 23 months) in column 5 if the sensitivity follows the pattern β_1, or in 2.14 years (or 25.7 months) in column 7 if the sensitivity follows pattern β_3.

Table 7.12 also shows that past screening interval Δ plays an important role in future screening: when one's past screening interval is longer, to maintain the same incidence probability p, she should come back a little bit earlier, and vice versa. For example, in the rows under MST = 5 years, and the columns under $\Delta = 1$ year, an individual who had *annual* (negative) prior screens and who wishes to keep the p below 0.1, can return 3.89, 4.07, and 4.24 years when sensitivity changes from β_1 to β_3; comparing with those who underwent *biannual* screening, the time is 3.69, 3.91, and 4.13 years under the columns $\Delta = 2$ years. Hence future screening time is shortened by 0.2, 0.16, and 0.11 years (or 2.4, 1.9, and 1.3 months) for participants with biannual exams in the past.

The mean sojourn time (MST) affects the next screening interval dramatically: longer MST (slowly growing tumor or low-risk people) means she can wait longer to take the next screening exams. However, it is impossible to predict the MST, even though people could be identified as high or low risk. Finally, lower probability of incidence p translates to shorter screening intervals in the future, which is consistent with our intuition. This incidence probability can be explained as risk tolerance; people who can tolerate higher risk can come back at a later time. Current age t_{K-1} also affects the next

TABLE 7.12
Scheduling time t^* when $(t_0, t_{K-1}) = (55, 61)$ or $(60, 66)$.

$(t_0, t_{K-1}) = (55, 61)$

	MST = 2 years								
	$\Delta = 1$ yr			$\Delta = 2$ yrs			$\Delta = 3$ yrs		
p	$^a\beta_1$	β_2	β_3	β_1	β_2	β_3	β_1	β_2	β_3
0.05	0.98	1.07	1.17	0.80	0.90	1.02	0.74	0.82	0.95
0.10	1.39	1.49	1.59	1.27	1.38	1.50	1.23	1.34	1.47
0.15	1.70	1.80	1.91	1.61	1.72	1.84	1.59	1.70	1.83
0.20	1.98	2.09	2.19	1.91	2.02	2.14	1.89	2.01	2.13
	MST = 5 years								
	$\Delta = 1$ yr			$\Delta = 2$ yrs			$\Delta = 3$ yrs		
p	β_1	β_2	β_3	β_1	β_2	β_3	β_1	β_2	β_3
0.05	2.90	3.07	3.23	2.66	2.87	3.09	2.48	2.70	2.96
0.10	3.89	4.07	4.24	3.69	3.91	4.13	3.55	3.79	4.05
0.15	4.67	4.85	5.02	4.49	4.71	4.94	4.37	4.62	4.87
0.20	5.36	5.55	5.72	5.20	5.43	5.65	5.10	5.35	5.59
	MST = 10 years								
	$\Delta = 1$ yr			$\Delta = 2$ yrs			$\Delta = 3$ yrs		
p	β_1	β_2	β_3	β_1	β_2	β_3	β_1	β_2	β_3
0.05	6.21	6.46	6.69	5.96	6.28	6.58	5.77	6.12	6.47
0.10	8.19	8.45	8.69	7.96	8.29	8.60	7.80	8.16	8.52
0.15	9.70	9.96	10.21	9.50	9.82	10.13	9.35	9.71	10.06
0.20	11.01	11.28	11.52	10.82	11.15	11.45	10.69	11.05	11.39

$(t_0, t_{K-1}) = (60, 66)$

	MST = 2 years								
	$\Delta = 1$ yr			$\Delta = 2$ yrs			$\Delta = 3$ yrs		
p	$^a\beta_1$	β_2	β_3	β_1	β_2	β_3	β_1	β_2	β_3
0.05	0.95	1.05	1.15	0.76	0.85	0.98	0.69	0.76	0.89
0.10	1.36	1.46	1.56	1.22	1.33	1.46	1.18	1.29	1.42
0.15	1.66	1.77	1.87	1.56	1.67	1.80	1.53	1.65	1.78
0.20	1.93	2.04	2.14	1.85	1.96	2.08	1.83	1.95	2.07
	MST = 5 years								
	$\Delta = 1$ yr			$\Delta = 2$ yrs			$\Delta = 3$ yrs		
p	β_1	β_2	β_3	β_1	β_2	β_3	β_1	β_2	β_3
0.05	2.82	2.98	3.15	2.55	2.76	2.99	2.33	2.55	2.82
0.10	3.76	3.94	4.10	3.53	3.75	3.98	3.35	3.60	3.87
0.15	4.48	4.66	4.83	4.28	4.50	4.73	4.13	4.38	4.64
0.20	5.12	5.30	5.47	4.93	5.16	5.38	4.81	5.06	5.31
	MST = 10 years								
	$\Delta = 1$ yr			$\Delta = 2$ yrs			$\Delta = 3$ yrs		
p	β_1	β_2	β_3	β_1	β_2	β_3	β_1	β_2	β_3
0.05	5.94	6.18	6.41	5.65	5.97	6.28	5.41	5.77	6.14
0.10	7.75	8.01	8.24	7.49	7.82	8.13	7.27	7.65	8.02
0.15	9.12	9.37	9.60	8.87	9.20	9.50	8.67	9.05	9.41
0.20	10.28	10.53	10.77	10.05	10.37	10.68	9.87	10.24	10.59

$^a\beta_i = \beta_i(s|Y) = [1 + \exp(-b_0 - b_1 \cdot \frac{s}{Y})]^{-1}, 0 \leq s \leq Y$, where the values of (b_0, b_1) equal to (0.85, 2.65), (1.40, 2.10), (2.20, 1.30) for $\beta_1, \beta_2, \beta_3$, respectively.

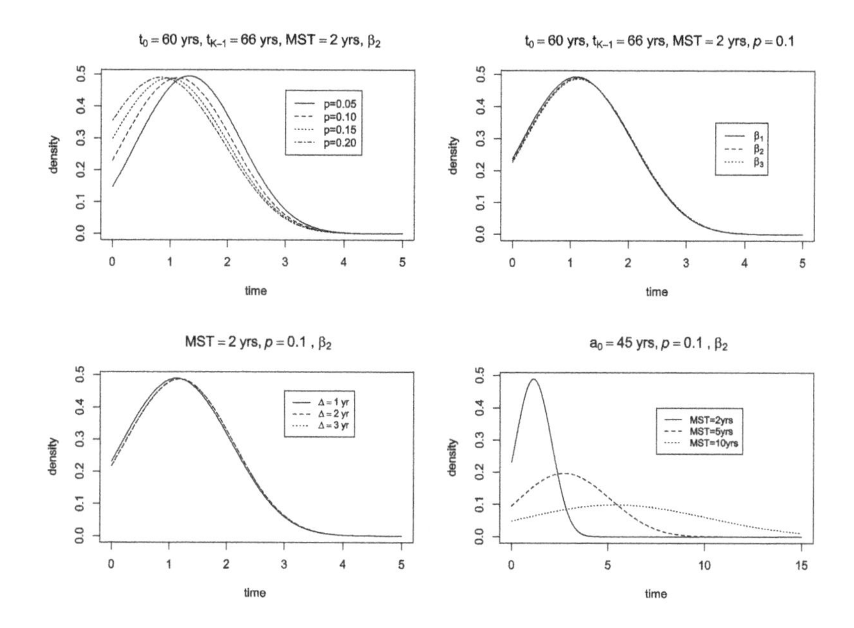

FIGURE 7.6
Lead time distribution under the four factors with $(t_0, t_{K-1}) = (60, 66)$.

screening time; usually, people at 66 should take the next exam earlier than those at 61 from our simulation.

We evaluated the lead time distribution for those who would be diagnosed with cancer at the future screening time t^* in Table 7.13. The estimated mean, median, mode, standard deviation, and 95% credible interval for the cohort $(t_0, t_{K-1}) = (55, 61)$ are listed in Table 7.13. We omitted the other age group $(t_0, t_{K-1}) = (60, 66)$ since the patterns are similar. Table 7.13 shows that the mean, median, and mode decrease as the incidence probability p increases; and they increase as the MST increases. They slightly change with sensitivity or past screening interval. The estimated standard deviation seems only changes with the MST, and it is almost the same under different p, or Δ or β_i. The 95% HPD interval won't change much for cohorts under the same mean sojourn time.

Using the density curve of the age cohort $(t_0, t_{K-1}) = (60, 66)$, Figure 7.6 illustrates how the lead time changes under the four factors using the optimal scheduling time t^*: the probability of incidence p, the sensitivity β, the historic screening interval Δ, and the MST. The density curves are all skewed to the right (with long tails), so the median and the mode are more reliable for the estimation of lead time than the mean. In the four panels of Figure 7.6, three factors are fixed, and only one factor is allowed to change. For example, the panel on the upper left corner shows how the PDF of the lead time changes with p when sensitivity is β_2, with MST = 2 years and the

TABLE 7.13
Estimated mean, median, mode, standard deviation, and 95% CI of the lead time under the optimal t^* when $(t_0, t_{K-1}) = (55, 61)$.

		$^a MST = 2$ **yrs,** β_1	
p	$\Delta = 1$ yr	$\Delta = 2$ yrs	$\Delta = 3$ yrs
0.05	1.43 1.37 1.30 0.75 (0, 2.71)	1.46 1.41 1.36 0.76 (0, 2.75)	1.48 1.43 1.38 0.76 (0, 2.77)
0.10	1.31 1.24 1.10 0.75 (0, 2.63)	1.33 1.27 1.15 0.76 (0, 2.65)	1.34 1.27 1.17 0.76 (0, 2.66)
0.15	1.24 1.15 0.95 0.75 (0, 2.58)	1.25 1.17 0.99 0.76 (0, 2.60)	1.26 1.18 1.00 0.76 (0, 2.60)
0.20	1.19 1.10 0.82 0.75 (0, 2.55)	1.20 1.11 0.85 0.75 (0, 2.56)	1.20 1.11 0.86 0.75 (0, 2.56)
		$^a MST = 2$ **yrs,** β_2	
p	$\Delta = 1$ yr	$\Delta = 2$ yrs	$\Delta = 3$ yrs
0.05	1.44 1.39 1.32 0.76 (0, 2.74)	1.48 1.44 1.39 0.76 (0, 2.78)	1.50 1.46 1.42 0.76 (0, 2.80)
0.10	1.32 1.25 1.13 0.76 (0, 2.65)	1.34 1.28 1.17 0.76 (0, 2.67)	1.35 1.29 1.19 0.76 (0, 2.68)
0.15	1.25 1.17 0.98 0.76 (0, 2.61)	1.26 1.19 1.01 0.76 (0, 2.62)	1.27 1.19 1.02 0.76 (0, 2.62)
0.20	1.20 1.11 0.85 0.76 (0, 2.58)	1.21 1.12 0.88 0.76 (0, 2.58)	1.21 1.13 0.88 0.76 (0, 2.59)
		$^a MST = 2$ **yrs,** β_3	
p	$\Delta = 1$ yr	$\Delta = 2$ yrs	$\Delta = 3$ yrs
0.05	1.44 1.40 1.33 0.76 (0, 2.75)	1.49 1.45 1.40 0.76 (0, 2.79)	1.51 1.47 1.43 0.76 (0, 2.80)
0.10	1.33 1.26 1.14 0.76 (0, 2.67)	1.35 1.29 1.18 0.76 (0, 2.68)	1.35 1.30 1.19 0.76 (0, 2.69)
0.15	1.26 1.18 1.00 0.76 (0, 2.62)	1.27 1.20 1.02 0.76 (0, 2.63)	1.27 1.20 1.03 0.76 (0, 2.63)
0.20	1.22 1.13 0.87 0.76 (0, 2.60)	1.22 1.14 0.89 0.76 (0, 2.60)	1.22 1.14 0.90 0.76 (0, 2.60)
		$^a MST = 5$ **yrs,** β_1	
p	$\Delta = 1$ yr	$\Delta = 2$ yrs	$\Delta = 3$ yrs
0.05	3.53 3.40 3.19 1.88 (0, 6.79)	3.55 3.43 3.23 1.89 (0, 6.82)	3.58 3.46 3.28 1.89 (0, 6.86)
0.10	3.25 3.07 2.71 1.89 (0, 6.59)	3.26 3.10 2.75 1.89 (0, 6.61)	3.29 3.12 2.80 1.89 (0, 6.63)
0.15	3.08 2.88 2.35 1.89 (0, 6.48)	3.10 2.90 2.39 1.89 (0, 6.50)	3.11 2.91 2.43 1.89 (0, 6.51)
0.20	2.97 2.74 2.03 1.89 (0, 6.41)	2.98 2.76 2.07 1.89 (0, 6.42)	2.99 2.77 2.11 1.89 (0, 6.43)
		$^a MST = 5$ **yrs,** β_2	
p	$\Delta = 1$ yr	$\Delta = 2$ yrs	$\Delta = 3$ yrs
0.05	3.56 3.43 3.24 1.89 (0, 6.83)	3.58 3.47 3.29 1.89 (0, 6.86)	3.61 3.50 3.34 1.90 (0, 6.89)
0.10	3.28 3.11 2.77 1.90 (0, 6.64)	3.30 3.14 2.81 1.90 (0, 6.66)	3.32 3.16 2.85 1.90 (0, 6.68)
0.15	3.12 2.92 2.42 1.90 (0, 6.53)	3.13 2.94 2.45 1.90 (0, 6.55)	3.14 2.95 2.49 1.90 (0, 6.56)
0.20	3.01 2.79 2.11 1.90 (0, 6.46)	3.02 2.80 2.15 1.90 (0, 6.47)	3.03 2.81 2.17 1.90 (0, 6.48)
		$^a MST = 5$ **yrs,** β_3	
p	$\Delta = 1$ yr	$\Delta = 2$ yrs	$\Delta = 3$ yrss
0.05	3.58 3.46 3.27 1.89 (0, 6.86)	3.60 3.49 3.31 1.89 (0, 6.89)	3.63 3.52 3.36 1.89 (0, 6.91)
0.10	3.30 3.15 2.82 1.90 (0, 6.68)	3.32 3.16 2.85 1.90 (0, 6.69)	3.33 3.18 2.88 1.90 (0, 6.70)
0.15	3.15 2.96 2.48 1.91 (0, 6.58)	3.16 2.97 2.50 1.91 (0, 6.58)	3.17 2.98 2.53 1.91 (0, 6.59)
0.20	3.05 2.83 2.19 1.91 (0, 6.51)	3.05 2.84 2.21 1.91 (0, 6.51)	3.06 2.85 2.23 1.91 (0, 6.52)
		$^a MST = 10$ **yrs,** β_1	
p	$\Delta = 1$ yr	$\Delta = 2$ yrs	$\Delta = 3$ yrs
0.05	7.06 6.81 6.39 3.77 (0, 13.62)	7.07 6.82 6.41 3.78 (0, 13.65)	7.09 6.85 6.44 3.78 (0, 13.68)
0.10	6.48 6.14 5.41 3.77 (0, 13.20)	6.50 6.16 5.44 3.78 (0, 13.22)	6.52 6.19 5.48 3.78 (0, 13.24)
0.15	6.13 5.72 4.65 3.77 (0, 12.93)	6.15 5.74 4.69 3.77 (0, 12.95)	6.16 5.76 4.72 3.77 (0, 12.97)
0.20	5.88 5.42 3.98 3.76 (0, 12.74)	5.90 5.44 4.02 3.76 (0, 12.76)	5.91 5.46 4.06 3.76 (0, 12.77)
		$^a MST = 10$ **yrs,** β_2	
p	$\Delta = 1$ yr	$\Delta = 2$ yrs	$\Delta = 3$ yrs
0.05	7.11 6.88 6.48 3.78 (0, 13.70)	7.13 6.90 6.51 3.78 (0, 13.72)	7.15 6.92 6.54 3.79 (0, 13.74)
0.10	6.55 6.22 5.53 3.79 (0, 13.29)	6.56 6.24 5.56 3.79 (0, 13.30)	6.58 6.26 5.59 3.80 (0, 13.32)
0.15	6.20 5.81 4.79 3.79 (0, 13.03)	6.22 5.82 4.82 3.79 (0, 13.05)	6.23 5.84 4.85 3.79 (0, 13.06)
0.20	5.96 5.51 4.13 3.78 (0, 12.85)	5.97 5.52 4.16 3.79 (0, 12.86)	5.98 5.54 4.19 3.79 (0, 12.87)
		$^a MST = 10$ **yrs,** β_3	
p	$\Delta = 1$ yr	$\Delta = 2$ yrs	$\Delta = 3$ yrs
0.05	7.16 6.93 6.55 3.79 (0, 13.75)	7.17 6.95 6.57 3.79 (0, 13.77)	7.19 6.97 6.60 3.79 (0, 13.78)
0.10	6.60 6.29 5.63 3.80 (0, 13.35)	6.61 6.30 5.65 3.80 (0, 13.36)	6.62 6.31 5.67 3.81 (0, 13.37)
0.15	6.26 5.88 4.91 3.81 (0, 13.11)	6.27 5.89 4.93 3.81 (0, 13.12)	6.28 5.90 4.95 3.81 (0, 13.12)
0.20	6.02 5.59 4.26 3.80 (0, 12.93)	6.03 5.59 4.28 3.80 (0, 12.94)	6.04 5.60 4.30 3.80 (0, 12.94)

historic screening interval $\Delta = 1$ year. It shows that the density curve of the lead time changes more with the incidence probability p and the MST (which are compatible with Table 7.13 results), but it changes less with the sensitivity function β_i and the historic screening interval Δ if a patient will follow the dynamic scheduling time t^* obtained in Table 7.12.

We then evaluated the probability of overdiagnosis if the optimal scheduling time t^* were adopted. The results are summarized in Table 7.14. Longer MST implies a much larger probability of overdiagnosis: it is below 1.1%, 4.1%, and 16.3% for the $(t_0, t_{K-1}) = (55, 61)$ group, and it is below 1.7%, 6.2%, and 22.6% for the $(t_0, t_{K-1}) = (60, 66)$ group if the MST is 2, 5, and 10 years correspondingly. The risk of overdiagnosis will slightly increase as the sensitivity increases when other factors are the same. These are compatible with our intuition. It is clear that the mean sojourn time plays the most important role in the estimation of overdiagnosis. And given someone would be diagnosed with cancer at a future time, probability of overdiagnosis would not change with the historic screening interval, but it would be monotonically increasing as the future screening time t increases. Comparing the two different age cohorts, the older age group $(t_0, t_{K-1}) = (60, 66)$ has a higher chance of overdiagnosis. Combing this information, longer MST and higher sensitivity usually mean that the future scheduling time t^* will be much larger, or a patient's age at the next screening time is much older, as shown in Table 7.13. Therefore, a higher risk of overdiagnosis may be caused by the confounding effects of advanced age, longer sojourn time, and higher sensitivity.

7.3.5 Application: Scheduling for heavy smokers based on the NLST-CT study

We applied the method to the National Lung Screening Trials computed tomography arm (NLST-CT) separately for two cohorts: male and female heavy smokers.

Using results in section 7.3.1, the probability of incidence is a function of the next screening time interval, the three key parameters, a person's current age t_{K-1}, and her past screening history. Wu et al 2022 estimated the three key parameters from the NLST-CT data using the same parametric models as that in the simulation equations (7.21) and (7.22).The unknown parameters in this model were $\theta = (b_0, b_1, \mu, \sigma^2, \lambda, \alpha)$. For each gender, using Markov Chain Monte Carlo (MCMC) with Gibbs sampler and a likelihood function, 6000 samples were generated; after 1000 burn-in and thinning every 50 iterations, a posterior sample of 100 from each chain was obtained. Running eight parallel chains with over-dispersed initial values provided 800 Bayesian posterior samples $\theta_j^*, j = 1, 2, \ldots, 800$ for each gender. For more details, see Wu et al 2022 [76].

We conducted Bayesian inference on hypothetical cohorts of asymptomatic women with initial screening age and current age $(t_0, t_{K-1}) = (55,\ 61)$, or $(60,\ 66)$, with different historic screening intervals $\Delta = 1, 2, 3$, and using

TABLE 7.14
Probability of overdiagnosis (in %) at t^* when (t_0, t_{K-1}) = (55, 61) or (60, 66).

$(t_0, t_{K-1}) = (55, 61)$

	$\Delta = 1$ yr			$\Delta = 2$ yrs			$\Delta = 3$ yrs		
MST = 2 years									
p	β_1	β_2	β_3	β_1	β_2	β_3	β_1	β_2	β_3
0.05	1.12	1.14	1.15	1.12	1.14	1.17	1.13	1.16	1.18
0.10	1.05	1.07	1.09	1.05	1.07	1.09	1.07	1.09	1.10
0.15	1.02	1.05	1.06	1.02	1.04	1.05	1.03	1.05	1.07
0.20	1.01	1.04	1.05	1.00	1.03	1.05	1.01	1.04	1.06
MST = 5 years									
p	β_1	β_2	β_3	β_1	β_2	β_3	β_1	β_2	β_3
0.05	3.67	3.80	3.87	3.62	3.72	3.84	3.61	3.72	3.82
0.10	3.67	3.81	3.88	3.62	3.73	3.86	3.61	3.72	3.86
0.15	3.73	3.83	3.97	3.68	3.79	3.91	3.68	3.79	3.91
0.20	3.83	3.93	4.04	3.78	3.90	4.01	3.77	3.89	4.01
MST = 10 years									
p	β_1	β_2	β_3	β_1	β_2	β_3	β_1	β_2	β_3
0.05	12.21	12.57	12.87	11.85	12.41	12.79	11.74	12.32	12.73
0.10	13.13	13.55	13.95	12.78	13.43	13.86	12.66	13.37	13.84
0.15	13.98	14.51	15.18	13.80	14.34	15.09	13.70	14.30	15.06
0.20	15.22	15.72	16.21	14.74	15.58	16.13	14.65	15.57	16.08

$(t_0, t_{K-1}) = (60, 66)$

	$\Delta = 1$ yr			$\Delta = 2$ yrs			$\Delta = 3$ yrs		
MST = 2 years									
p	[a]β_1	β_2	β_3	β_1	β_2	β_3	β_1	β_2	β_3
0.05	1.75	1.80	1.82	1.76	1.81	1.84	1.77	1.82	1.85
0.10	1.66	1.69	1.71	1.67	1.70	1.72	1.68	1.71	1.73
0.15	1.60	1.63	1.66	1.61	1.64	1.66	1.61	1.64	1.67
0.20	1.57	1.62	1.65	1.58	1.61	1.65	1.57	1.61	1.66
MST = 5 years									
p	β_1	β_2	β_3	β_1	β_2	β_3	β_1	β_2	β_3
0.05	5.67	5.80	5.98	5.59	5.76	5.89	5.56	5.74	5.89
0.10	5.63	5.77	6.00	5.57	5.74	5.88	5.55	5.72	5.87
0.15	5.68	5.85	5.98	5.64	5.81	5.96	5.61	5.78	5.94
0.20	5.83	6.00	6.14	5.68	5.96	6.11	5.66	5.95	6.11
MST = 10 years									
p	β_1	β_2	β_3	β_1	β_2	β_3	β_1	β_2	β_3
0.05	18.09	18.91	19.38	17.80	18.40	19.23	17.57	18.21	19.12
0.10	19.16	20.15	20.60	18.84	19.52	20.51	18.67	19.33	20.45
0.15	20.43	21.01	21.57	19.71	20.83	21.48	19.53	20.71	21.40
0.20	21.36	21.98	22.57	21.15	21.85	22.48	20.48	21.74	22.39

$p = 0.01, 0.1, 0.15$, and 0.2 as the incidence probability. We use the 800 posterior samples from each gender to make Bayesian inference on optimal scheduling time/age. For each posterior sample θ_j^*, using $P(I_K|I_K \cup D_K, H_K, \theta_j^*) = \alpha$, a scheduling time t_j^* $(j = 1, 2, \ldots, 800)$ can be found. The calculated posterior mean optimal time and its standard deviation (in years) based on the 800 t_j^* are summarized in Table 7.15.

For a 61-year-old male/female heavy smoker for lung cancer screening, using the NLST-CT data, one should come back at 1.01 (1.25), 0.95 (1.22), or 0.95 (1.21) years to maintain a 90% early detection if his/her past screening interval was 1, 2, or 3 years according to Table 7.15. Apparently, male heavy smokers need to come back earlier than their female counterparts. The upcoming screening time interval t^* is slightly decreasing with a person's current age if the other parameters are the same, and it is increasing with the incidence probability p. The t^* is negatively correlated with the past screening interval Δ: smaller Δ means a slightly larger t^*; i.e., one can come back at a later time if s/he has frequent negative screen results in the past; on the other hand, a larger Δ in the past means that one should come back for screening a little earlier. This follows the same pattern as found in the simulation study.

We further investigated how the lead time and the probability of overdiagnosis would change in different scenarios for the above cohorts. Using each pair of the 800 posterior samples θ_j^* and its corresponding t_j^*, one lead time distribution can be obtained. And the predictive posterior distribution of the lead time is

$$f_L^{NLST-CT}(l) \approx \frac{1}{n}\sum_{i=1}^{n} f_L^{NLST-CT}(l|\theta_j^*, t_j^*).$$

Then we calculate the mean, median, mode, and standard deviation of the lead time density $f_L^{NLST-CT}(l)$. The results are listed in Table 7.16.

Similarly, the probability of overdiagnosis was calculated using each of the 800 posterior samples θ_j^* and the corresponding t_j^*. Then we calculate the mean and percentiles of the probability of overdiagnosis based on the 800 cases. The results are listed in Table 7.17. Note that the probability of true-early-detection is one minus the probability of overdiagnosis, and they share the same standard deviation.

From Table 7.16, the mean lead time slightly changes between 0.91 and 1.11 years for males and 0.87 and 1.06 years for females; the median lead time changes between 0.80 and 1.01 years for males, 0.78 and 0.97 years for females; and the mode of lead time (the highest point on the density curve) changes between 0.55 and 0.94 years for males, 0.58 and 0.91 years for females. The standard deviation is about 0.67 for males and 0.62 for females. We can see that the lead time distribution changes with p if the other elements are the same: when p increases, the mean, median, and mode of lead time decrease. In other words, the mean/median/mode of the lead time seems to be negatively correlated with the p. The mean, median, and mode of lead time slightly increases as the past screening interval Δ increases from 1 to 2 years, and it

TABLE 7.15
Application: Posterior mean scheduling time t^* (95% CI) using NLST-CT data.

$(t_0, t_{K-1}) = (55, 61)$

	Female			Male		
$p\backslash\Delta$	1.0	2.0	3.0	1.0	2.0	3.0
0.05	0.95(0.76,1.18)	0.88(0.59,1.15)	0.87(0.54,1.15)	0.69(0.51,0.89)	0.60(0.19,0.86)	0.59(0.16,0.85)
0.10	1.25(1.07,1.47)	1.22(1.02,1.43)	1.21(1.01,1.43)	1.01(0.83,1.18)	0.95(0.73,1.15)	0.95(0.72,1.16)
0.15	1.47(1.20,1.73)	1.45(1.19,1.70)	1.44(1.19,1.69)	1.25(1.05,1.42)	1.21(1.04,1.39)	1.21(1.03,1.37)
0.20	1.66(1.32,2.03)	1.64(1.30,1.98)	1.64(1.32,1.99)	1.46(1.26,1.69)	1.43(1.24,1.62)	1.43(1.22,1.61)

$(t_0, t_{K-1}) = (60, 66)$

	Female			Male		
$p\backslash\Delta$	1.0	2.0	3.0	1.0	2.0	3.0
0.05	0.94(0.74,1.17)	0.85(0.53,1.14)	0.84(0.47,1.13)	0.68(0.49,0.87)	0.57(0.16,0.84)	0.56(0.11,0.80)
0.10	1.23(1.06,1.45)	1.20(1.00,1.41)	1.19(0.97,1.40)	0.99(0.82,1.15)	0.93(0.66,1.12)	0.92(0.64,1.13)
0.15	1.45(1.19,1.70)	1.42(1.19,1.66)	1.42(1.18,1.66)	1.22(1.07,1.42)	1.18(0.99,1.35)	1.18(0.97,1.34)
0.20	1.63(1.31,1.99)	1.61(1.31,1.97)	1.61(1.32,1.95)	1.43(1.24,1.64)	1.40(1.21,1.58)	1.39(1.20,1.57)

TABLE 7.16
Application: Estimated mean, median, mode (with standard deviation) of the lead time at the future t^* using the NLST-CT data (in years).

Female heavy smokers			
p	$\Delta = 1.0$	$\Delta = 2.0$	$\Delta = 3.0$
	$t_0 = 55, t_{K-1} = 61$		
0.05	1.03 0.95 0.86 (0.62)	1.06 0.97 0.90 (0.62)	1.06 0.97 0.91 (0.62)
0.10	0.95 0.86 0.76 (0.62)	0.96 0.87 0.77 (0.62)	0.96 0.87 0.77 (0.62)
0.15	0.91 0.82 0.68 (0.62)	0.91 0.82 0.69 (0.62)	0.91 0.82 0.69 (0.62)
0.20	0.88 0.79 0.61 (0.61)	0.88 0.79 0.62 (0.61)	0.88 0.79 0.62 (0.61)
	$t_0 = 60, t_{K-1} = 66$		
0.05	1.03 0.95 0.86 (0.62)	1.06 0.98 0.91 (0.62)	1.06 0.98 0.91 (0.62)
0.10	0.95 0.86 0.75 (0.62)	0.96 0.87 0.76 (0.62)	0.96 0.87 0.77 (0.62)
0.15	0.90 0.81 0.66 (0.62)	0.91 0.81 0.67 (0.62)	0.91 0.81 0.67 (0.62)
0.20	0.87 0.78 0.58 (0.61)	0.88 0.78 0.59 (0.61)	0.88 0.78 0.59 (0.61)

Male heavy smokers			
p	$\Delta = 1.0$	$\Delta = 2.0$	$\Delta = 3.0$
	$t_0 = 55, t_{K-1} = 61$		
0.05	1.09 0.99 0.89 (0.67)	1.11 1.01 0.93 (0.67)	1.11 1.01 0.93 (0.67)
0.10	1.00 0.89 0.74 (0.67)	1.01 0.91 0.77 (0.67)	1.01 0.91 0.77 (0.67)
0.15	0.95 0.84 0.64 (0.66)	0.96 0.84 0.66 (0.66)	0.96 0.85 0.66 (0.66)
0.20	0.92 0.80 0.56 (0.66)	0.92 0.81 0.57 (0.66)	0.92 0.81 0.57 (0.66)
	$t_0 = 60, t_{K-1} = 66$		
0.05	1.09 0.99 0.90 (0.67)	1.11 1.01 0.94 (0.67)	1.11 1.01 0.94 (0.67)
0.10	1.00 0.89 0.74 (0.67)	1.01 0.91 0.78 (0.67)	1.02 0.91 0.78 (0.67)
0.15	0.95 0.83 0.64 (0.66)	0.95 0.84 0.66 (0.66)	0.95 0.84 0.66 (0.66)
0.20	0.91 0.80 0.55 (0.66)	0.92 0.80 0.56 (0.66)	0.92 0.80 0.56 (0.66)

is almost the same when Δ equals to 2 or 3 years. The lead time distribution barely changes for the two age cohorts of each gender, showing that the current age seems not important in the lead time distribution. The mean (median, mode) lead time of male heavy smokers is slightly longer than their female counterparts. the standard deviation of the lead time is comparatively small.

For overdiagnosis, the average probability of overdiagnosis is between 0.73–0.84% (1.26–1.44%) for the 61-years-old female (male) group; and it increases to 1.08–1.24% (1.73–1.98%) for the 66 years old female (male) group. The corresponding C.I. increases as well from Table 7.17. In general, based on the NLST-CT study, the risk of overdiagnosis for heavy smokers is very low, although it slightly increases with age, gender (of males), and the past screening interval Δ. The probability of overdiagnosis among the screen-detected is very small, less than 2% for all cases.

TABLE 7.17
Application: Mean probability of overdiagnosis with 95% CI (in percentage) at t^* using the NLST-CT data.

Female heavy smokers			
p	$\Delta = 1.0$	$\Delta = 2.0$	$\Delta = 3.0$
		$t_0 = 55, t_{K-1} = 61$	
0.05	0.827 (0.479, 1.252)	0.838 (0.454, 1.230)	0.839 (0.441, 1.220)
0.10	0.776 (0.460, 1.189)	0.780 (0.422, 1.156)	0.781 (0.422, 1.157)
0.15	0.749 (0.450, 1.151)	0.751 (0.420, 1.121)	0.751 (0.420, 1.122)
0.20	0.737 (0.396, 1.082)	0.737 (0.396, 1.081)	0.737 (0.396, 1.081)
		$t_0 = 60, t_{K-1} = 66$	
0.05	1.213 (0.660, 1.807)	1.231 (0.611, 1.759)	1.233 (0.662, 1.807)
0.10	1.142 (0.670, 1.761)	1.149 (0.613, 1.708)	1.150 (0.613, 1.710)
0.15	1.102 (0.577, 1.626)	1.105 (0.577, 1.629)	1.106 (0.577, 1.631)
0.20	1.084 (0.579, 1.608)	1.085 (0.609, 1.635)	1.085 (0.609, 1.636)

Male heavy smokers			
p	$\Delta = 1.0$	$\Delta = 2.0$	$\Delta = 3.0$
		$t_0 = 55, t_{K-1} = 61$	
0.05	1.424 (0.893, 2.037)	1.435 (0.896, 2.027)	1.435 (0.896, 2.029)
0.10	1.343 (0.839, 1.973)	1.351 (0.822, 1.948)	1.352 (0.822, 1.952)
0.15	1.294 (0.746, 1.879)	1.300 (0.798, 1.926)	1.301 (0.800, 1.926)
0.20	1.260 (0.739, 1.843)	1.263 (0.739, 1.837)	1.263 (0.739, 1.837)
		$t_0 = 60, t_{K-1} = 66$	
0.05	1.958 (1.229, 2.806)	1.971 (1.230, 2.792)	1.970 (1.230, 2.793)
0.10	1.844 (1.142, 2.709)	1.857 (1.138, 2.692)	1.857 (1.161, 2.717)
0.15	1.781 (1.092, 2.660)	1.792 (1.093, 2.652)	1.792 (1.093, 2.657)
0.20	1.731 (1.009, 2.540)	1.736 (1.009, 2.540)	1.737 (1.009, 2.541)

7.4 Bibliographic notes

The idea of using the probability of incidence to schedule the upcoming exam came to me in 2006 and I wrote a grant application on this (unfunded). However, I was using the $P(I_K)$ alone at that time. Later, I did some numerical simulations and found out that the $P(I_K)$ was so small that the next exam could be waiting forever.

The first draft of the method assumed that the current age equals the last screening age, i.e., $a_0 = t_{K-1}$. It was finished in 2017, with the application to the HIP study (Wu and Kafadar 2022[69]). I gave a few conference presentations on this paper, including the 2016 Joint Statistical Meeting (JSM), the 2018 International Conference on Health Policy Statistics (ICHPS), and the

4th International Conference on Big Data and Information Analytics (2018). However, it is not accepted for publication yet. We have published a JSM conference proceeding paper applying the same method to the NLST-CT data (Wu and Kafadar 2019 [68]). There are two editorial articles on this topic, which were published in Wu 2016 [57] and Wu 2019 [58].

Then I extended the method to the more general situation when $a_0 \geq t_{K-1}$, and the derivation of the conditional probability of incidence was also simplified. The second paper was accepted recently [61]. That was the method presented in section 7.2. The methods in section 7.3 are recently developed, and the draft is ready for submission [60].

7.5 Solution for some exercises

Exercise 7.1:

(a)

$$\begin{aligned} P(H_2) &= 1 - \int_0^{a_0} w(x)dx + (1-\beta_0)(1-\beta_1)\int_0^{t_0} w(x)Q(a_0-x)dx \\ &\quad + (1-\beta_1)\int_{t_0}^{t_1} w(x)Q(a_0-x)dx + \int_{t_1}^{a_0} w(x)Q(a_0-x)dx. \end{aligned}$$

(b)

$$\begin{aligned} P(A_2) &= 1 - \int_0^{t_2} w(x)dx \\ &\quad + (1-\beta_0)(1-\beta_1)(1-\beta_2)\int_0^{t_0} w(x)Q(t_2-x)dx \\ &\quad + (1-\beta_1)(1-\beta_2)\int_{t_0}^{t_1} w(x)Q(t_2-x)dx \\ &\quad + (1-\beta_2)\int_{t_1}^{t_2} w(x)Q(t_2-x)dx. \end{aligned}$$

Exercise 7.2:

(a)

$$\begin{aligned} P(H_K) &= 1 - \int_0^{a_0} w(x)dx + \int_{t_{K-1}}^{a_0} w(x)Q(a_0-x)dx \\ &\quad + \sum_{i=0}^{K-1}(1-\beta_i)\cdots(1-\beta_{K-1})\int_{t_{i-1}}^{t_i} w(x)Q(a_0-x)dx. \end{aligned}$$

(b)

$$
\begin{aligned}
P(A_K) &= 1 - \int_0^{t_K} w(x)dx \\
&+ \sum_{j=0}^{K} (1-\beta_j)\cdots(1-\beta_K) \int_{t_{j-1}}^{t_j} w(x)Q(t_K - x)dx.
\end{aligned}
$$

Exercise 7.5:

(a)

$$
\begin{aligned}
P(H_K) &= 1 - \int_0^{t_{K-1}} w(x)dx \\
&+ \sum_{i=0}^{K-1} \int_{t_{i-1}}^{t_i} w(x) \int_{t_{K-1}-x}^{\infty} q(t) \left\{ \prod_{j=i}^{K-1} [1-\beta(t_j - x|t)] \right\} dtdx;
\end{aligned}
$$

(b)

$$
\begin{aligned}
P(A_K) &= 1 - \int_0^{t_K} w(x)dx \\
&+ \sum_{i=0}^{K} \int_{t_{i-1}}^{t_i} w(x) \int_{t_K-x}^{\infty} q(t) \left\{ \prod_{j=i}^{K} [1-\beta(t_j - x|t)] \right\} dtdx.
\end{aligned}
$$

Bibliography

[1] Stuart G. Baker. Analysis of survival data from a randomized trial with all-or-none compliance: Estimating the cost-effectiveness of a cancer screening program. *Journal of the American Statistical Association*, 93:929–934, 1998.

[2] B. D. Badgwell, S. H. Giordano, Z. Z. Duan, I, Bedrosian, S. Fang, H. M. Kuerer, S. E. Singletary, K. K. Hunt, G. N. Nortobagyi, and G. Babiera. Mammography before diagnosis among women age 80 years and older with breast cancer. *Journal of Clinical Oncology*, 26:2482–2488, 2008.

[3] Donald A. Berry, Cornelia J. Baines, Michael Baum, Kay Dickersin, Suzanne W. Fletcher, Peter C. Gøtzsche, Karsten Juhl Jørgensen, Bernard Junod, Jan Maehlen, Lisa M. Schwartz, H. Gilbert Welch, Steven Woloshin, Hazel Thornton, and Per-Henrik Zahl. Flawed inferences about screening mammography's benefit based on observational data. *Journal of Clinical Oncology*, 27:639–640, 2009.

[4] Bradley Carlin and Thomas Louis. *Bayesian Methods for Data Analysis*. CRC Press, 2008.

[5] George Casella and Roger L. Berger. *Statistical Inference, 2nd Ed.* Cengage Learning, 2001.

[6] W. Y. Chen, P. R. Annamreddy, and L. T. Fan. Modeling growth of a heterogeneous tumor. *Journal of Theoretical Biology*, 221:205–227, 2003.

[7] Yinlu Chen, Guy Brock, and Dongfeng Wu. Estimating key parameters in periodic breast cancer screening-application to the canadian national breast screening study data. *Cancer Epidemiology*, 34(4):429–433, 2010.

[8] Yuting Chen, Diane Erwin, and Dongfeng Wu. Over-diagnosis in lung cancer screening using the mskc-lcsp data. *Journal of Biometrics and Biostatistics*, 5(201), 2014.

[9] Ronald Christensen, Wesley O. Johnson, Adam J. Branscum, Timothy E. Hanson, and Timothy Christensen Hanson. *Bayesian Ideas and Data Analysis: An Introduction for Scientists and Statisticians*. CRC Press, 2010.

[10] Timothy R. Church, Jack S. Mandel, and Fred Ederer. Fecal occult blood screening in the Minnesota study: Sensitivity of the screening test. *Journal of the National Cancer Institute*, 89:1440–1457, 1997.

[11] D. R. Cox and D. Oakes. Analysis of survival data, 1984.

[12] D. Wu, S. N. Rai, and A. Seow. Estimation of preclinical state onset age and sojourn time for heavy smokers in lung cancer. *Statistics and Its Interface*, 15(3):349–358, 2022.

[13] O. Davidov and M. Zelen. Overdiagnosis in early detection programs. *Biostatistics*, 5:603–613, 2004.

[14] Nicholas E. Day and Stephan D. Walter. Simplified models of screening for chronic disease: Estimation procedures from mass screening programmes. *Biometrics*, 40:1–13, 1984.

[15] D. M. Eddy. *Screening for Cancer: Theory, Analysis and Design.* Prentice Hall, Englewood Cliffs, New Jersey, 1980.

[16] R. S. Fontana, D. R. Sanderson, L. B. Woolner, W. E. Miller, P. E. Bernatz, W. S. Payne, and W. F. Taylor. The Mayo Lung Project for early detection and localization of bronchogenic carcinoma: A status report. *Chest*, (5):511–522, 1975.

[17] US Preventive Services Task Force. Screening for cervical cancer: US preventive services task force recommendation statement. *JAMA*, 319(6):588–594, 2018.

[18] US Preventive Services Task Force. Screening for lung cancer US preventive services task force recommendation statement. *JSMA*, 325(10):962–970, 2021.

[19] Andrew Gelman, John Carlin, Hal Stern, David Dunson, Aki Vehtari, and Donald Rubin. *Bayesian Data Analysis.* CRC Press, 2013.

[20] Peter Hoff. *A First Course in Bayesian Statistical Methods.* Springer, 2009.

[21] Hyejeong Jang, Seongho Kim, and Dongfeng Wu. Bayesian lead time estimation for the Johns Hopkins Lung Project data. *Journal of Epidemiology and Global Health*, 3(3):157–163, 2013.

[22] Karen Kafadar and Philip C. Prorok. A data-analytic approach for estimating lead time and screening benefit based on survival curves in randomized cancer screening trials. *Statistics in Medicine*, 13(5–7):569–586, 1994.

[23] Karen Kafadar and Philip C. Prorok. Computer simulation of randomized cancer screening trials to compare methods of estimating lead time and benefit time. *Computational Statistics and Data Analysis*, 23(2):263–291, 1996.

[24] Karen Kafadar and Philip C. Prorok. Alternative definitions of comparable case groups and estimates of lead time and benefit time in randomized cancer screening trials. *Statistics in Medicine*, 22(1):83–111, 2003.

[25] Sarah K. Kendrick, Shesh N. Rai, and Dongfeng Wu. Simulation study for the sensitivity and mean sojourn time specific lead time in cancer screening when human lifetime is a competing risk. *Journal of Biometrics and Biostatistics*, 6(237), 2015.

[26] Seongho Kim, Hyejeong Jang, Dongfeng Wu, and Judith Abrams. A bayesian nonlinear mixed-effects disease progression model. *Journal of Biometrics and Biostatistics*, 6(5), 2015.

[27] Seongho Kim and Dongfeng Wu. Estimation of sensitivity depending on sojourn time and time spent in preclinical state. *Statistical Methods in Medical Research*, 25(2):728–740, 2016.

[28] Seongho Kim, Dongfeng Wu, and Diane Erwin. Efficacy of dual lung cancer screening by chest x-ray and sputum cytology using Johns Hopkins Lung Project data. *Journal of Biometrics and Biostatistics*, 3(139), 2012.

[29] K. J. Jorgensen and P. C. Gotzsche. Overdiagnosis in publicly organized mammography screening programmes: Systematic review of incidence trends. *British Medical Journal*, 2009.

[30] Sandra J. Lee and Marvin Zelen. Scheduling periodic examinations for the early detection of disease: Applications to breast cancer. *Journal of the American Statistical Association*, 93(444):1271–1281, 1998.

[31] Ruiqi Liu, Jeremy Gaskins, Ritendranath Mitra, and Dongfeng Wu. A review of estimation of key parameters and lead time in cancer screening. *Revista Colombiana de Estadística*, 40(2):263–278, 2017.

[32] Ruiqi Liu, Beth Levitt, Tom Riley, and Dongfeng Wu. Bayesian estimation of the three key parameters in CT for the National Lung Screening Trial data. *Journal of Biometrics and Biostatistics*, 6(263), 2015.

[33] Ruiqi Liu, Adriana Perez, and Dongfeng Wu. The lead time distribution in the National Lung Screening Trial study. *Journal of Healthcare Informatics Research*, 2:353–366, 2018.

[34] Ruiqi Liu, Dongfeng Wu, and Shesh N Rai. Estimation of the lead time distribution for individuals with screening history. *Statistics and Its Interface*, 14(2):131–149, 2021.

[35] Dianhong Luo, Alexander C. Cambon, and Dongfeng Wu. Evaluating long term effect of fobt in colon cancer screening. *Cancer Epidemiology*, 36:e54–e60, 2012.

[36] A. B. Miller, C. J. Baines, T. To, and C. Wall. Canadian national breast screening study 1: Breast cancer detection and death rates among women aged 40 to 49 years. *Canadian Medical Association Journal*, 147:1459–1476, 1992.

[37] A. B. Miller, C. J. Baines, T. To, and C. Wall. Canadian national breast screening study 2: Breast cancer detection and death rates among women aged 50 to 59 years. *Canadian Medical Association Journal*, 147:1477–1488, 1992.

[38] NCI. Seer fast stats results, 2015. http://seer.cancer.gov/statfacts/html/lungb.html.

[39] G. Parmigiani. Timing medical examinations via intensity functions. *Biometrika*, 84:803–816, 1997.

[40] G. Parmigiani, S. Skates, and M. Zelen. Modeling and optimization in early detection programs with a single exam. *Biometrics*, 58:30–36, 2002.

[41] P. H. Zahl, J. Mahlen, and H. G. Welch. The natural history of invasive breast cancers detected by screening mammography. *Arch internal Medicine*, 168:2311–2316, 2008.

[42] Philip C. Prorok. Bounded recurrence times and lead time in the design of a repetitive screening program. *Journal of Applied Probability*, 19(1):10–19, 1982.

[43] Farhin Rahman and Dongfeng Wu. Inference of sojourn time and transition density using the NLST x-ray screening data in lung cancer. *Medical Research Archives*, 9(5), 2021.

[44] L. A. G. Ries, M. P. Eisner, C. L. Kosary, B. F. Hankey, A. B. Miller, L. Clegg, and B. K. Edwards. Seer cancer statistics review, 1973–1999. Technical report, National Cancer Institute, Bethesda, Maryland, 2002.

[45] Marc D. Ryser, Jane Lange, Lurdes Y. T. Inoue, Ellen S. O'Meara, Charlotte Gard, Diana L. Miglioretti, Jean-Luc Bulliard, Andrew F. Brouwer, E. Shelley Hwang, and Ruth B. Etzioni. Estimation of breast cancer overdiagnosis in a U.S. breast screening cohort. *Annals of Internal Medicine*, 175(4): 471–478, 2022.

[46] S. Zackrisson, I. Andersson, L. Janzon, J. Manjer, and J. P. Garne. Rate of over-diagnosis of breast cancer 15 years after end of Malmö mammographic screening trial: Follow-up study. *BMJ*, 332:689–692, 2006.

[47] S. Shapiro, W. Venet, P. Strax, and L. Venet. *Periodic Screening for Breast Cancer: The Health Insurance Plan Project and Its Sequelae, 1963–1986.* Johns Hopkins University Press, 1988.

[48] Yu Shen, Dongfeng Wu, and Marvin Zelen. Testing the independence of two diagnostic tests. *Biometrics*, 57(4):1009–1017, 2001.

[49] Yu Shen and Marvin Zelen. Parametric estimation procedures for screening programmes: Stable and nonstable disease models for multimodality case finding. *Biometrika*, 86(3):503–515, 1999.

[50] Justin Shows and Dongfeng Wu. Inferences for the lead time in breast cancer screening trials under a stable disease model. *Cancers*, 3(2):2131–2140, 2011.

[51] Huub Straatman, Petronella G. M. Peer, and Andre L. M. Verbeek. Estimating lead time and sensitivity in a screening program without estimating the incidence in the screened group. *Biometrics*, 53(1):217–229, 1997.

[52] S. W. Duffy, E. Lynge, H. Jonsson, S. Ayyaz, and A. H. Olsen. Complexities in the estimation of overdiagnosis in breast cancer screening. *British Journal of Cancer*, 99:1176–1178, 2008.

[53] The National Lung Screening Trial Research Team. The national lung screening trial: Overview and study design. *Radiology*, 258(1):243–253, 2011.

[54] Stephan D. Walter and Nicholas E. Day. Estimation of the duration of a preclinical disease state using screening data. *American Journal of Epidemiology*, 118(6):865–886, 1983.

[55] Dengzhi Wang, Beth Levitt, Tom Riley, and Dongfeng Wu. Estimation of sojourn time and transition probability of lung cancer for smokers using the plco data. *Journal of Biometrics and Biostatistics*, 8(360), 2017.

[56] Dongfeng Wu. Overdiagnosis in screening: Does it make sense? *Journal of Biometrics and Biostatistics*, 3(110), 2012.

[57] Dongfeng Wu. Clinical impact: When to schedule for the upcoming screening exam? *Journal of Biometrics and Biostatistics*, 7(291), 2016.

[58] Dongfeng Wu. Scheduling mammogram and physical exam for a healthy woman. *Annals of Women's Health*, 9(1), 2019.

[59] Dongfeng Wu. When to initiate cancer screening exam? *Statistics and Its Interface*, 15(4):503–514, 2022.

[60] Dongfeng Wu. Dynamic scheduling for the upcoming cancer screening exam when sensitivity is a function of sojourn time. Methods in section 7.3 is based on this draft, 2023.

[61] Dongfeng Wu. A probability method to schedule the upcoming exam for asymptomatic individuals in cancer screening. *Statistics and Its Interface*, 2023. accepted on 1/16/2023.

[62] Dongfeng Wu. When to initiate a screening exam if sensitivity is a function of sojourn time? Methods in section 6.3 is based on this draft, 2023.

[63] Dongfeng Wu, Ricolindo L. Cariño, and Xiaoqin Wu. When sensitivity is a function of age and time spent in the preclinical state in periodic cancer screening. *Journal of Modern Applied Statistical Methods*, 7(1):297–303, 2008.

[64] Dongfeng Wu, Diane Erwin, and Seongho Kim. Projection of long-term outcomes using x-rays and pooled cytology in lung cancer screening. *Open Access Medical Statistics*, 1:13–19, 2011.

[65] Dongfeng Wu, Diane Erwin, and Gary L. Rosner. Estimating key parameters in FOBT screening for colorectal cancer. *Cancer Causes and Control*, 20(1):41–46, 2009.

[66] Dongfeng Wu, Diane Erwin, and Gary L. Rosner. A projection of benefits due to fecal occult blood test for colorectal cancer. *Cancer Epidemiology*, 33(3):212–215, 2009.

[67] Dongfeng Wu, Diane Erwin, and Gary L. Rosner. Sojourn time and lead time projection in lung cancer screening. *Lung Cancer*, 72(3):322–326, 2011.

[68] Dongfeng Wu and Karen Kafadar. Scheduling of the upcoming screening exam using CT in lung cancer. In *2019 Proceedings of the American Statistical Association, International Chinese Statistical Association Section*, pages 2177–2186. American Statistical Association, 2019.

[69] Dongfeng Wu and Karen Kafadar. Dynamic scheduling for the upcoming exam in periodic cancer screening. Submitted, 2022.

[70] Dongfeng Wu, Karen Kafadar, and Shesh N. Rai. Inference of long-term screening outcomes for individuals with screening histories. *Statistics and Public Policy*, 5(1):1–10, 2018.

[71] Dongfeng Wu, Karen Kafadar, and Gary L Rosner. Inference of long term effects and overdiagnosis in periodic cancer screening. *Statistica Sinica*, 24(2):815–831, 2014.

[72] Dongfeng Wu, Karen Kafadar, Gary L. Rosner, and Lyle D. Broemeling. The lead time distribution when lifetime is subject to competing risks in cancer screening. *The International Journal of Biostatistics*, 8(1), 2012.

[73] Dongfeng Wu, Ruiqi Liu, Beth Levitt, Riley Tom, and Kathy B. Baumgartner. Evaluating long-term outcomes via computed tomography in lung cancer screening. *Journal of Biometrics and Biostatistics*, (1), 2016.

[74] Dongfeng Wu and Adriana Perez. A limited review of over-diagnosis methods and long term effects in breast cancer screening. *Oncology Reviews*, 5:143–147, 2011.

[75] Dongfeng Wu and Adriana Perez. *Colorectal Cancer-From Prevention to Patient Care*, Chapter 24: Modeling and inference in screening: Exemplification with the faecal occult blood test, pages 473–490. InTech, 2012.

[76] Dongfeng Wu, N. Rai, Shesh, and Seow Albert. Estimation of preclinical state onset age and sojourn time for heavy smokers in lung cancer. *Statistics and Its Interface*, 15(3):349–358, 2022.

[77] Dongfeng Wu and Gary L Rosner. *Frontiers in Computational and Systems Biology*, Chapter 10: Probability modeling and statistical inference in periodic cancer screening, pages 203–218. Springer, London, 2010.

[78] Dongfeng Wu and Gary L Rosner. A projection of true-early-detection, no-early-detection, over-diagnosis and not-so-necessary probabilities in tumor screening. In *2010 Proceedings of the American Statistical Association Biopharmaceutical Section*, pages 1144–1157, 2010.

[79] Dongfeng Wu, Gary L. Rosner, and Lyle Broemeling. Mle and bayesian inference of age-dependent sensitivity and transition probability in periodic screening. *Biometrics*, 61(4):1056–1063, 2005.

[80] Dongfeng Wu, Gary L. Rosner, and Lyle D. Broemeling. Bayesian inference for the lead time in periodic cancer screening. *Biometrics*, 63(3):873–880, 2007.

[81] Dongfeng Wu, Gary L. Rosner, and Broemeling Lyle D. Inference for the lead time in cancer screening. In *2006 Proceedings of the American Statistical Association, Biometrics Section*, pages 427–433, 2006.

[82] Dongfeng Wu and Kim Seongho. Problems in the estimation of the key parameters using MLE in lung cancer screening. *Journal of Clinical Research and Reports*, 5(3), 2020.

[83] Dongfeng Wu and Kim Seongho. Inference of onset age of preclinical state and sojourn time for breast cancer. *Medical Research Archives*, 10(2), 2022.

[84] Dongfeng Wu, Xiaoqin Wu, Ioana Banicescu, and Ricolindo L. Cariño. Simulation procedure in periodic cancer screening trials. *Journal of Modern Applied Statistical Methods*, 4(2):522–527, 2005.

[85] Jian-Lun Xu, Richard M. Fagerstrom, and Philip C. Prorok. Estimation of post-lead-time survival under dependence between lead-time and post-lead-time survival. *Statistics in Medicine*, 18:155–162, 1999.

[86] Jian-Lun Xu and Philip C. Prorok. Non-parametric estimation of the post-lead-time survival distribution of screen-detected cancer cases. *Statistics in Medicine*, 14:2715–2725, 1995.

[87] M. Zelen and M. Feinleib. On the theory of screening for chronic diseases. *Biometrika*, 56(3):601–614, 1969.

[88] Marvin Zelen. Optimal scheduling of examinations for the early detection of disease. *Biometrika*, 80(2):279–293, 1993.

Index

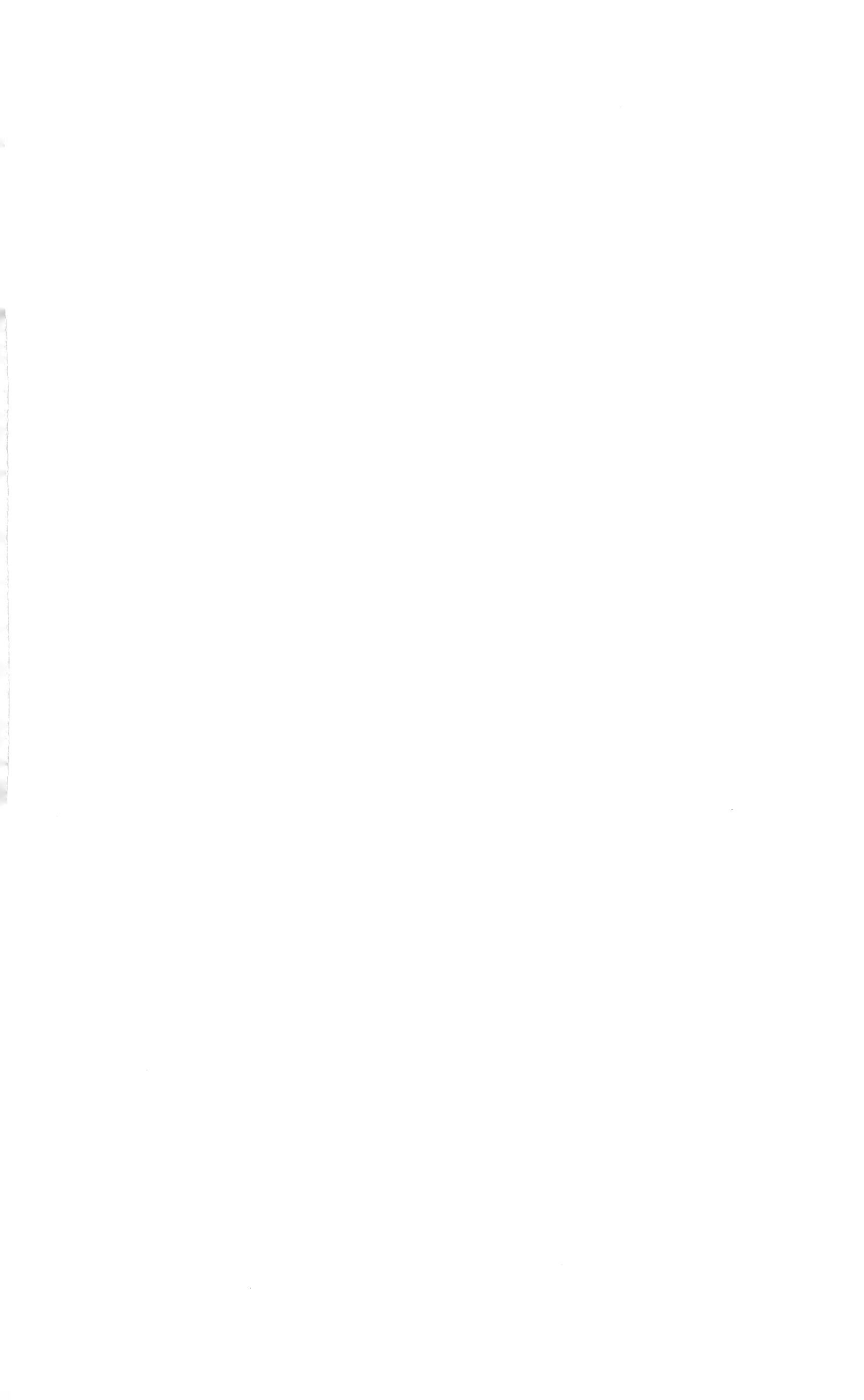